2015

The Year Book of HAND AND UPPER LIMB SURGERY®

Editors-in-Chief

Jeffrey Yao, MD

Associate Professor, Robert A. Chase Hand & Upper Limb Center, Department of Orthopaedic Surgery, Redwood City, California

Julie Adams, MD

Associate Professor, Orthopedic Surgery, Mayo Clinic, Austin, Minnesota

ELSEVIER

MOSBY

ELSEVIER
MOSBY

VP Global Medical Reference: Mary E. Gatsch
Senior Clinics Editor: Jennifer Flynn-Briggs
Developmental Editor: Colleen Viola
Production Supervisor, Electronic Year Books: Donna M. Skelton
Electronic Article Manager: Mike Sheets
Illustrations and Permissions Coordinator: Dawn Vohsen

2015 EDITION

Composition by TNQ Books and Journals Pvt Ltd, India

Editorial Office:
Elsevier
Suite 1800
1600 John F. Kennedy Blvd.
Philadelphia, PA 19103-2899

International Standard Serial Number: 1551-7977
International Standard Book Number: 978-0-323-35545-2

Contributing Editors

Joshua M. Abzug, MD
Assistant Professor, University of Maryland School of Medicine; Director, University of Maryland Brachial Plexus Clinic; Director of Pediatric Orthopedics, University of Maryland Medical Center; Deputy Surgeon-in-Chief, University of Maryland Children's Hospital, Department of Orthopedics, Timonium, Maryland

Andrea Atzei, MD
Hand Surgery Unit, Casa di Cura "Giovanni XXIII," Monastier di Treviso, Treviso, Italy

Philip Blazar, MD
Associate Professor, Department of Orthopaedic Surgery, Brigham and Women's Hospital, Boston, Massachusetts

John T. Capo, MD
Professor, Department of Orthopaedics, NYU-Hospital for Joint Diseases, New York, New York; Chief of Hand Surgery, Jersey City Medical Center, Jersey City, New Jersey

Emilie Cheung, MD
Associate Professor, Chief, Shoulder and Elbow Service, Department of Orthopedic Surgery, Stanford University Medical Center, Redwood City, California

Harvey Chim, MD
Assistant Professor of Clinical Surgery, Division of Plastic Surgery, University of Miami Miller School of Medicine, Miami, Florida

Matthew Seung Suk Choi, MD
Associate Professor, Chief, Department of Plastic and Reconstructive Surgery, Hanyang University Guri Hospital, Guri, Gyunggi-do, Korea

Alphonsus KS Chong, MD
Head and Senior Consultant, Department of Hand and Reconstructive Microsurgery; Assistant Professor, Department of Orthopaedic Surgery, Yong Loo Lin School of Medicine, National University Hospital, Singapore

Akin Cil, MD
Associate Professor of Orthopedics, University of Missouri-Kansas City, Kansas City, Missouri

Susan J. Clark, OTR/L, CHT
Certified Hand Therapist, Stanford University Medical Center, Redwood City, California

Catherine Curtin, MD
Assistant Professor, Robert A. Chase Hand & Upper Limb Center, Division of Plastic Surgery, Stanford University Medical Center, Stanford, California

Piotr Czarnecki, MD, PhD
Hand Surgery Department, Poznan University of Medical Sciences, Poznan, Poland

Johnny Elfar, MD
Associate Professor, Department of Orthopaedic Surgery, Division of Sports Medicine and Hand Surgery, University of Rochester Medical Center, Rochester, New York

Glenn Gaston, MD
Fellowship Director, OrthoCarolina Hand Fellowship; Chief of Hand Surgery, Carolinas Medical Center, Department of Orthopedic Surgery, Charlotte, North Carolina

Jacqueline A. Geissler, MD
Faculty at Hennepin County Medical Center, Orthopaedic Department, Minneapolis, Minnesota

Michael B. Gottschalk, MD
NYU-Hospital for Joint Diseases Hand Fellow, New York, New York

Ruby Grewal, MD, MSc, FRCS
Associate Professor, Roth|McFarlane Hand and Upper Limb Centre, St Joseph's Health Centre, London, Ontario, Canada

Warren C. Hammert, MD
Professor of Orthopaedic Surgery and Plastic Surgery, Chief, Division of Hand Surgery, Department of Orthopaedics and Rehabilitation, University of Rochester Medical Center, Rochester, New York

Jan Ragnar Haugstvedt, MD, PhD
Senior Consultant, Hand Surgery, Department of Orthopedics Østfold Hospital Trust, Norway

Mike Hayton, BSc(Hons) MBChB FRCS(orth) FFSEM(uk)
Consultant Orthopaedic Hand Surgeon, The Wrightington Hospital, Lancashire, United Kingdom

Cherrie Heinrich, MD, FACS
Department of Plastic Surgery, Regions Hospital, St. Paul, Minnesota

Vincent R. Hentz, MD
Professor of Surgery, Robert A. Chase Hand & Upper Limb Center, Division of Plastic Surgery, Stanford University Medical Center, Stanford, California

Guillaume Herzberg, MD, PhD
Hôpital Édouard Herriot, Orthopaedic Surgery – Shoulder & Elbow, Wrist, Hand, Lyon, France

Pak-Cheong Ho, MD, MBBS, FRCS, FHKCOS, FHKAM (Orthopeadics)
Consultant & Chief, Clinical Professor (Honorary), Division of Hand & Microsurgery, Department of Orthopaedic & Traumatology, Prince of Wales Hospital, Chinese University of Hong Kong, Hong Kong, China

Nathan A. Hoekzema, MD
Assistant Professor, UCSF - Fresno, Community Regional Medical Center, Department of Orthopaedic Surgery, Fresno, California

Jerry I. Huang, MD
Associate Professor, Program Director, UW Combined Hand Fellowship, Department of Orthopaedics and Sports Medicine, University of Washington Medical Center, Seattle, Washington

Thomas B. Hughes, MD
Clinical Associate Professor of Orthopaedic Surgery, University of Pittsburgh School of Medicine; Orthopaedic Specialists, UPMC, Pittsburgh, Pennsylvania

Sidney M. Jacoby, MD
Associate Professor in Orthopaedic Surgery, Thomas Jefferson University Hospital, The Philadelphia Hand Center, P.C., Philadelphia, Pennsylvania

Ryosuke Kakinoki, MD, PhD
Professor of Hand Surgery & Microvascular Reconstructive Surgery, Department of Orthopaedic Surgery, Faculty of Medicine, Kindai University, Osaka, Japan

Michael W. Kessler, MD
Chief - Division of Hand & Elbow Surgery, Assistant Professor, Department of Orthopaedic Surgery, MedStar Georgetown University Hospital, Washington, DC

Elspeth Kinnucan, MD
Kaiser Permanente, Roseville, California

Sonja Kranz, OT, CHT
Department of Physical Medicine and Rehabilitation, Mayo Clinic, Rochester, Minnesota

Leo T. Kroonen, MD
Hand and Upper Extremity Surgery, Southern California Permanente Medical Group, San Diego, California

Amy L. Ladd, MD
Editor-in-Chief, Emeritus, Yearbook of Hand & Upper Limb Surgery; Professor of Orthopaedic Surgery & Plastic Surgery, Robert A. Chase Hand & Upper Limb Center at Stanford University, Palo Alto, California

Ericka Lawler, MD
Clinical Assistant Professor, University of Iowa, Iowa City, Iowa

Jeffrey Macalena, MD
Assistant Professor, Department of Orthopaedic Surgery, University of Minnesota, Minneapolis, Minnesota

Corey McGee, PhD, OTR/L, CHT
Instructor, Program in Occupational Therapy, University of Minnesota - Rochester, Rochester, Minnesota

Kai Megerle, MD
Assistant Professor, Department of Plastic Surgery and Hand Surgery, Technical University of Munich, Munich, Germany

Amy T. Moeller, MD
Assistant Professor, Department of Orthopaedic Surgery, University of Minnesota, Minneapolis, Minnesota

Peter M. Murray, MD
Professor and Chair, Department of Orthopedic Surgery; Consultant, Orthopedic Surgery and Neurosurgery, Mayo Clinic, Jacksonville, Florida

Virginia H. O'Brien, OTD, OTR/L, CHT
Hand Therapy Residency Coordinator, Fairview Hand Center, University Orthopaedics Therapy Center, University of Minnesota Medical Center, Fairview, Minneapolis, Minnesota

Jose A. Ortiz, Jr., MD
Assistant Clinical Professor of Orthopedics, Mayo Clinic College of Medicine, Chief of Staff, Orthopedic Center, Hand and Upper Extremity Service, Eau Claire, Wisconsin

Rick F. Papandrea, MD
Partner, Orthopaedic Associates of Wisconsin, Waukesha, Wisconsin

Jason Saillant, MD
The Philadelphia Hand Center, P.C., King of Prussia, Pennsylvania

Steven S. Shin, MD
Chief of Hand Surgery, Kerlan-Jobe Orthopaedic Clinic, Los Angeles, California

Juan Pablo Simone, MD
Shoulder and Elbow Surgeon, Hospital Aleman, Buenos Aires, Argentina

David J. Slutsky, MD
The Hand and Wrist Institute; Assistant Professor, Department of Orthopedics, Harbor-UCLA Medical Center, Torrance, California

Philipp N. Streubel, MD
Assistant Professor, Hand, Elbow and Shoulder Surgery, Department of Orthopaedic Surgery University of Nebraska Medical Center, Omaha, Nebraska

Jin Bo Tang, MD
Professor and Chair, Department of Hand Surgery, Affiliated Hospital of Nantong University, Chair, Hand Surgery Research Center, Nantong University, Jiangsu, China

Jonathan Tueting, MD
Chief, Hand and Upper Extremity Surgery, Department of Orthopedics and Rehabilitation Medicine, University of Wisconsin School of Medicine and Public Health, Madison, Wisconsin

David Zelouf, MD
Assistant Clinical Professor, Department of Orthopaedic Surgery, Thomas Jefferson University Hospital and The Philadelphia Hand Center, King of Prussia, Pennsylvania

Dan Zlotolow, MD
Associate Professor, Department of Orthopaedic Surgery, Shriners Hospital for Children, Philadelphia, Pennsylvania

Table of Contents

Journals Represented

Journals represented in this Year Book are listed below.

Acta Anaesthesiologica Scandinavica
American Journal of Emergency Medicine
American Journal of Sports Medicine
Annals of Plastic Surgery
Arthroscopy
Bone and Joint Journal
British Journal of Radiology
British Journal of Sports Medicine
Clinical Neurology and Neurosurgery
Clinical Orthopaedics and Related Research
European Journal of Plastic Surgery
Hand
Injury
Journal of Athletic Training
Journal of Bone and Joint Surgery (American)
Journal of Bone Mineral Research
Journal of Hand Surgery (American)
Journal of Hand Therapy
Journal of Orthopaedic and Sports Physical Therapy
Journal of Orthopaedic Research
Journal of Orthopaedic Trauma
Journal of Pediatric Orthopedics
Journal of Plastic, Reconstructive & Aesthetic Surgery
Journal of Ultrasound in Medicine
Journal of Vascular Surgery
Medicine
Microsurgery
New England Journal of Medicine
Orthopedics
Plastic and Reconstructive Surgery
Skeletal Radiology
World Journal of Surgery
World Neurosurgery

Standard Abbreviations

The following terms are abbreviated in this edition: acquired immunodeficiency syndrome (AIDS), cardiopulmonary resuscitation (CPR), central nervous system (CNS), cerebrospinal fluid (CSF), computed tomography (CT), deoxyribonucleic acid (DNA), electrocardiography (ECG), health maintenance organization (HMO), human immunodeficiency virus (HIV), intensive care unit (ICU), intramuscular (IM), intravenous (IV), magnetic resonance (MR) imaging (MRI), ribonucleic acid (RNA), and ultrasound (US).

Note

The Year Book of Hand and Upper Limb Surgery® is a literature survey service providing abstracts of articles published in the professional literature. Every effort is made to assure the accuracy of the information presented in these pages. Neither the editors nor the publisher of the YEAR BOOK OF HAND AND UPPER LIMB SURGERY® can be responsible for errors in the original materials. The editors' comments are their own opinions. Mention of specific products within this publication does not constitute endorsement.

To facilitate the use of the YEAR BOOK OF HAND AND UPPER LIMB SURGERY® as a reference tool, all illustrations and tables included in this publication are now identified as they appear in the original article. This change is meant to help the reader recognize that any illustration or table appearing in the YEAR BOOK OF HAND AND UPPER LIMB SURGERY® may be only one of many in the original article. For this reason, figure and table numbers will often appear to be out of sequence within the YEAR BOOK OF HAND AND UPPER LIMB SURGERY®.

Introduction

We are proud to bring you the 31st edition of the YEAR BOOK OF HAND AND UPPER LIMB SURGERY. It is our honor to continue a Mayo Clinic and Stanford University collaborative editorial tradition begun by Drs James Dobyns and Robert Chase and continued by Drs Peter Amadio and Vincent Hentz, and most recently by Drs Richard Berger, Amy Ladd, James Chang, and Scott Steinmann.

After 3 years of an editorial board, this year, the YEAR BOOK has transitioned to two editors: Dr Jeffrey Yao and Dr Julie Adams. Certainly, however, the YEAR BOOK would not be possible without the valuable input of the contributing editors. Our contributing editors, from all over the world, are all recognized experts in the field of hand and upper extremity surgery and generously shared their expertise with the readers of the YEAR BOOK. Likewise, we would like to thank Colleen Viola from Elsevier for her tireless and enthusiastic work to troubleshoot and to bring this edition to fruition. We hope you continue to enjoy the cutting edge and thoughtful commentaries on this year's publications in the field of hand and upper limb surgery!

Julie Adams, MD

Jeffrey Yao, MD

1 Hand and Wrist Arthritis

The Biomechanical Stability of Salvage Procedures for Distal Radioulnar Joint Arthritis

Douglas KC, Parks BG, Tsai MA, et al (MedStar Union Memorial Hosp, Baltimore, MD; George Washington Univ Med Ctr, DC)

J Hand Surg Am 39:1274-1279, 2014

Purpose.—To test distal forearm stability after 3 surgical procedures for distal radioulnar joint (DRUJ) arthritis.

Methods.—We tested 11 cadaver limbs with the DRUJ intact, after distal ulna–matched hemiresection, after Darrach distal ulna resection, and after unlinked total DRUJ arthroplasty. We evaluated distal forearm stability in neutral rotation, full pronation, and full supination in unweighted and 1-kg–weighted conditions. We measured dorsal/palmar translation and convergence/divergence of the distal radius relative to the ulna.

Results.—Under neutral rotation, whether weighted or unweighted, matched hemiresection and Darrach specimens demonstrated significant radioulnar convergence relative to intact specimens. Weighted and unweighted, DRUJ arthroplasty demonstrated similar radioulnar convergence to intact. Weighted and unweighted, only Darrach specimens showed significant radius-palmar translation compared with intact, hemiresected, and DRUJ arthroplasty. In pronation, no testing scenario, either weighted or unweighted, demonstrated statistically significant radioulnar convergence relative to intact state. In unweighted pronation, palmar translation of the radius was significantly different from the intact state for all surgical scenarios and the Darrach was significantly worse than the other procedures. In weighted pronation, palmar translation of the radius was significantly different from the intact state for all surgical scenarios and the matched hemiresection was significantly better than the other procedures. In supination, weighted and unweighted, Darrach specimens had significant radioulnar convergence relative to intact. Either weighted or unweighted, the hemiresection and arthroplasty groups demonstrated similar radioulnar convergence relative to intact. Unweighted, all scenarios demonstrated similar dorsal translation of the radius. Weighted, the Darrach group showed significant radius-dorsal translation relative to intact specimens.

Conclusions.—For tested procedures, DRUJ arthroplasty overall was biomechanically superior to the other conditions except that we found greater stability in the hemiresected group in weighted pronation.

Clinical Relevance.—Knowledge of baseline biomechanical characteristics of DRUJ arthritis procedures will aid surgical decision-making and patient counseling.

▶ There is no universal solution to a structurally or functionally invalid distal radioulnar joint (DRUJ). The importance of the distal ulna in providing a stable and yet highly mobile anchorage for the forearm bone and ulnar carpus is repeatedly emphasized in the literature. Taking away the ulnar head will produce laxity of the radioulnar ligaments, ulnocarpal ligament complex, and possibly the interosseous ligament. The consequence is forearm instability and ulnocarpal and even radiocarpal instability. However, simple resection of the ulnar head remains a popular procedure worldwide because of its simplicity and the longstanding reputation. It gets rid of the culprit of pain in DRUJ arthritis with high certainty. Although distal ulnar stump instability can be shown at rest in almost 100% of patients undergoing the Darrach procedure, not all of them will have symptoms. Many factors influence the occurrence of instability pain such as age, functional status, hand dominance, the amount of bone resection, and probably most importantly, the soft-tissue reconstruction to preserve or augment the stability of the ulnar stump.

The authors compared the stability of 3 methods of reconstruction for DRUJ salvage in the sagittal and frontal planes. The study was purely based on the intrinsic stability of the various skeletal constructs without an attempt to rebuild the soft-tissue constraints. Even the DRUJ capsule and skin were not closed. As described by the authors, under this worst-case scenario (which probably won't happen in real life), the DRUJ total arthroplasty offered the best stability in all planes among the 3 choices, with the exception of palmar translation of the radius under weighted pronation. The difference was particularly marked in neutral rotation. As the authors humbly concluded, knowledge of the baseline biomechanical characteristics of DRUJ arthritis procedures helped surgical decision-making and patient counseling. The study design is, however, constrained by several factors. (1) The ulna is transfixed to the humerus with an external fixator, thus, eliminating the natural adduction, abduction, and flexion extension of the ulna upon forearm rotation. (2) Pronation and supination motion was produced by a passive pull on the pronator teres and biceps brachii tendon, respectively. The effect of the pronator quadratus and supinator muscle was not taken into account. Both muscles originate from the ulna and may have a more direct impact on the biomechanical behavior of the radius after ulnar head resection. (3) The soft tissue envelope was not repaired.

The Darrach procedure is still my treatment of choice, especially in older patients with relatively lower functional demands. The key to success is a meticulous reconstruction of the soft-tissue constraints. I prefer a proximally based half slip of the extensor carpi ulnaris (ECU) tendon passed through the distal end of ulna stump and sutured back to its intact half in physiological tension. This internal splinting provides a reliable active dynamic stabilization of the stump on active gripping when the ECU muscle is activated. This compares favorably to the conventional passive tenodesis methods.

P. C. Ho, MD

Long-Term Results of Arthroscopic Wrist Synovectomy in Rheumatoid Arthritis

Lee HI, Lee KH, Koh KH, et al (Univ of Ulsan College of Medicine, Gangneung, Korea; SungKyunKwan Univ School of Medicine, Seoul, Korea; Inje Univ Ilsan Paik Hosp, Goyang, Korea)
J Hand Surg Am 39:1295-1300, 2014

Purpose.—To investigate the effects of arthroscopic wrist synovectomy on the clinical course of rheumatoid arthritis in a large series with long-term follow-up.

Methods.—We performed arthroscopic synovectomy on 56 wrists in 49 patients with rheumatoid arthritis. At a mean follow-up of 7.9 years (range, 5–12 y), we evaluated pain and patient satisfaction using a visual analog scale and assessed overall function using the Mayo wrist score. Radiographic stage was graded according to Larsen stage. We determined clinical outcomes on the recurrence of wrist synovitis, which we evaluated by symptoms of pain and swelling and physical examination. Preoperative variables were statistically analyzed to find factors that could influence the results.

Results.—The mean visual analog scale score for wrist pain decreased from 6.3 to 1.7, and the mean Mayo wrist score (evaluated in 39 wrists) improved from 48 (range, 5–70) to 76 (range, 55–100). The mean visual analog scale score for patient satisfaction was 7.9. At final followup, synovitis was controlled in 42 wrists (75%) and recurred in the others. The mean Larsen stage progressed from 2.2 to 3.3. Analysis of preoperative variables revealed no factors that significantly affected clinical outcomes in terms of sex, age, duration of wrist symptom, preoperative serologic inflammatory markers, or Larsen stage.

Conclusions.—Arthroscopic synovectomy of the wrist can provide pain relief and functional improvement with control of synovitis in 75% of rheumatoid wrists that have not responded to medication.

Type of Study/Level of Evidence.—Therapeutic IV.

► The authors presented the long-term results of arthroscopic synovectomy on 56 wrists in 49 patients of rheumatoid arthritis at an average follow-up of 7.9 years. This is by far the largest study with the longest follow-up information on this area in the literature. The authors used the recurrence rate of synovitis as the primary outcome and reported a low incidence of 25% after a single operation over an extended period. The clinical outcome did not correlate with many factors, including symptom duration, preoperative inflammatory parameters, and Larsen stage. Although there was a trend of radiologic deterioration in 70% of the cohort, there was again no correlation with the pain and clinical outcome. This result aligns with the common observation in many arthritic conditions that poor radiologic appearance does not necessarily equate to disabling pain and poor function. The culprit of the pain often lies on the activity of the synovial proliferation, which, in turn, produces various noxious lysosomal factors that directly induce pain and inflammation. Mechanical factors such as stability and load transmission may not have the critical role as in posttraumatic arthritis. Thus, it may not be surprising to see good control of pain even in advanced Larsen stages. The best indication for arthroscopic synovectomy is always on those patients with monoarticular or oligoarticular disease in which wrist symptoms predominate and the disease is not at the peak of the activity. A successful surgery will lessen or even obviate the need for further medication control and, thus, saves the patient from its potential side effects.

Since 1997 in our institute, we have routinely performed arthroscopic synovectomy for inflammatory arthritis of the wrist and hand uncontrolled by medication for more than 6 months. In a recent review (unpublished data) of our results of 39 wrist arthroscopic synovectomies in 30 patients with rheumatoid arthritis operated on between 1997 and 2002, we obtained similar results as those of the current study. At an average follow-up of 13 years (6–17.5 years), the Visual Analog Scale pain score, Wrist Total Performance Score, and grip strength were significantly improved compared with baseline. Our group involved more advanced cases, with 61.5% being Larsen grade III and IV. All except 3 early cases were completed under portal site local anesthesia or intravenous anesthesia. This offers unique anesthetic advantage for rheumatoid patients. Satisfactory results were shown in both early and late arthritis. Arthroscopic synovectomy of the wrist as a minimally invasive surgery should have a definite role in the management of rheumatoid disease, even in the new era of biologic treatment.

P. C. Ho, MD

Comparison of Arthroplasties With or Without Bone Tunnel Creation for Thumb Basal Joint Arthritis: A Randomized Controlled Trial

Vermeulen GM, Spekreijse KR, Slijper H, et al (Erasmus MC Univ Med Ctr, Rotterdam, The Netherlands; Dept of Rehabilitation Medicine, Rotterdam, The Netherlands; Xpert Clinic Hilversum, The Netherlands)

J Hand Surg Am 39:1692-1698, 2014

Purpose.—To compare the results for treatment of basal thumb osteoarthritis with and without the use of a bone tunnel at the base of the first metacarpal.

Methods.—Women aged 40 years or older with stage IV osteoarthritis were randomized to 1 of 2 treatments. Patients were evaluated preoperatively and postoperatively at 3 and 12 months by assessing pain, outcome function measures, range of motion, strength, time to return to work or activities, satisfaction with the results, and complication rate.

Results.—A total of 79 patients were enrolled in this study. Three months after surgery, Patient-Rated Wrist and Hand Evaluation pain and total scores were significantly improved in the bone tunnel group compared with the tunnel-free group. At 12 months, however, we found no significant differences for all outcome scores between groups. In addition, we observed no significant differences between groups in strength, duration to return to work or activities, patient satisfaction, and complication rates.

Conclusions.—After the bone tunnel technique, patients have better function and less pain 3 months after surgery than do those in the non—bone tunnel group, which indicates faster recovery. However, 12 months after surgery, the functional outcome was similar. Because of faster recovery, we prefer the bone tunnel technique in the treatment of stage IV osteoarthritis.

Type of Study/Level of Evidence.—Therapeutic I.

▶ This article compares a Littler—Eaton—Burton—Pellegrini tendinous interposition with one-half of the flexor carpi radialis (FCR) and bone tunnels with a Weilby wraparound using the abductor pollicis longus around the FCR for the treatment of pantrapezial arthritis. The former may be considered if we subscribe to the classic Littler school of reconstruction, an anatomic reconstruction of suspensory and stabilizing ligaments. The latter may, in theory, be more of an interposition procedure. The authors found that the bone tunnel patients had better outcome scores in the early phase, and thus this is their preferred procedure.

This is a reasonable assumption, but not, in my research experience, based on anatomic restoration. The APL wraparound I have found often causes attritional rupture of the FCR and may explain the longer rehabilitation reported in this article. The myriad operations for thumb carpometacarpal arthritis suggest we have much more to learn: better treatment options are needed for end-stage disease, early-stage disease, and, importantly, prevention. We keep going!

A. Ladd, MD

Effect of Carpometacarpal Joint Osteoarthritis, Sex, and Handedness on Thumb *In Vivo* Kinematics

Hamann N, Heidemann J, Heinrich K, et al (German Sport Univ Cologne, Germany; Joint Centre Brühl, Germany)

J Hand Surg Am 39:2161-2167, 2014

Purpose.—To investigate the influence of trapeziometacarpal (TMC) osteoarthritis (OA) on the 3-dimensional motion capability of the TMC and thumb metacarpophalangeal (MCP) joints. In order to examine other factors affecting the thumb's motion kinematics, we further aimed to address the influence of sex and handedness on the motion capability of normal TMC and MCP joints.

Methods.—We included 18 healthy subjects (9 women, 9 men; 8 dominant hands, 10 nondominant hands) and 18 women with stage II/III TMC

OA. A motion analysis system using surface markers was used to quantify the thumb's 3-dimensional opposition–reposition kinematics. The range of motion of the thumb's TMC and MCP joints in flexion–extension, abduction–adduction, and pronation–supination were determined.

Results.—TMC OA led to a loss in abduction–adduction in the TMC joint (38° in controls, 26° in TMC OA subjects), although neither flexion–extension nor pronation–supination were affected. At the MCP joint, the TMC OA subjects showed a 48% reduction in abduction–adduction (32° controls, 16° TMC OA subjects) and 42% reduction in pronation–supination (34° in controls, 20° in TMC OA subjects) than the healthy controls. Ranges of motion of the healthy TMC and MCP joints were similar in dominant and nondominant hands as well as in women and men.

Discussion.—The study demonstrated that stage II/III TMC OA restricts the motion of the TMC joint in abduction–adduction and of the MCP joint in abduction–adduction and pronation–supination. Thumb motion capability was unaffected by sex and handedness.

Clinical Relevance.—Osteoarthritis-induced loss of TMC motion did not reflect a generalizable clinical parameter, rather, it seemed to distinctly affect the TMC and the MCP joints and their motion planes and directions. As neither sex nor handedness influenced the motion capabilities of the healthy thumb, kinematic factors contributing to TMC OA may develop at a later age.

▶ The authors present a well-designed study comparing men and women suffering from stage II/III trapeziometacarpal osteoarthritis with a control group of healthy subjects. Their goal was to determine whether gender and/or handedness affected the motion capability of normal trapeziometacarpal and metacarpophalangeal joints. The authors used a previously validated 3-dimensional motion capture system to evaluate trapeziometacarpal and metacarpophalangeal range of motion in the planes of flexion–extension, pronation–supination, and abduction–adduction. The authors' hypothesis was that in patients with painful motion at the trapeziometacarpal joint, the metacarpophalangeal joint would compensate with greater range of motion. The results of the investigation showed that the patients with trapeziometacarpal osteoarthritis had significantly smaller range of motion in the trapeziometacarpal joint and the metacarpophalangeal joint during abduction–adduction and only decreased motion at the metacarpophalangeal joint in pronation–supination. There were no differences in healthy patients' motion at the metacarpophalangeal or trapeziometacarpal joints, regardless of gender or handedness. I was surprised by the findings in this analysis, as we are classically taught that patients with trapeziometacarpal arthritis who lack palmar abduction frequently become hypermobile at the metacarpophalangeal joint, leading to hyperextension. This study provides interesting insight into motion at one of the joints in the hand most commonly that is associated with osteoarthritis. With improving technology, it is clear that further investigation is required to determine whether gender-related mobility differences or variability in joint articulation morphology account for the development of trapeziometacarpal osteoarthritis.

M. Kessler, MD

Disability in Patients with Trapeziometacarpal Joint Arthrosis: Incidental Versus Presenting Diagnosis

Becker SJE, Makarawung DJS, Spit SA, et al (Massachusetts General Hosp, Boston)

J Hand Surg Am 39:2009-2015, 2014

Purpose.—To test the hypothesis that there is no difference in trapeziometacarpal (TMC) joint arthrosis–related symptoms and disability between patients seeking treatment for symptoms of TMC arthrosis and those with incidental TMC joint arthrosis.

Methods.—We compared 64 patients presenting for care of TMC joint arthrosis with 64 with incidental TMC joint arthrosis. For both groups, the diagnosis was based on crepitation on examination. Bivariate and multivariate analyses assessed factors associated with symptoms and disability related to TMC joint arthrosis.

Results.—In bivariate analysis, patients presenting for care of TMC joint arthrosis had significantly more symptoms and disability from TMC joint arthrosis than those with incidental TMC joint arthrosis. The best multivariate linear regression model for fewer TMC joint arthrosis–related symptoms and disability included patients with incidental TMC joint arthrosis, male sex, no other painful conditions, less catastrophic thinking, and fewer depressive symptoms and explained 74% of the variability. Having incidental TMC joint arthrosis (25%) and more adaptive coping strategies (less catastrophic thinking; 5%) were the most important contributors to fewer symptoms and less disability.

Conclusions.—Future studies are merited to determine whether training in better coping strategies (eg, less catastrophic thinking and fewer depressive symptoms) can decrease symptoms and disability in patients with TMC joint arthrosis.

Type of Study/Level of Evidence.—Prognostic III.

► This prospective cohort study compared 2 groups of patients: 64 presenting with incidental, asymptomatic trapeziometacarpal (TMC) arthrosis and 64 presenting for care of the TMC arthrosis. The diagnosis was made clinically on the basis of crepitus, and radiographs were not used. A statistical analysis was then performed looking for differences between the 2 groups. Metrics included the QuickDASH, pain intensity score, PHQ-9 (Patient Health Questionnaire, a measure of depressive symptoms), PCS (Pain Catastrophizing Scale), and PSEQ (Patient Self-Efficacy questionnaire). Statistical analysis revealed that patients presenting for care had significantly more symptoms from TMC joint arthrosis and thumb-related activity than patients with incidental TMC joint arthrosis. Similar findings were also noted when comparing QuickDASH scores between the 2 groups. Patients presenting for treatment also exhibited greater catastrophic thinking, lower pain self-efficacy, and more depressive symptoms than those who did not present for TMC arthrosis. Patients who did not present for TMC arthrosis were more likely to exhibit lower DASH scores, be of male sex, have no other painful conditions, exhibit less catastrophic thinking, and demonstrate greater pain self-efficacy scores. Also, patients with passive but not static MP joint hyperextension had significantly less disability compared with those without passive MP joint hyperextension.

Dr Ring, based on this cohort as well as previous publications, once again points out that mood and coping strategies are the strongest correlates of symptoms and disability, suggesting that an "optimal mindset" can facilitate adaptation to TMC joint arthrosis. Dr Ring continues to further our understanding of our patients' perception of pain and disability. He continues to champion the concept that our patients need better coping strategies, with less catastrophic thinking and fewer depressive symptoms. I've often wondered why many individuals with clinically severe TMC joint arthrosis report minimal to no symptoms, whereas others with far less severe arthrosis are much more symptomatic. I do think this article sheds some light on this very issue, and I certainly agree that patients with high QuickDASH scores who report that they are depressed tend to be more symptomatic and exhibit fewer signs. The article is quite interesting and thought provoking, although from a practical standpoint, it does not necessarily help me manage my patients who exhibit poor coping strategies and depression. In such a patient, I favor a conservative approach, and I have had some success with limited physiotherapy and modifications to activities of everyday living, along with other nontraditional modalities such as acupuncture. Surgical intervention in such a patient should clearly be a last resort. Lastly, I do agree with the conclusions of this study but would also suggest that progressive stiffness in the setting of severe TMC arthrosis, as well as decreased activity level, may contribute to fewer symptoms, particularly as one ages.

D. Zelouf, MD

The Effect of Pisiform Excision on Wrist Function

van Eijzeren J, Karthaus RP (Medisch Spectrum Twente Hosp, Enschede, The Netherlands)

J Hand Surg Am 39:1258-1263, 2014

Purpose.—To investigate the effect of pisiform excision on wrist function compared with age- and sex-matched control subjects.

Methods.—The authors evaluated the charts of 11 consecutive patients who had undergone pisiform excision. Nine of these patients could be included and clinically examined, and results were compared with 9 matched controls. Measurements included range of motion, strength measurements, neurological examination, and questionnaires.

Results.—Extension in the operated wrist was reduced in patients compared with controls. The Disabilities of the Arm, Shoulder, and Hand and Michigan Hand Outcomes Questionnaires were significantly different between patients and controls. All other entities were equal between groups. Subjectively, patients experienced impairments in function of the operated wrist, but these could not be identified objectively.

Conclusions.—Although great care must be taken in handling the surrounding soft tissue, pisiform excision is a well-tolerated, safe treatment for pain in the pisotriquetral joint resulting from arthrosis and not controlled by nonsurgical means.

Type of Study/Level of Evidence.—Therapeutic III.

► This retrospective study compares several parameters and validated instruments in control subjects versus a handful of subjects who underwent pisiform excision. The major weakness of the article is that no preoperative comparisons are made to postoperative outcome. But 3 points are worth noting. Pisiform excised subjects had persistent lack of wrist extension, but preexisting ulnar nerve symptoms essentially resolved with surgery. The authors also highlight that pisotriquetral arthritis is often missed: This is the most important feature of the study and also reflects my own experience. We often allude to mysterious things that can go awry on the wrist's ulnar side; the "low back pain of the wrist," a "black hole," etc—that is, things which are hard to diagnose or often missed. Pisotriquetral arthritis is another entity to add to the list of potential causes of ulnar-sided wrist pain.

A. Ladd, MD

Proximal Row Carpectomy Versus Scaphoid Excision and Intercarpal Arthrodesis: Intraoperative Assessment and Procedure Selection

Zinberg EM, Chi Y (Wayne State Univ School of Medicine, Detroit, MI)

J Hand Surg Am 39:1055-1062, 2014

Purpose.—To demonstrate the relative frequency of degenerative changes of the radiolunate and capitolunate joints in osteoarthritis of the wrist as seen by direct visualization, and to demonstrate the disparity between findings on preoperative radiographs and direct visualization.

Methods.—We reviewed 18 consecutive patients who underwent either a proximal row carpectomy (PRC) or a scaphoid excision and 4-corner arthrodesis (SEFCA) for symptomatic degenerative arthritis of the wrist. In each case, the articular surfaces of the radiolunate and capitolunate joints were inspected intraoperatively; based on the relative degree of degenerative changes, either a PRC or an SEFCA was performed. We compared preoperative radiographs and the predicted procedure based on them with intraoperative findings and the procedure actually performed.

Results.—Of 18 wrists, 15 had more severe degenerative changes on the proximal articular surface of the lunate than on the capitate head and underwent a PRC; the remaining 3 had more severe changes on the capitate head than on the proximal surface of the lunate and underwent an SEFCA. In contrast, preoperative radiographs in 13 of the 18 cases revealed degenerative changes at the capitolunate joint and minimal or no changes at the radiolunate joint. An SEFCA was the predicted procedure in all 13, but was performed in 3. The remaining 10 underwent a PRC.

Conclusions.—Preoperative radiographs did not correlate well with intraoperative findings in the assessment of degenerative changes at the radiolunate and capitolunate joints, with changes at the radiolunate joint often underestimated. Our findings contradict the widely held contention that the radiolunate joint is consistently spared in osteoarthritis. The lunate fossa of the radius appears to be consistently spared, but not the proximal surface of the lunate. We recommend intraoperative assessment of the articular surfaces, rather than preoperative radiographs, for selection of the surgical procedure.

Type of Study/Level of Evidence.—Therapeutic IV.

► The authors present a retrospective study on the reliability of standard X-rays for preoperative selection of salvage procedure for the treatment of arthritic wrist.

At surgery, direct evaluation of the articular cartilage of the radiolunate and capitolunate joints showed a gross disparity of findings compared with radiographic assessment. Consequently, in more than half of the patients in the series, the procedure had to be changed from the initial preoperative planning, which was based on radiographs. The most striking finding of this study was the high frequency of moderate to severe and extensive degenerative changes at the proximal surface of the lunate (83%), contradicting the expected sparing of this joint in stage III scaphoid nonunion advanced collapse/scaphoid lunate advanced collapse (SNAC/SLAC) wrists. Therefore, 77% of surgeries in this series were converted from scaphoid excision and 4-corner arthrodesis (SEFCA) to proximal row carpectomy (PRC). According to these findings, it seems appropriate to introduce, as the authors suggest, 2 subdivisions to Krakauer et al's classification of stage III (IIIA wrists), with greater degeneration at the radiolunate joint considered candidates for PRC and IIIB wrists, with greater degeneration at the capitolunate joint, considered candidates for SEFCA. I believe that this study should significantly change the method of preoperative selection for the treatment of the SNAC/SLAC wrist toward the assessment by direct visualization of the severity and extension of the degenerative changes. Personally, I prefer to perform a preliminary arthroscopic staging of the wrist, after which I discuss my operative plan with the patient to obtain his or her informed consent for either PRC or SEFCA.

Regrettably, a limitation of this study was that the distal surface of the lunate was not inspected. I would favor further studies that focus on the degeneration of the distal surface of the lunate (and the whole midcarpal joint) to define any possible stage of the SNAC/SLAC wrist in which to perform midcarpal sparing intercarpal fusions (ie, radioscapholunate fusion), thus preserving the advantages of a well-functioning "dart-throwing motion" of the wrist.

A. Atzei, MD

Silicone Proximal Interphalangeal Joint Arthroplasty for Primary Osteoarthritis Using a Volar Approach

Proubasta IR, Lamas CG, Natera L, et al (Hosp Sant Pau, Barcelona, Spain)
J Hand Surg Am 39:1075-1081, 2014

Purpose.—To evaluate the short-term clinical and radiographic outcome of a silicone proximal interphalangeal (PIP) joint implant using a volar approach in patients with primary osteoarthritis.

Methods.—We retrospectively reviewed 36 proximal PIP joints that were replaced with Avanta silicone implants in 26 patients. Inclusion criteria were diagnosis of primary osteoarthrtitis of the PIP joint and failure to respond to conservative treatment. Clinical asessment included range of motion, patient satisfaction, and pain scores. The *Quick*—Disabilities of the Arm, Shoulder, and Hand questionnaire was administered at final follow-up. Radiographs were reviewed for alignment and implant fracture. Complications were also recorded.

Results.—After an average follow-up of 18 months (range, 12—60 mo), pain relief was markedly reduced in all patients, decreasing from a mean score of 7.2 preoperatively to 0.4 postoperatively. The arc of active motion of the PIP joint improved from 33° to 72°. Satisfaction averaged 4.8 on a 5-point Likert scale, and all patients stated they would repeat the surgery. The median final average *Quick*—Disabilities of the Arm, Shoulder, and Hand score was 7 (range, 4—12). Radiograph review showed 2 implant fractures at 1 and 2 years after surgery, respectively, but without clinical changes. The average deformity in the coronal plane changed from 12° (range, 8° to 18°) preoperatively to 4° (range, 3° to 8°) postoperatively, whereas the average flexion contracture changed from 18° (range, 10° to 30°) to 0° (all patients achieved full active extension). No other complications were observed. No revision surgery has been needed to date.

Conclusions.—The volar approach to PIP joint silicone arthroplasty offers the advantages of maintaining the integrity of the extensor mechanism, providing pain relief, and improving postoperative range of motion with minimal complications. However, further research is needed to determine the long-term efficacy of this implant.

Type of Study/Level of Evidence.—Therapeutic IV.

▶ The present study reports the results after proximal interphalangeal (PIP) joint arthroplasty with silicone implants using a volar approach. Even though there have been several publications on this topic, the present paper differs from previous works in the following ways:

1. Use of Avanta implants: most papers dealing with volar approach use Swanson implants or surface replacement devices.
2. The inclusion of only primary osteoarthritis makes the patient group truly homogeneous. Previous works have also included several other etiologies, rendering the study population heterogeneous.

The authors found marked reduction of pain in all operated patients, and a high satisfaction rate among the patients, with all patients stating that they would repeat the operation. The authors reported a reduction of deformity in the coronal plane and a full release of the flexion contracture in all patients. More interesting, improvement of active range of motion from 33 degrees to 72 degrees was found. Implant fracture occurred in 2 of 36 arthroplasties. None of them, however, required reoperation. Swan-neck deformity, a potential complication inherent to the volar approach, was not observed in this series.

It is remarkable that the active arc of motion of the PIP joint improved significantly. This is in contrast to previous comparable investigations. The authors believe that this improvement is due to the use of the palmar approach and the design of the Avanta implants, which have a sharp-angled border between stems and hinge area, and the center of flexion in these devices is palmar to the joint's longitudinal axis.

Even though the findings of this article need to be verified by long-term studies, we can summarize that PIP joint arthroplasty with Avanta implants using a volar approach may be favorable in patients with primary osteoarthritis.

M. Choi, MD

Osteochondral Resurfacing With Proximal Row Carpectomy: 8-Year Follow-Up

Fowler JR, Tang PC, Imbriglia JE (Univ of Pittsburgh, PA; Allegheny Health Network, Pittsburgh, PA; Hand & Upper Ex Center (JEI), Wexford, PA)

Orthopedics 37:e856-e859, 2014

Degenerative arthrosis of the proximal row remains a challenging problem for both patients and surgeons. Proximal row carpectomy is a motion-preserving treatment option, with studies documenting acceptable long-term outcomes. Proximal row carpectomy is an attractive option because there is no need for fusion to occur between the carpal bones, as in 4-corner fusion. As a result, laborers and smokers may be able to return to work more quickly. However, capitate chondrosis traditionally has been considered a contraindication to proximal row carpectomy. The goal of this study was to review the long-term follow-up of patients who underwent osteochondral resurfacing of capitate chondrosis performed in the same setting as proximal row carpectomy. Final follow-up was obtained in 5 of 8 (63%) patients at an average of 101 months (range, 99-102) after surgery. Grip strength improved at each time point, but wrist flexion and extension decreased. The average Mayo Wrist Score was 74 (range, 65-85) and remained stable or improved in all patients between the 18-month visit and the final visit. The Disabilities of the Arm, Shoulder and Hand (DASH) score was unchanged at final follow-up compared with 18-month follow-up ($P = .7$). This study found that osteochondral resurfacing of the capitate in the setting of proximal row carpectomy for patients with capitate chondrosis offers good outcomes compared with standard proximal row carpectomy in patients without capitate chondrosis on patient-directed outcome tools (DASH, Mayo Wrist Score) at long-term follow-up of 101 months.

▶ The authors present a long-term (average 8 years) follow-up retrospective review of 5 patients treated with a modified proximal row carpectomy (PRC) including osteochondral resurfacing for Outerbridge II–IV chondrosis of the capitate (less than 10 mm in diameter). The osteochondral graft was harvested from the lunate. The authors conclude that this modified PRC offers good outcomes compared with standard PRC.

Despite the strengths of a carefully designed study with enough follow-up, there are some drawbacks that the reader should be aware of. The number is small, the etiologies of collapses are not available, the original shape of the capitate according to Viegas was not considered, and the average Mayo score at follow-up is fair. Three of the 5 patients continued to have moderate pain, and 3 had severe capitate-radius arthrosis. Pain was progressive from the 18-month visit to the final follow-up in 3 patients.

This technique is an elegant and technically easy way to cope with an arthritic head of the capitate when performing a PRC. However, more clinical evidence is needed to know whether the surgeon should use it on a large scale or go to a 4-corner fusion.

I routinely perform standard PRC for carpal collapse stage II. Biologic resurfacing of the capitate is appealing for a stage III, but before more evidence is provided, I still prefer 4-corner fusion, especially for heavy male individuals. However, the functional needs of any particular patient may influence the final decision.

G. Herzberg, MD

Rigid versus semi-rigid orthotic use following TMC arthroplasty: A randomized controlled trial

Prosser R, Hancock MJ, Nicholson L, et al (Sydney Hand Therapy & Rehabilitation Centre, Australia; Univ of Sydney, New South Wales, Australia; et al)

J Hand Ther 27:265-271, 2014

Introduction.—The trapeziometacarpal (TMC) joint of the human thumb is the second most common joint in the hand affected by osteoarthritis. TMC arthroplasty is a common procedure used to alleviate symptoms. No randomized controlled trials have been published on the efficacy of different postoperative orthotic regimes.

Method.—Fifty six participants who underwent TMC arthroplasty were allocated to either rigid orthotic or semi-rigid orthotic groups. Both groups started an identical exercise program at two weeks following surgery. Outcome measures were assessed by an assessor blinded to group allocation. The primary outcome was the Patient Rated Wrist and Hand Evaluation (PRWHE) and secondary outcomes included the Michigan Hand

Questionnaire (MHQ), thumb palmar abduction, first metacarpophalangeal extension and three point pinch grip. Measures were taken preoperatively, at six weeks, three months and one year post-operatively. Between-group differences were analyzed with linear regression.

Results.—Both groups performed equally well. There was no significant between-group difference for PRWHE scores (0.47, CI −11.5 to 12.4), including subscales for pain and function, or for any of the secondary outcomes at one year follow-up.

Conclusion.—We found no difference in outcomes between using a rigid or semi-rigid orthosis after TMC arthroplasty. Patient comfort, cost and availability may determine choice between orthoses in clinical practice.

Level of Evidence.—1b RCT.

▶ This randomized controlled study was set up to determine the benefits of 2 types of orthotics used after trapeziometacarpal (TMC) arthroplasty. The assumption was that early motion with the use of a semirigid orthosis may lead to improved outcomes. The authors did a nice job describing the rigid orthosis and the semirigid orthosis that they custom fabricated to use in their study with 56 postoperative patients that were randomly assigned to the 2 groups. They used standardized outcome measures, range-of-motion measurements, and pinch strength to compare the 2 groups. Their data demonstrated that the rigid orthosis was no better or worse than the semirigid orthosis regarding outcomes.

This study allows the therapist to use clinical reasoning with orthotic application post-TMC arthroplasty. Because both types of orthotics (semirigid and rigid) had comparable outcomes, the therapist is free to determine which type of orthosis would be most beneficial to the patient, allowing the greatest comfort and function for the patient while providing the appropriate amount of protection. Other considerations would be ease of fabrication for the therapist, availability of materials, and cost. The authors stated that the semirigid orthosis may be more cost-effective because the rigid component could be removed at the proper time postoperatively and the patient would have light support with the neoprene thumb and wrist component. However, in our clinic, we modify the rigid thumb spica orthosis to a hand-based thumb orthosis simply by remolding the thermoplast, which is also quite cost-effective. Therapists will most likely have an appropriate orthosis they are comfortable making and modifying, either rigid or semirigid, which this article affirms.

I appreciate having a good-quality study to reference that gives outcome-based evidence concerning the use of orthotics in TMC arthroplasty.

S. J. Clark, OTR/L, CHT

2 Dupuytren's Contracture

Multiple Collagenase Injections Are Safe for Treatment of Dupuytren's Contractures

Gajendran VK, Hentz V, Kenney D, et al (Stanford Univ, Redwood City, CA)
Orthopedics 37:e657-e660, 2014

The authors report the case of a 65-year-old, right-hand-dominant man who had severe Dupuytren's disease with multiple cords and flexion contractures of the metacarpophalangeal and proximal interphalangeal joints of both hands and underwent repeated collagenase injections for treatment. Collagenase has been shown to be safe and effective in the treatment of Dupuytren's contractures when administered as a single dose, but the results of multiple injections over a prolonged period are unknown. Antibodies to collagenase develop in all patients after several treatments, raising concerns about safety and efficacy as a result of sensitization from repeated exposures. The antibodies generated as a result of repeated exposure to collagenase could theoretically render it less effective with time and could also lead to immune reactions as severe as anaphylaxis. The authors present the case of a single patient who experienced continued correction of his contractures with only minor and self-limited adverse reactions after administration of 12 collagenase doses through 15 injections during a 4-year period. Over time, the injections continued to be effective at correcting metacarpophalangeal joint contractures, but less effective at correcting proximal interphalangeal joint contractures. The patient did eventually require a fasciectomy, but the safety and modest success of the repeated collagenase injections shows promise for a less invasive treatment with a better risk profile than open fasciectomy. Although further studies are needed, repeated administration of collagenase appears to be safe and modestly effective for severe Dupuytren's contractures, although a fasciectomy may ultimately be required in the most severe cases.

▶ Gajendran et al report a case that raises many questions about the role of mixed clostridial collagenase, Xiaflex, (CCH) in treating Dupuytren's contracture. Their case is a patient who was treated with 12 doses of CCH over 5 years to treat bilateral contractures in 5 fingers. The patient had no unusual or severe adverse reaction, and the medication seemed to be effective even at the 12th dose, which was actually distributed at 3 different sites (an off-label use). This case raises the issues of cost of treatment, the use of biologic treatment over years and multiple doses, and the ultimate role of CCH in the surgeon's armamentarium for treating Dupuytren's contracture.

Many other factors in addition to cost come into play when choosing among the Dupuytren's contracture treatment options, including patient preference, degree of contracture and impact on the patient, recurrence, and complication rates. However, cost is an important consideration, and there are limited or no data on the relative costs of treatment with CCH compared with needle aponeurotomy and open surgery. The cost analysis is likely to be very different for an individual with disease in 5 fingers compared with those with less diffuse disease. Although this patient received about half of the doses of medication under a clinical trial, the retail cost of the medication alone for these 12 doses would have reached $39 000 at $3250 a dose.

The use of repeated doses of large proteins as medications is relatively new, and the outcomes in terms of effectiveness and serious adverse reactions based on immunologic response are still to be determined for this relatively new medication. The authors comment on the use of Botulinum toxin, a similar injected large protein, which has been in use for a much longer period. Whether the safety and efficacy profiles of CCH will change with multiple doses over long periods is an open question that needs to be answered with studies over longer periods.

Perhaps most compelling is the suggestion by this case report that patients with severe disease may be treated as if they had chronic disease managed by a medical model rather than a surgical one. The contractures are managed by a medication until refractory to medical treatment and then by surgical fasciectomy (as this patient had for his right small finger). Although we are a long way from arriving at that model (as peptic ulcer disease has), this report suggests we have taken a step in that direction.

P. Blazar, MD

Steroid Injection and Needle Aponeurotomy for Dupuytren Disease: Long-Term Follow-Up of a Randomized Controlled Trial

McMillan C, Binhammer P (Sunnybrook Health Sciences Centre, Toronto, Ontario, Canada)

J Hand Surg Am 39:1942-1947, 2014

Purpose.—To compare long-term outcomes and retreatment rates for patients with Dupuytren disease who underwent needle aponeurotomy (NA) combined with a series of triamcinolone acetonide injections or underwent NA alone as part of a prior randomized controlled trial.

Methods.—During this follow-up study, 44 of 47 participants in the original study were examined as needed between 6 and 53 months from their initial procedure. Those who had not been reassessed within 18 months of the original NA were asked to return for follow-up. The average total active extension deficit (TAED) of previously treated joints was compared between groups 7 to 12, 13 to 24, 25 to 36, and 37 to

48 months following treatment. Timing of retreatment (if performed) was recorded.

Results.—Forty-four participants returned for assessment an average of 4.8 times over 53 months. Mean TAED was significantly less in needle aponeurotomy triamcinolone injection patients at 6 months and between 13 and 24 months. Sixty-two percent of NA group patients and 30% of needle aponeurotomy triamcinolone injection patients returned for a second treatment on the same digit(s) (retreatment). This difference was not significant. Mean time to retreatment and mean TAED immediately prior to retreatment did not differ significantly between groups. Kaplan-Meier survival estimates demonstrated a significantly higher percentage of NA group patients expected to return for retreatment by 24 but not by 36 months. Younger age, more than one joint treated at the initial NA, and TAED severity throughout the follow-up period were associated with earlier retreatment.

Conclusions.—Serial triamcinolone injections combined with NA was associated with lower TAED for up to 24 months. A larger study would more accurately quantify the potential benefits of combining triamcinolone injections with NA for treatment of Dupuytren disease.

Type of Study/Level of Evidence.—Therapeutic III.

▶ The authors present intermediate-term follow-up of a previously published randomized control trial to determine the benefit of triamcinolone injections in patients undergoing needle aponeurotomy (NA) for Dupuytren contracture. The previous study demonstrated significantly lower total active extension deficit (TAED) at 6 months in the triamcinolone group. The authors followed 44 of the original 47 patients on an average 4.8 times between 7 and 53 months. Based on a Kaplan–Meier survival analysis, the percentage of NA patients needing retreatment was higher at 12, 24, and 36 months in the patients who did not have triamcinolone. There was also a significantly higher TAED at 24 months in the NA only group (70 vs 27 degrees). The main limitation of the study was the use of participant-driven follow-up rather than prospective trial of routine visits at 12, 24, and 36 months and an inherent selection bias from this.

Based on previous published reports and correspondence with other hand surgeons who have performed a large number of NA procedures, I currently perform triamcinolone injections at the end of my NA procedures but do not perform this as a series of injections as described by the authors here. The triamcinolone injections seem to have the added benefit of softening the residual cords and nodules. Anecdotally, it also appears to decrease swelling and inflammation from the procedure. A randomized prospective trial comparing NA and NA with triamcinolone with yearly follow-up up to 3 or 4 years would be an important future study.

J. Huang, MD

Prospective Randomized Controlled Trial Comparing 1- Versus 7-Day Manipulation Following Collagenase Injection for Dupuytren Contracture

Mickelson DT, Noland SS, Watt AJ, et al (Univ of Washington, Seattle)

J Hand Surg Am 39:1933-1941, 2014

Purpose.—To compare the efficacy, tolerance, and safety of manual manipulation at day 7 to day 1 following collagenase *Clostridium histolyticum* (CCH) injection for Dupuytren contracture.

Methods.—Eligible patients were randomized to manipulation at day 1 versus day 7 following CCH injection. Preinjection, premanipulation, postmanipulation, and 30-day follow-up metacarpophalangeal (MCP) and proximal interphalangeal (PIP) joint contractures were measured. Pain scores were recorded at each time point. Data were stratified per cohort based on primary joint treated (MCP vs PIP). Means were compared using paired and unpaired *t*-tests.

Results.—Forty-three patients with 46 digits were eligible and were randomized to 1-day (22 digits) and 7-day (24 digits) manipulation. For MCP joints, there were no significant differences in flexion contractures between 1- and 7-day cohorts for initial (47° vs 46°), postmanipulation (0° vs 2°), or 30-day follow-up (1° vs 2°) measurements. Premanipulation, the residual contracture was significantly lower in the 7-day group (23° vs 40°). For PIP joints, there were no significant differences between 1- and 7-day cohorts for initial (63° vs 62°), premanipulation (56° vs 52°), postmanipulation (13° vs 15°), or 30-day (14° vs 16°) measurements. There were no significant differences in pain or skin tears between the 2 groups. No flexor tendon ruptures were observed.

Conclusions.—The effectiveness of CCH in achieving correction of Dupuytren contractures was preserved when manipulation was performed on day 7, with no differences in correction, pain, or skin tears. These data suggest that manipulation can be scheduled at the convenience of the patient and surgeon within the first 7 days after injection.

Type of Study/Level of Evidence.—Therapeutic I.

▶ The authors have demonstrated the benefit of a treatment algorithm that most of heavy collagenase users have already adopted, that is, going off-label in terms of the interval between injection and manipulation. Many clinician-users have schedules that do not involve consecutive clinic or office days. Early on, they modified the industry and US Food and Drug Administration (FDA) recommendations to suit their own specific work schedule. Soon after FDA release, I asked the same question as did the authors because I saw my Stanford hand patients 1 morning a week. In 2012, I began injecting on Monday morning and manipulating the following Monday. After 25 injections, I looked at the results, comparing them to a previous 25 injections in which the manipulation followed injection by the industry- and FDA-recommended 24 hours. My results were essentially the same as those reported in this study except I had better results in proximal interphalangeal joint contractures in the 1-week group. A notable number of patients had already ruptured their cords and did not need my manipulation. At 1 week, their hands were much less swollen and tender, which reduced the anxiety of those patients who needed manipulation. This experience was published in the February 2014 volume of *Hand Clinics*.[1]

V. R. Hentz, MD

Reference

1. Hentz VR. Collagenase injections for treatment of Dupuytren disease. *Hand Clin.* 2014;30:25-32.

Patterns of Dupuytren Disease in Fingers: Studying Correlations with a Multivariate Ordinal Logit Model

Lanting R, Nooraee N, Werker PMN, et al (Univ of Groningen, The Netherlands)

Plast Reconstr Surg 134:483-490, 2014

Background.—Dupuytren disease affects fingers in a variable fashion. Knowledge about specific disease patterns (phenotype) based on location and severity of the disease is lacking.

Methods.—In this cross-sectional study, 344 primary affected hands with Dupuytren disease were physically examined. The Pearson correlation coefficient between the coexistence of Dupuytren disease in pairs of fingers was calculated, and agglomerative hierarchical clustering was applied to identify possible clusters of affected fingers. With a multivariate ordinal logit model, the authors studied the correlation on severity, taking into account age and sex, and tested hypotheses on independence between groups of fingers.

Results.—The ring finger was most frequently affected by Dupuytren disease, and contractures were seen in 15.1 percent of affected rays. The severity of thumb and index finger, middle and ring fingers, and middle and little fingers was significantly correlated. Occurrences in pairs of fingers were highest in the middle and ring fingers and lowest in the thumb and index finger. Correlation between the ring and little fingers and a correlation between fingers from the ulnar and radial sides could not be demonstrated.

Conclusions.—Rays on the ulnar side of the hand are predominantly affected. The middle finger is substantially correlated with other fingers on the ulnar side, and the thumb and index finger are correlated; however, there was no evidence that the ulnar side and the radial side were correlated in any way, which suggests that occurrence on one side of the hand does not predict Dupuytren disease on the other side of the hand.

Clincial Question/Level of Evidence.—Risk, III (Table 5).

▶ The authors examined many patients with Dupuytren disease and mapped the location of the proliferative tissue, according to which areas of the hand

TABLE 5.—Predicted Occurrences of Dupuytren Disease with 95% Confidence Intervals in Single and Combinations of Fingers for Men and Women Separately at Age 65 Years

Fingers*	Occurrence, % (95% CI) Men	Women
One or two fingers		
1	30.9 (25.6–36.4)	26.1 (20.8–31.6)
2	12.8 (8.8–17.4)	10.4 (6.8–14.9)
3	53.8 (47.8–60.1)	48.7 (41.3–54.3)
4	77.3 (73.0–81.1)	72.9 (67.5–77.8)
5	59.5 (53.0–65.1)	53.6 (46.7–59.9)
1, 2	5.4 (3.0–8.3)	3.7 (1.9–6.3)
1, 3	19.4 (14.8–24.1)	14.9 (10.5–19.9)
1, 4	24.5 (19.4–29.6)	19.4 (14.0–25.1)
1, 5	20.2 (15.6–25.1)	15.6 (11.2–20.8)
2, 3	7.4 (4.3–11.0)	5.3 (2.8–8.3)
2, 4	8.3 (5.1–12.0)	5.8 (3.1–9.4)
2, 5	8.2 (5.0–12.0)	5.9 (3.1–9.3)
3, 4	46.2 (39.7–53.0)	39.7 (32.8–46.7)
3, 5	35.5 (29.4–41.5)	29.2 (23.1–35.5)
4, 5	45.9 (39.5–51.8)	38.7 (31.5–45.8)
Three or more fingers		
1, 2, 3	3.7 (1.9–5.8)	2.4 (1.1–4.0)
1, 2, 4	3.9 (2.0–6.2)	2.4 (1.0–4.5)
1, 2, 5	3.9 (2.1–6.2)	2.5 (1.2–4.5)
1, 3, 4	16.3 (11.9–21.0)	12.1 (7.9–16.7)
1, 3, 5	13.3 (9.4–17.7)	9.5 (6.1–14.0)
1, 4, 5	15.5 (11.5–20.0)	11.2 (7.2–16.1)
2, 3, 4	5.7 (3.1–8.9)	3.8 (1.8–6.4)
2, 3, 5	5.4 (2.9–8.5)	3.6 (1.7–6.2)
2, 4, 5	5.6 (3.2–8.5)	3.7 (1.7–6.5)
3, 4, 5	29.5 (23.4–35.4)	23.2 (17.3–29.5)
1, 2, 3, 4	2.8 (1.4–4.7)	1.7 (0.7–3.1)
1, 2, 3, 5	2.8 (1.3–4.6)	1.7 (0.7–3.1)
1, 2, 4, 5	2.7 (1.4–4.5)	1.6 (0.6–3.2)
1, 3, 4, 5	11.0 (7.6–15.2)	7.5 (4.5–11.7)
2, 3, 4, 5	4.1 (2.1–6.7)	2.6 (1.0–4.6)
1, 2, 3, 4, 5	2.1 (1.0–3.5)	1.2 (0.4–2.3)

*1, thumb; 2, index; 3, middle, 4, ring; 5, little.

Reprinted from Lanting R, Nooraee N, Werker PMN, et al. Patterns of Dupuytren Disease in Fingers: Studying Correlations with a Multivariate Ordinal Logit Model. Plast Reconstr Surg. 2014;134:483-490.

and fingers were involved. Their goal was to fill in gaps of knowledge regarding disease-specific patterns, termed "phenotypes"—for example, index-thumb presentation or middle finger-small finger presentation. Understanding the methodology requires the reader to possess an advanced degree in statistics because the text is made difficult to understand by frequent use of terms such as "probits," "logits," "agglomerative hierarchical clustering," and "bootstrapping," terms that may be jargon to the statistician but are likely meaningless to the average interested reader. Here is where a good editor would have asked the authors to provide a brief sentence or two to educate the reader, but perhaps the editor was himself or herself a statistician. Nonetheless, the findings correlate with previous studies of incidence per finger and extend the understanding by generating likely pair or triplet phenotypes, occurrences that are not just the product of disease being, for example, most common in the ring finger, with a significant correlation between the thumb and the index finger, the middle and ring fingers, and the middle and little fingers (Table 5). Surprisingly, there was no significant correlation between ring and little finger after factoring for the high incidence of ring disease.

V. R. Hentz, MD

3 Tendon

The Detrimental Effects of Systemic Ibuprofen Delivery on Tendon Healing Are Time-Dependent

Connizzo BK, Yannascoli SM, Tucker JJ, et al (Univ of Pennsylvania, Philadelphia; et al)
Clin Orthop Relat Res 472:2433-2439, 2014

Background.—Current clinical treatment after tendon repairs often includes prescribing NSAIDs to limit pain and inflammation. The negative influence of NSAIDs on bone repair is well documented, but their effects on tendon healing are less clear. While NSAIDs may be detrimental to early tendon healing, some evidence suggests that they may improve healing if administered later in the repair process.

Questions/Purposes.—We asked whether the biomechanical and histologic effects of systemic ibuprofen administration on tendon healing are influenced by either immediate or delayed drug administration.

Methods.—After bilateral supraspinatus detachment and repair surgeries, rats were divided into groups and given ibuprofen orally for either Days 0 to 7 (early) or Days 8 to 14 (delayed) after surgery; a control group did not receive ibuprofen. Healing was evaluated at 1, 2, and 4 weeks postsurgery through biomechanical testing and histologic assessment.

Results.—Biomechanical evaluation resulted in decreased stiffness and modulus at 4 weeks postsurgery for early ibuprofen delivery (mean ± SD [95% CI]: 10.8 ± 6.4 N/mm [6.7–14.8] and 8.9 ± 5.9 MPa [5.4–12.3]) when compared to control repair (20.4 ± 8.6 N/mm [16.3–24.5] and 15.7 ± 7.5 MPa [12.3–19.2]) ($p = 0.003$ and 0.013); however, there were no differences between the delayed ibuprofen group (18.1 ± 7.4 N/mm [14.2–22.1] and 11.5 ± 5.6 MPa [8.2–14.9]) and the control group. Histology confirmed mechanical results with reduced fiber reorganization over time in the early ibuprofen group.

Conclusions.—Early administration of ibuprofen in the postoperative period was detrimental to tendon healing, while delayed administration did not affect tendon healing.

Clinical Relevance.—Historically, clinicians have often prescribed ibuprofen after tendon repair, but this study suggests that the timing of ibuprofen administration is critical to adequate tendon healing. This research necessitates future clinical studies investigating the use of ibuprofen for pain control after rotator cuff repair and other tendon injuries.

▶ The authors evaluated the use of ibuprofen and the effects of it on tendon healing in 3 groups of rats: those given ibuprofen immediately after repair of a simulated rotator cuff tear (detachment of the supraspinatus) for 7 days, those given ibuprofen in a delayed fashion beginning 8 days after repair, and a control group who did not have ibuprofen. After death at 1, 2, or 4 weeks after surgery, biomechanical testing was performed to evaluate strength of repair, and histology was performed.

More hematomas and neovascularity were seen in all of those given ibuprofen, and early administration of ibuprofen was deleterious to tendon repair as evidenced by biomechanical testing. The authors should be congratulated on their work to evaluate the effect of ibuprofen administration on tendon healing in the early and late course. As surgeons experience pressure to decrease use of narcotic analgesics and encourage our patients to use alternative medications, we should carefully consider the potential effects on our surgical repairs. The data suggest that later administration of ibuprofen is accompanied by less deleterious results on tendon healing; however, it is worrisome that, compared with the control, there was still a higher incidence of hematomas and of vascularity with delayed ibuprofen administration over control.

J. E. Adams, MD

Parathyroid Hormone 1–34 Enhances Extracellular Matrix Deposition and Organization During Flexor Tendon Repair

Lee DJ, Southgate RD, Farhat YM, et al (Univ of Rochester Med Ctr, NY)

J Orthop Res 33:17-24, 2015

Parathyroid hormone (PTH) 1–34 is known to enhance fracture healing. Tendon repair is analogous to bone healing in its dependence on the proliferation and differentiation of mesenchymal stem cells, matrix formation, and tissue remodeling. We hypothesized that PTH 1–34 enhances tendon healing in a flexor digitorum longus (FDL) tendon repair model. C57Bl/6J mice were treated with either intraperitoneal PTH 1–34 or vehicle-control (PBS). Tendons were harvested at 3–28 days for histology, gene expression, and biomechanical testing. The metatarsophalangeal joint range of motion was reduced 1.5–2-fold in PTH 1–34 mice compared to control mice. The gliding coefficient, a measure of adhesion formation, was 2–3.5-fold higher in PTH 1–34 mice. At 14 days post-repair, the tensile strength was twofold higher in PTH 1–34 specimens, but at 28 days there were no differences. PTH 1–34 mice had increased fibrous tissue deposition that correlated with elevated expression of collagens and fibronectin as seen on quantitative PCR. PTH 1—34 accelerated the deposition of reparative tissue but increased adhesion formation.

▶ This is a well-designed study that investigated the effect of parathyroid hormone 1-34 on tendon-healing biology and adhesion formation. Not surprisingly, it enhanced production of the extracellular matrix in an animal model, but at the same time, it increased adhesion formation rather drastically. The gliding coefficient of the treated tendon was twice that of the untreated tendon 2 weeks after surgery. In the past, quite a few molecules were tested by different investigators. So far, many studies yielded a similar result: increasing both collagen production and adhesions of the treated tendon. In this study, the treatment only transiently increased tensile strength of the healing tendons. Based on the findings in this report, parathyroid hormone 1-34 has not shown benefits greater than those molecules tested previously.

One can assume many molecules that enhance tissue growth would promote tendon healing, but our goal is to find a method to increase tendon-healing strength at multiple time points after surgery, while not increasing adhesion formation around the tendon. Thus far, few methods tested experimentally have fulfilled this requirement, and no clinical trials have proven their efficacy. Finding a method that powerfully enhances tendon healing and does not increase collagen deposition over the tendon surface (which leads to adhesions) is a much sought-after goal.

J. B. Tang, MD

CORR® ORS Richard A. Brand Award for Outstanding Orthopaedic Research: Engineering Flexor Tendon Repair With Lubricant, Cells, and Cytokines in a Canine Model

Zhao C, Ozasa Y, Reisdorf RL, et al (Mayo Clinic, Rochester, MN; et al)
Clin Orthop Relat Res 472:2569-2578, 2014

Background.—Adhesions and poor healing are complications of flexor tendon repair.

Questions/Purposes.—The purpose of this study was to investigate a tissue engineering approach to improve functional outcomes after flexor tendon repair in a canine model.

Methods.—Flexor digitorum profundus tendons were lacerated and repaired in 60 dogs that were followed for 10, 21, or 42 days. One randomly selected repair from either the second or fifth digit in one paw in each dog was treated with carbodiimide-derivatized hyaluronic acid, gelatin, and lubricin plus autologous bone marrow stromal cells stimulated with growth and differentiation factor 5; control repair tendons were not treated. Digits were analyzed by adhesion score, work of flexion, tendon-pulley friction, failure force, and histology.

Results.—In the control group, 35 of 52 control tendons had adhesions, whereas 19 of 49 treated tendons had adhesions. The number of repaired tendons with adhesions in the control group was greater than the number in the treated group at all three times ($p = 0.005$). The normalized work of flexion in treated tendons was 0.28 (± 0.08), 0.29 (± 0.19), and 0.32 (± 0.22) N/mm/° at Day 10, Day 21, and Day 42 respectively, compared with the untreated tendons of 0.46 (± 0.19) at Day 10 (effect size, 1.5; $p = 0.01$), 0.77 (± 0.49) at Day 21 (effect size, 1.4; $p < 0.001$), and 1.17 (± 0.82) N/mm/° at Day 42 (effect size, 1.6; $p < 0.001$). The friction data were comparable to the work of flexion data at all times. The repaired tendon failure force in the untreated group at 42 days was 70.2 N (± 8.77), which was greater than the treated tendons 44.7 N (± 8.53) (effect size, 1.9; $p < 0.001$). Histologically, treated repairs had a smooth surface with intrinsic healing, whereas control repairs had surface adhesions and extrinsic healing.

Conclusions.—Our study provides evidence that tissue engineering coupled with restoration of tendon gliding can improve the quality of tendon healing in a large animal in vivo model.

Clinical Relevance.—Tissue engineering may enhance intrinsic tendon healing and thus improve the functional outcomes of flexor tendon repair.

▶ This is a continuing investigation building on the work over the past decades by the Mayo group on tendon repair biomechanics and the cellular and chemical modulation of tendon healing. I commend the authors on their great contribution to the advancement of this field and their innovative approach to solving difficult problems in tendon healing. Of great promise in future application to real-world practice are the following: (1) cell implementation between the 2 stumps of the lacerated tendons and (2) the creation of a carbodiimide-derivatized gelatin, hyaluronic acid, and lubricin-modified tendon gliding surface. Both have great potential to enhance tendon healing and reduce adhesion formation. I look forward to seeing their translation to clinical practice with possible benefits to direct tendon suture repair and tendon grafting.

I believe biological modulation is a promising field that may yield exciting advancements in this field. The structure of the tendon is unique in that it contains few cells in contrast to its dense and rich extracellular matrix, and it has poor vascular supply.

In the results of this study, however, it is worth noting that at day 42 (week 7), the breaking strength of the repaired tendon with cell patch treatment was significantly (about 30%) weaker than the untreated control. At week 7, the strength in the untreated control tendon was increased greatly compared with day 10 and week 3, but this was not seen in the treated tendon. This is a serious concern. In other words, the proposed treatment prevented a much-needed increase in the healing strength after week 3. Therefore, additional measures should be taken to combat this problem.

My colleagues and I have been developing growth factor-based gene therapy using adeno-associated virus (AAV) vectors to enhance tendon healing strength and decrease adhesions. Using AAV2-anti-transforming growth factor-beta-microRNA in a chicken model, we were able to decrease the adhesions of the tendon and work of flexion of the operated digits. However, we detected a decrease in the healing strength in the first a few weeks after surgery. Our group faces a similar challenge: how to decrease adhesion formation while achieving a healed strength identical to the untreated tendon. This is a key question for future investigations.

J. B. Tang, MD

Primary Flexor Tendon Repair in Zones 1 and 2: Early Passive Mobilization Versus Controlled Active Motion

Frueh FS, Kunz VS, Gravestock IJ, et al (Univ Hosp Zurich, Raemistrasse, Switzerland; Univ of Zurich, Switzerland) *J Hand Surg Am* 39:1344-1350, 2014

Purpose.—To compare early passive mobilization (EPM) with controlled active motion (CAM) after flexor tendon surgery in zones 1 and 2.

Methods.—We performed a retrospective analysis of collected data of all patients receiving primary flexor tendon repair in zones 1 and 2 from 2006 to 2011, during which time 228 patients were treated, and 191 patients with 231 injured digits were eligible for study. Exclusion criteria were replantation, finger revascularization, age younger than 16 years, rehabilitation by means other than EPM or CAM, and missing information regarding postoperative rehabilitation. This left 132 patients with 159 injured fingers for analysis. The primary endpoint was the comparison of total active motion (TAM) values 4 and 12 weeks after surgery between the EPM and the CAM protocols. The analysis of TAM measurements under the rehabilitation protocols was conducted using *t*-tests and further linear modeling. We defined rupture rate and the assessment of adhesion/infection as secondary endpoints.

Results.—There was a statistically significant difference between the TAM values of the EPM and the CAM protocols 4 weeks after surgery. At 12 weeks, however, there was no significant difference between the 2 protocols. Older age and injuries with finger fractures were associated with lower TAM values. Rupture rates were 5% (CAM) and 7% (EPM), which were not statistically different.

Conclusions.—This study showed a favorable effect of CAM protocol on TAM 4 weeks after surgery. The percent rupture rate was slightly lower in the patients with CAM than in the patients with EPM regime. Further studies are required to confirm our results and to investigate whether faster recovery of TAM is associated with shorter time out of work.

Type of Study/Level of Evidence.—Therapeutic III.

▶ This is an excellent clinical study that compares rupture rates of zone 1 and 2 primary digital flexor tendon repair after either early active or early passive finger mobilization. The striking finding is that tendons had a lower risk of repair rupture after early active finger mobilization than after early passive mobilization. Although the difference in percent rupture rate is statistically insignificant, it appears certain that early active digital motion does not produce greater rupture rates compared with early passive motion.

It should be noted that in this report, all flexor tendons were repaired with a 4-strand core suture using a 3-0 or 4-0 suture, plus a circumferential locking peripheral suture using a 6-0 suture. The early active protocol that the authors began to use in 2011 features many important components of a protocol I proposed previously.[1] The reported rupture rate (5%) with the early active motion protocol is reasonable and consistent with the results of other investigators. Based on analysis of a large number of patients, the study found favorable outcomes of early active motion after primary tendon repair using a multistrand core suture, which indicates that the practice is safe and that its outcomes may be better than those of early passive motion.

I now use early active motion in almost all patients with zone 1, 2, or 3 repairs. I must stress that the tendon should be repaired with at least a 4-strand core suture. I use a 6-strand repair for all FDP tendon repairs and feel that a 6-strand repair resists gap formation much better than a 4-strand repair. I have had no repair ruptures over the past several years, using early active motion after a strong core suture repair. I believe that early active motion will grow in popularity, and I must stress 4 key points regarding surgery and early motion: (1) a strong core suture repair should be executed with some tension across the suture lines; (2) ensure proper management of the major pulleys, including venting the entire A4 pulley or a part of the A2 pulley, to free tendon gliding if necessary; (3) perform the digital extension-flexion test, preferably with local anesthesia,[2] and (4) partial (one-third to two-thirds) range of active digital flexion in the first 3 weeks after full range of passive motion increases finger elasticity. Following a protocol with these considerations should favor a successful repair.

J. B. Tang, MD

References

1. Tang JB. Indications, methods, postoperative motion and outcome evaluation of primary flexor tendon repairs in zone 2. *J Hand Surg Eur Vol.* 2007;32:118-129.
2. Lalonde DH, Martin AL. Wide-awake flexor tendon repair and early tendon mobilization in zones 1 and 2. *Hand Clin.* 2013;29:207-213.

Reattachment of Flexor Digitorum Profundus Avulsion: Biomechanical Performance of 3 Techniques

Brar R, Owen JR, Melikian R, et al (Virginia Commonwealth Univ, Richmond; OrthoCarolina Hand Ctr, Charlotte, NC)
J Hand Surg Am 39:2214-2219, 2014

Purpose.—To investigate whether inclusion of the volar plate in repair of flexor digitorum profundus avulsions increases the strength of the repair and resists gapping.

Methods.—Cadaveric fingers (n = 18) were divided into 3 equal groups. The first technique involved 2 micro-suture anchors only (A). The second used only volar plate repair (VP). The third group was a hybrid, combining a micro-suture anchor with volar plate augmentation (AVP). Specimens were loaded cyclically to simulate passive motion rehabilitation before being loaded to failure. Clinical failure was defined as 3 mm of gapping, and physical failure as the highest load associated with hardware failure, suture breakage, anchor pullout, or volar plate avulsion.

Results.—Gapping throughout cycling was significantly greater for the A group than VP and AVP with no difference detected between VP and AVP groups. Gapping exceeded 3 mm during cycling of 3 A specimens, but in none of the VP or AVP specimens. Load at clinical and physical failure for A was significantly lower than for VP and AVP, whereas no difference was detected between VP and AVP.

Conclusions.—In this cadaveric model, incorporating the volar plate conferred a significant advantage in strength, increasing the mean load to physical failure by approximately 100 N.

Clinical Relevance.—According to previous biomechanical studies, current reconstructive strategies for flexor digitorum profundus zone I avulsions are not strong enough to withstand active motion rehabilitation. We demonstrated the potential use of volar plate augmentation and the prospective advantageous increase in strength in this cadaveric model. In vivo performance and effects on digital motion are not known.

► This well-designed and executed biomechanical study examined 3 techniques for the repair of flexor digitorum profundus (FDP) zone I injuries using a human cadaveric model. Technique A repaired the FDP directly to the bone in the distal phalanx using suture anchors; technique B repaired the FDP to the volar plate with suture; and technique C used a hybrid repair of the tendon to bone with anchors and also to the volar plate with suture. After establishing the technique and validating the model in 4 cadavers, the authors used the index, middle, and ring fingers in 6 cadavers to perform each repair technique while randomizing the technique to each type of finger. Biomechanical testing was performed by cyclically loading the distal interphalangeal joints to simulate passive motion using a MTS system with a digital camera to evaluate gap formation at the repair site. Load to failure testing was also performed after 500 cycles and was recorded as the highest load achieved without hardware failure, suture breakage, anchor pullout, or volar plate avulsion.

None of the repairs physically failed during cyclic testing. There were significant differences in both gap formation and load to failure testing in FDP repair using only suture anchors when compared with those that incorporated the volar plate into the repair using either technique. The authors concluded that including the volar plate in FDP repairs improves strength and may allow for more aggressive therapy protocols. This study contributes meaningful biomechanical data that supports an operative technique that I learned during training. Future in vivo studies could contribute even more to our understanding and potentially allow conclusions to be made regarding the local tissue effects and healing potential using this technique.

J. Tueting, MD

Wide-Awake Extensor Indicis Proprius to Extensor Pollicis Longus Tendon Transfer

Lalonde DH (Dalhousie Univ, Saint John, New Brunswick, Canada)

J Hand Surg Am 39:2297-2299, 2014

This article provides video and narration to describe the technical details of how to inject local anesthesia and perform the extensor indicis proprius to extensor pollicis longus tendon transfer in patients with wide-awake local anesthesia and no tourniquet. Lidocaine for anesthesia and epinephrine for hemostasis are the only 2 medications given to the patient. Sedation and the tourniquet are not required. Wide-awake patients are comfortable, cooperative, and educable, and are able to help the surgeon set the correct tension for the transfer. They flex and extend the thumb before the skin is closed to make sure the transfer is not too tight or too loose. It helps that they remember seeing the thumb move nicely during the surgery when they are in postoperative hand therapy.

► The wide-awake extensor indicis proprius (EIP) to extensor pollicis longus (EPL) transfer described by the author, in theory, affords the recipients the opportunity to initiate learning and sensorimotor cortical reorganization earlier rather than later. This approach also likely better enables the surgeon to more accurately measure the effects of the tension used when establishing the transfer. If not enough, the muscle-tendon unit is made actively insufficient, and thumb extension lag is resultant, and if too much, the muscle-tendon unit is made passively insufficient, resulting in limited tendon excursion and restrictions in composite thumb flexion/opposition. For the correct candidate, this approach also eliminates the need for and side effects of tourniquet, regional blocks, sedation, and anesthesia.

Bezuhly et al,[1] through the use of a case-series design, report positive outcomes among 6 patients who underwent the wide-awake procedure in that thumb range of motion resolved to that equivalent to the patients' unaffected side. To date, however, there are no controlled trials to establish that surgical or rehabilitative outcomes are any different for those undergoing wide-awake compared with more traditional approaches to EIP—EPL transfers. Any improved outcomes may well be owing to the feedback offered to the surgeon during surgery but not necessarily to patient learning. It could be that any benefit of early learning is diminished by the inability to carry over such learning during the postoperative immobilization period described in the literature of 3—6 weeks. This finding is supported by evidence that there is reduced density in the contralateral cortex's sensorimotor strip after an average of 16 days of upper limb cast immobilization.[2]

The carryover of learning, however, might be facilitated by early mobilization protocols[3] when appropriate. In those instances in which early mobilization is not permissible, learning might be maintained through the use of mirror box treatment.[4]

This surgical approach may afford fewer potential complications, improved surgical outcomes, and better rehabilitation outcomes when compared with other approaches; however, at this time, additional empirical evidence is needed.

C. McGee, PhD, OTR/L, CHT

References

1. Bezuhly M, Sparkes GL, Higgins A, Neumeister MW, Lalonde DH. Immediate thumb extension following extensor indicis proprius-to-extensor pollicis longus tendon transfer using the wide-awake approach. *Plast Reconstr Surg*. 2007;119: 1507-1512.
2. Langer N, Hänggi J, Müller NA, Simmen HP, Jäncke L. Effects of limb immobilization on brain plasticity. *Neurology*. 2012;78:182-188.
3. Germann G, Wagner H, Blome-Eberwein S, Karle B, Wittemann M. Early dynamic motion versus postoperative immobilization in patients with extensor indicis proprius transfer to restore thumb extension: a prospective randomized study. *J Hand Surg Am*. 2001;26:1111-1115.
4. Rostami HR, Arefi A, Tabatabaei S. Effect of mirror therapy on hand function in patients with hand orthopaedic injuries: a randomized controlled trial. *Disabil Rehabil*. 2013;35:1647-1651.

Rehabilitation of a patient following hand replantation after near-complete distal forearm amputation

Sturm SM, Oxley SB, Van Zant RS (St. Mary's Med Ctr, Huntington, WV; Huntington Physical Therapy Rehabilitation Specialists, WV; Univ of Findlay, OH)

J Hand Ther 27:217-224, 2014

Study Design.—Case report.

Introduction.—Reports of comprehensive rehabilitation following hand replantation are limited.

Purpose of the Study.—To describe hand therapy of a patient following hand replantation.

Methods.—Right hand dominant 55 year-old male assessed 9 days following left hand replantation to treat distal forearm amputation. Patient presented with dorsal blocking orthotic. Initial status: AROM digits and thumb 0–20° extension, 0–40° flexion; absent light touch sensation; 0–1/5 hand strength. Patient underwent 70 hand therapy sessions over 13 months focusing on A/PROM, therapeutic exercise, neuromuscular re-education, and modalities to address functional limitations.

Results.—Hand therapy discharge status: AROM digits and thumb form composite fist, thumb opposition to digit 3, light touch sensation (monofilament) 4.03 (digits 2, 4) and 4.17 (digits 1, 3, 5); 3- to 4–/5 hand strength.

Discussion.—Hand therapy allowed for near complete functional return of the hand following replantation.

Conclusion.—Comprehensive Hand therapy aided restoration of adequate sensation and strength for functional use of the replanted hand.

Level of Evidence.—4.

▶ This case report is a thorough discussion of the intense and lengthy hand therapy rehabilitation intervention for one man after amputation of the distal left forearm after hand replantation over a span of 14 months. The report gives excellent detail of 3 episodes of care after the initial replantation and 2 subsequent surgeries. The challenge of this case was the lack of evidence in the literature on which to plan the interventions. The therapists discuss how they met this challenge by the melding of known rehabilitation protocols for each portion of the case: bone healing, tendon, arterial, venous and muscle healing, management of edema, and monitoring sensation loss and reinnervation, along with maintaining the movement and function of the noninjured but adjacent joints—the shoulder and the elbow—all of this at the proper time and force, with the proper orthoses and exercises to support the repaired tissues. In addition, it is important to engage the patient in this process: educating him at each stage, analyzing his needs, gaining his participation and focusing rehabilitation on his basic current needs, and looking to future functional abilities and occupational needs to ensure he continued to be engaged.

The therapists used a psychometrically sound functional scale, the Patient-Specific Functional Scale, to measure function in the second and third episodes of care. The authors report that a more broad scale of overall disability would have been useful in the rehabilitation planning and report of progress throughout the case.

For each episode of care, the therapists note proper orthotic intervention, edema control, range of motion, tendon gliding, stiffness reduction, and sensory re-education were important foci of each stage of his rehabilitation. A generally good functional outcome was realized for this case with regard to patient-reported function, grip strength, and fair sensibility. The positive functional result is reported to be related to the type of amputation, proximity to a specialty hospital and the postoperative rehabilitation team, and diligence over time. This excellent case report lays the groundwork for positive intervention for the complex case of a person with a transplanted hand.

V. H. O'Brien, OTD, OTR/L, CHT

Percutaneous Trigger Thumb Release in Children: Neither Effective Nor Safe

Masquijo JJ, Ferreyra A, Lanfranchi L, et al (Dept of Pediatric Orthopaedics, Sanatorio Allende, Córdoba, Argentina; ABC Med Ctr, Mexico City)

J Pediatr Orthop 34:534-536, 2014

Background.—Although percutaneous trigger thumb release has been extensively used in adults, the technique is not widespread in children. The purpose of this study was to evaluate the efficacy and safety of percutaneous trigger thumb release in the pediatric age group.

Methods.—Twenty consecutive thumbs of 15 patients scheduled for surgical release of the A1 pulley were included in this cohort. Each patient received first the percutaneous release (PR) followed by an open release (OR) and served as self-controls. Thumb extension was assessed immediately before PR, after PR, and finally after OR, using a goniometer. Extent of the A1 pulley release, iatrogenic injury to the digital nerve and vessels, and flexor tendon laceration was assessed after PR. The distance between the PR and the digital nerve was measured in millimeters. Comparison between thumb extension after PR and OR was made using a paired *t* test.

Results.—Preoperative range of motion averaged −45.2 ± 21.7 degrees loss of extension (range, −80 to −10 degrees), decreased to −4 ± 8 degrees loss of extension (range, −25 to 0 degrees) after PR, and to 0 degrees after OR. Clinically, release was complete in 14 cases (70%) and partial in 6 cases (30%). Once the thumb was approached, we confirmed that A1 pulley was completely cut in 4 cases (20%), to >75% in 2 cases (10%), and between 50% and 75% in the remaining 14 cases (70%). There were no neurovascular iatrogenic injuries. Mean distance between the needle and the digital nerve was 2.45 ± 0.9 mm (range, 1 to 4 mm). Lacerations to the flexor tendons were observed in 80% of the cases.

Conclusions.—We do not recommend PR in the pediatric thumb given the risk of neurovascular iatrogenic injury or incomplete A1 pulley release.

Level of Evidence.—Level II therapeutic study—prospective comparative study.

▶ It is unlikely that a study of this type would have made it through an Institutional Review Board in the United States, but hopefully the data will convince those who would consider performing a percutaneous trigger thumb release in children to think twice. Although thankfully no neurovascular injuries occurred, the digital nerve was on average less than 3 mm from the needle insertion site. Eighty percent of tendons were also partially lacerated. This is a substantial risk for a procedure that has only a 70% clinical and 20% anatomic success rate. Open trigger thumb release via a transverse incision at the thumb metacarpophalangeal joint crease leaves little to no scar, can be accomplished in less than 5 minutes, and allows for visualization of the entire A1 pulley. Tendon and nerve laceration remains a risk for the open procedure, and the risk of these complications is likely underestimated. We recommend visualizing both neurovascular bundles during the open release to limit the risk of injury.

D. A. Zlotolow, MD

The Biophysical Characteristics of Human Composite Flexor Tendon Allograft for Upper Extremity Reconstruction

DeGeorge BR Jr, Rodeheaver GT, Drake DB (Univ of Virginia Med Ctr, Charlottesville)

Ann Plast Surg 72:S184-S190, 2014

Introduction.—Devastating volar hand injuries with significant damage to the skin and soft tissues, pulley structures and fibro-osseous sheath, flexor tendons, and volar plates pose a major problem to the reconstructive hand surgeon. Despite advances in tendon handling, operative technique, and postoperative hand rehabilitation, patients who have undergone flexor tendon reconstruction are often plagued by chronic pain, stiffness, and decreased range of motion with resultant decreased ability to work and poor quality of life. In this article, we expand the technique of human composite flexor tendon allografts (CFTAs), pioneered by Dr E.E. Peacock, Jr, which consist of both the intrasynovial and extrasynovial flexor digitorum superficialis and flexor digitorum profundus tendons and their respective fibro-osseous sheath consisting of the digital pulley structures, periosteum, and volar plates procured from cadaveric donors with the use of modern tissue processing techniques.

Methods.—Human cadaveric CFTAs were procured and divided into 2 groups—unprocessed CFTAs and processed CFTAs, which are cleansed and sterilized to a sterility assurance level of 10^{-6}. Physical length and width relationships as well as tensile strength and gliding resistance assessments were recorded pre-tissue and post-tissue processing. The histologic properties of the composite allografts were assessed before and after tissue processing.

Results.—There was no significant difference with respect to physical properties of the composite allografts before or after tissue processing. The processed composite allografts demonstrated equivalent maximum load to failure and elastic modulus compared to unprocessed tendons. The gliding resistance of the composite tendon allografts was not significantly different between the 2 groups.

Conclusions.—The use of CFTAs addresses the issues of adhesion formation and lack of suitable donor material by providing a source of intrasynovial tendon in its unaltered fibro-osseous sheath without donor morbidity. This approach represents an important step toward designing an ideal material for complex flexor tendon reconstruction, which takes advantage of an intrasynovial flexor tendon in its native fibro-osseous sheath without the need for additional donor morbidity using a construct which can be engineered to have minimal tissue reactivity, negligible potential for disease transmission, and improved tendon healing properties versus standard tendon allograft.

▶ Extrasynovial tendon autografts are the standard for flexor tendon grafting. The potential for morbidity and the lack of synovial sheaths in these donor tendons make them less than ideal choices. In severe hand injuries with loss of flexor tendon tissue, the requirement for tendon tissue may outstrip its availability.

A suitable alternative to the autograft would be most helpful to the hand and reconstructive surgeon. This alternative is an extension in concept of the banked bone allografts and synthetic bone substitutes being used for bone grafting. Work by multiple groups has focused on the development of synthetic tendon substitutes and the use of tendon allografts for such purposes. Synthetic substitutes have yet to achieve the kind of material and biological properties required for clinical tendon reconstruction. Allografts could be a better alternative if issues such as disease transmission, immune reaction, and preservation of mechanical properties are successfully addressed.

It is this last concern toward which this work is directed. The authors characterized composite flexor tendon allografts (CFTA) after processing for acellularization and sterilization. As described in the abstract, the CFTAs consist of not just intrasynovial tendon but also the fibro-osseous sheath, allowing reconstruction of the complete flexor apparatus using the whole allograft. Additionally, there is the possibility for parts of it to be used for more specific defects. They demonstrate that the processing process did not adversely affect the important biomechanical properties such as maximum load to failure and elastic modulus. In addition, gliding resistance of the allografts was maintained. Their work and findings parallel those of other groups who have also done similar work, albeit with differing tendon composition and sterilization techniques.[1]

Their findings provide promise that CFTAs can be a viable alternative to human autografts for flexor tendon grafting. The report shows that at the point of preservation, many of the important aspects of tendon material properties can be maintained. However, it still needs to be shown that these properties can be maintained with storage and how these processed tissues will respond to the biological effects after implantation.

A. Chong, MD

Reference

1. Pridgen BC, Woon CY, Kim MY, et al. Flexor tendon tissue engineering: acellularization of human flexor tendons with preservation of biomechanical properties and biocompatibility. *Tissue Eng Part C Methods*. 2011;17:819-828.

Long-Term Outcomes Following a Single Corticosteroid Injection for Trigger Finger

Wojahn RD, Foeger NC, Gelberman RH, et al (Washington Univ School of Medicine, Saint Louis, MO)

J Bone Joint Surg Am 96:1849-1854, 2014

Background.—The outcomes of corticosteroid injection for trigger finger are well documented only with short-term follow-up. The purpose of this investigation was to determine the long-term effectiveness of a single injection and to examine predictors of success up to ten years after injection.

Methods.—This case series analyzed 366 first-time corticosteroid injections in flexor tendon sheaths from January 2000 to December 2007 with a minimum follow-up duration of five years. Two hundred and forty patients (66%) were female, 161 patients (44%) had multiple trigger fingers, and eighty-eight patients (24%) had diabetes at the time of injection. The primary outcome of treatment failure was defined as subsequent injection or surgical trigger finger release of the affected digit. Medical records were reviewed, and any patients without documented failure or a return office visit in 2012 to 2013 were contacted by telephone regarding symptom recurrence and the need for additional treatment. Kaplan-Meier analyses with log-rank test and Cox regression analysis assessed the effect of baseline patient and disease characteristics on injection success.

Results.—Forty-five percent of patients demonstrated long-term treatment success after a single injection. In the final regression model, the interaction of sex and the number of trigger fingers was the single predictor of treatment success. Exploring this association revealed a ten-year success rate of 56% for female patients presenting for the first time with a trigger finger compared with 35% in male patients presenting for the first time with a trigger finger, 39% in female patients with multiple trigger fingers, and 37% in male patients with multiple trigger fingers. Eighty-four percent of treatment failures occurred within the first two years following injection. Patient age, symptom type, and undifferentiated diabetes status were not predictive of treatment success.

Conclusions.—Female patients presenting with their first trigger finger have the highest rate of long-term treatment success after a single corticosteroid injection. Patients who continue to experience symptom relief two years after injection are likely to maintain long-term success.

► This level IV retrospective study analyzed the long-term result of a single corticosteroid injection in a population of 366 patients undergoing their first injection for a trigger digit. Treatment failure was defined as a subsequent injection or surgical release. All patients with treatment failure or follow-up of at least 5 years were included in the study. Of a potential 475 participants, 366 completed follow-up with no missing data. The authors report that 200 patients (54.6%) had treatment failure requiring repeat injection or surgical release, and 166 patients (45.4%) did not require further treatment. Seven patients (1.9%) exhibited no improvement and were counted as immediate treatment failure. Of the 200 patients with treatment failure, 128 (65%) required repeat injection, and 65 (33%) underwent surgical release. Thus, 65 of 366 patients (18%) required surgery. Female patients responded better than male patients (49.2% vs 38.1% success), and patients with multiple trigger digits fared worse than those with 1 trigger digit (38.5% vs 50.7% success). Most treatment failures occurred within the first 2 years (84%), and contrary to other studies, diabetes mellitus did not appear to increase the likelihood of treatment failure.

In summary, this retrospective study with good long-term follow-up in a large number of patients continues to support the use of a corticosteroid injection in patients presenting for treatment of a trigger digit. This study does contradict previous studies reporting less success in diabetic patients, but the study did note a higher incidence of multiple trigger digits in those with diabetes mellitus. It appeared, however, that diabetes was not an independent risk factor for treatment failure.

The authors are to be commended for contacting a large number of patients and providing us with useful information. I continue to recommend corticosteroid injections to my patients presenting for treatment of trigger digits. I have noted that most patients improve and exhibit less frequent and less bothersome triggering, but on physical examination, a mild but definite degree of triggering remains evident in many patients. It appears that in such a patient, the improvement after the injection is often "enough," and their ongoing symptoms are tolerable and do not necessitate surgery.

D. Zelouf, MD

Percutaneous First Annular Pulley Release for Trigger Digits: A Systematic Review and Meta-Analysis of Current Evidence

Zhao J-G, Kan S-L, Zhao L, et al (Tianjin Med Univ, China)

J Hand Surg Am 39:2192-2202, 2014

Purpose.—To determine the overall success rate and potential influencing factors within the current evidence for percutaneous first annular pulley release.

Methods.—We searched PubMed, EMBASE, and the Cochrane Library for all clinical studies of percutaneous release. The rates of successful procedure and complication were extracted and analyzed. We charted the overall success rate on a forest plot with 95% confidence intervals. Data of success rates were analyzed in 5- and 10-year intervals to determine whether the rate of success had increased chronologically. We then performed 3 subgroup analyses according to instrument type (needles vs knife blades), cortisone use (cortisone vs noncortisone), and sonography guidance (sonography vs non-sonography guidance). Pooled success rates were calculated in the subgroups and compared using chi-square test.

Results.—A total of 34 studies involving 2,114 percutaneous procedures were included in this systematic review and meta-analysis. The total success rate was 94%. There was a trend toward increasing number of publications in the past 20 years. We found a statistically significant trend showing that overall success rates had increased over time. Chi-square test revealed that percutaneous release with sonography guidance had a significantly higher success rate than non-sonography guidance. There were no significant differences in other subgroup analyses including instrument type and cortisone use.

Conclusions.—Percutaneous release is an effective and safe procedure for the treatment of trigger digit. It has become progressively popular in recent years, with a trend toward increased overall success. Sonography might be a helpful tool for maximizing success. The success rates were not affected by instruments and cortisone use.

Type of Study/Level of Evidence.—Therapeutic IV.

▶ This article studied the success rate and trend of percutaneous trigger finger release over 2 decades. It was an exhaustive review and meta-analysis of 34 studies in the literature that looked at 2114 percutaneous trigger finger releases, following strict guidelines (of the Preferred Reporting Items for Systematic Reviews and Meta-Analysis). Independent reviews were performed by 2 investigators, and a third was used if necessary when a discrepancy existed. The findings of this study are important in that they indicate an increasing trend in and success rate of the percutaneous trigger finger release procedure, with or without the use of cortisone or ultrasonography.

I do not perform percutaneous trigger finger releases in my practice. I was trained only in the open release, preferably under local anesthesia, so that I am able to ask the patient to actively flex and extend the finger after the release to make sure the triggering was resolved. In a small number of cases, I have found that the triggering did not resolve with release of the first annular pulley alone; sometimes part of the second annular pulley or proximal pseudo-sheath will need to be incised, and sometimes a significant flexor tenosynovectomy needs to be performed, and sometimes a debridement of significant fraying of the flexor digitorum superficialis tendon needs to be performed. A retinacular cyst might also be seen through the open approach, something that would not have been appreciated with percutaneous release. For these reasons, I prefer the open release.

S. S. Shin, MD, MMSc

Trigger Finger: Assessment of Surgeon and Patient Preferences and Priorities for Decision Making

Döring A-CD, Hageman MGJS, Mulder FJ, et al (Massachusetts General Hosp, Boston)

J Hand Surg Am 39:2208-2213.e2, 2014

Purpose.—To test the null hypothesis that there are no differences in the priorities and preferences of patients with idiopathic trigger finger (TF) and hand surgeons.

Methods.—One hundred five hand surgeons of the Science of Variation Group and 84 patients with TF completed a survey about their priorities and preferences in decision making regarding the management of TF. The questionnaire was structured according the Ottawa Decision Support Framework for the development of a decision aid.

Results.—Patients desired orthotics more and surgery less than physicians. Patients and physicians disagreed on the main advantage of several treatment options for TFs and on disadvantages of the treatment options.

Patients preferred to decide for themselves after receiving advice, whereas physicians preferred a shared decision. Patients preferred booklets, and physicians opted for Internet and video decision aids.

Conclusions.—Comparing patients and hand surgeons, there were some differences in treatment preferences and perceived advantages and disadvantages regarding idiopathic TF—differences that might be addressed by a decision aid.

Clinical Relevance.—Information that helps inform patients of their options based on current best evidence might help them understand their own preferences and values, reduce decisional conflict, limit surgeon-to-surgeon variations, and improve health.

▶ This study addresses an increasingly important aspect of practice for the hand surgeon: patient preferences. There is a well-described methodology to assess and understand patient preferences and drivers affecting care choice. The authors chose to study patient and provider preferences for the treatment of trigger finger, a common condition with several reasonable treatment options. Their results were quite informative with patients more interested in orthotics and less interested in surgery compared with surgeons. Both groups felt a steroid injection was the most desirable treatment option. Another interesting finding was that patients preferred a model in which they were given the information and decided the treatment themselves. In contrast, surgeons preferred a shared decision-making process. More patients wanted information presented by an expert in the field in a booklet format. This article provided an important view of the differences and areas of agreements between physicians and patients on trigger finger treatments and decision aids. This study of a common hand condition with many reasonable treatment options provides a useful view into patients' preferences and is an article that hand surgeons should read. Understanding patient preferences can improve communication and ultimately patient satisfaction and quality of care.

C. Curtin, MD

The Efficacy of 95-Hz Topical Vibration in Pain Reduction for Trigger Finger Injection: A Placebo-Controlled, Prospective, Randomized Trial

Park KW, Boyer MI, Calfee RP, et al (Washington Univ School of Medicine, St Louis, MO)

J Hand Surg Am 39:2203-2207, 2014

Purpose.—To determine whether vibratory stimulation would decrease pain experienced by patients during corticosteroid injection for trigger finger.

Methods.—A total of 90 trigger finger injections were randomized to 1 of 3 cohorts. With the injection, patients received no vibration (control group), ultrasound vibration (sham control group), or vibration (experimental group). We used a commercial handheld massaging device to provide a vibratory stimulus for the experimental group. We obtained visual analog scale (VAS) pain scores before and after injection to assess anticipated pain and actual pain experienced.

Results.—Anticipated pain and actual pain did not differ significantly among groups. Anticipated VAS pain scores were 45, 48, and 50 and actual VAS pain scores were 56, 56, and 63 for the vibration, control, and sham control groups, respectively. When normalized using anchoring VAS pain scores for "stubbing a toe" or "paper cut," no between-group differences remained in injection pain scores.

Conclusions.—Concomitant vibratory stimulation does not reduce pain experienced during corticosteroid injections for trigger finger.

Type of Study/Level of Evidence.—Therapeutic I.

▶ Use of vibration devices for pain control has been described in dermatologic injections as well as botulinum injections in the face. The concept is based on the "gate theory" of pain. By stimulating the pain receptors with the vibration device, the patients would have a diminished response to the actual injections. The authors performed a randomized study to determine the efficacy of a vibration device in reducing the pain experienced during a corticosteroid injection for trigger fingers. Previously, physicians have used vapo-coolant sprays as well as anesthetic creams while performing these injections. The vibration device chosen was the AcuVibe Softtouch, an inexpensive massager that is commercially available. The authors did not find that vibration anesthesia provided any benefits in reducing pain with steroid injections. Overall, this is a well-designed randomized study with a control group and a sham control. The authors do not recommend use of vibration device for trigger injections. Rather, other modalities such as verbal reassurance, use of vapo-coolant sprays (ethyl chloride), and anesthetic creams can be considered in anxious patients who are needle-phobic.

J. I. Huang, MD

Treatment preferences for trigger digit by members of the American Association for Hand Surgery

Pruzansky JS, Goljan P, Lundmark DP, et al (The Philadelphia Hand Ctr, PA)

Hand 9:529-533, 2014

Background.—Trigger digit is a common pathology encountered by hand surgeons, but there is a lack of evidence-based guidelines. We investigated the treatment preferences of hand surgeons and explored whether geographic location, type of residency training, or clinical experience is associated with differences in practice.

Methods.—An online survey was distributed via email by the American Association for Hand Surgery to 615 members. The survey consisted of 17 questions related to conservative and operative management of trigger digits.

Results.—One hundred thirty-nine unique responses were received (22.6%). Geographic distribution of respondents encompassed the entire USA and was not associated with variations in practice. Of the respondents, 56.8% were trained in orthopedic surgery while 37.4% had plastic surgery training. In regards to duration of practice, 8.6% were in practice for up to 5 years, 29.5% for 6–15 years, 33.8% for 16–25 years, and 28.1% for more than 25 years. Notably, the great majority of respondents preferred corticosteroid injections for initial treatment. Those who were willing to give three or more injections prior to surgery were more likely to be plastic surgeons in practice for 16 years or more. A large minority of surgeons utilized splinting in their conservative management. Orthopedic surgeons were more likely to perform tenolysis during pulley release and more likely to use monitored anesthesia care.

Conclusions.—Variation exists between the treatment algorithms of hand surgeons when managing a trigger digit. Some of these differences may be attributable to the type of training or the duration of clinical practice.

▶ This is an interesting study regarding treatment norms of trigger finger, but it does not answer many questions to guide decision making.

It is worth noting that more mature surgeons provide more injections before offering surgery. This is likely secondary to their experience with complications, good results with injections, and a fuller surgery schedule that encourages conservative treatment of benign conditions.

It is also interesting that local anesthetic is more commonly used by plastic surgeons, given their experience with the technique and their greater experience with in-office procedures. Remarkably, there are some surgeons still advocating general anesthesia for trigger-finger surgery. It is something that orthopedic surgeons should take note of. In the current practice climate, costs will be scrutinized more closely, and the use of local anesthetic for simple procedures such as A1 pulley release can significantly decrease costs by eliminating anesthesiologists, recovery time, medications, and preoperative testing.

Finally, I am surprised by the persistence of tenolysis in the practice patterns of hand surgeons, particularly orthopedically trained hand surgeons. This practice is not supported by the literature in the majority of cases (except in inflammatory arthritis) and points to the need for more randomized studies to clearly show the indications, results, and complications of this additional procedure.

I typically advocate that my patients attempt a corticosteroid injection. If they experience prolonged relief (>6 months) but their symptoms recur, I would push them to try a second injection. In cases in which patients have incomplete relief or brief relief of symptoms, I feel that surgical treatment is likely the best course. After 2 injections, I counsel them that they are likely not avoiding surgery, rather delaying it with an additional injection. In some cases, delay is welcome, and patients attempt a third injection, whereas others prefer the higher reliability of surgical release.

T. Hughes, MD

Standard versus over-tensioning in the transfer of extensor indicis proprius to extensor pollicis longus for chronic rupture of the thumb extensor

Jung S-W, Kim C-K, Ahn B-W, et al (Sungkyunkwan Univ School of Medicine, Changwon-si, South Korea)

J Plast Reconstr Aesthet Surg 67:979-985, 2014

Purpose.—The purpose of this study was to evaluate the functional outcomes of the over-tensioning technique compared with those of the standard tensioning technique in the transfer of extensor indicis proprius (EIP) to extensor pollicis longus (EPL) for the chronic rupture of the thumb extensor.

Methods.—Data were collected from patients who underwent tendon transfer using EIP between March 2003 and August 2011. 23 were treated with the standard tensioning technique and 25 patients (Group B) with the over-tensioning technique. While standard tension was maintained with the thumb in full extension and the wrist in 30° of flexion, over-tension was maintained with the thumb in full extension and the wrist in the neutral position. All patients were assessed for total range of motion, elevation and flexion deficit, the thumb grip and pinch strength, and the thumb and the index extension strength compared to the unaffected side, EIP–EPL evaluation as suggested by Lemmen et al. and Disabilities of the Arm, Shoulder, and Hand questionnaire (DASH).

Results.—Group A: total range of motion 115°, elevation deficit 2.0 cm, combined flexion deficit 1.0 cm, thumb extension strength 75%, thumb grip strength 91%, and pinch strength 87%. Functional outcomes were 13 excellent, 6 good, 3 fair, and 1 poor. Median DASH score was 21.3 points. Group B total range of motion 125°, elevation deficit 1.0 cm, combined flexion deficit 1.5 cm, thumb extension strength 85%, thumb grip strength 88%, and pinch strength 83%. Functional outcomes were 16 excellent, 7 good, 2 fair, and 0 poor. Median DASH score was 19.8 points. There are significant differences in the range of motion, elevation deficit, and extension strength of thumb between the two groups ($p = .001$, $p = .001$, and $p = .028$, respectively).

Conclusion.—While the functional outcomes of both groups were favorably acceptable in a majority of the patients, there were significant differences in aspects of range of motion, elevation deficit, and strength of the thumb between both groups.

Level of Evidence.—Case–control study, Level III.

▶ This is a well-written article that provides the reader with a good overview of the details of extensor indicis proprius to extensor pollicis longus tendon transfer. The authors demonstrate good functional results in the 2 techniques of tensioning used, favoring the over-tensioning group. In my practice, I also tend to over tension the transfer. I am of the opinion that, over the first few months of rehabilitation, some of the over tensioning is lost by the stronger flexor mechanism stretching out the transfer resulting in the correct balancing. The recent interest in "wide-awake" surgery under local infiltration anesthesia has the added advantage of tensioning the transfer with the patient awake and actively moving the thumb to ensure correct tensioning, and this technique should be encouraged.

M. Hayton, MD

Relative Motion Splint: Active Motion After Extensor Tendon Injury and Repair

Merritt WH (Univ of Virginia, Charlottesville)
J Hand Surg Am 39:1187-1194, 2014

The relative motion splint was initially developed to facilitate postoperative rehabilitation after repair of extensor tendon injuries at the dorsum of the hand and forearm. It has subsequently been used for rehabilitation of sagittal band injuries and after repair of closed attrition extensor tendon ruptures in rheumatoid arthritis. This is much less awkward than other braces and can readily be worn during normal past-time and work activities. This so-called immediate controlled active motion splinting protocol has also more recently been applied to both operative and nonsurgical rehabilitation for boutonniere deformity.

▶ Dr Merritt has written a comprehensive review of the use, benefits, and efficacy of relative motion splinting, also known as immediate controlled active motion splinting. He thoroughly describes the rationale for each use of the splint and then goes on to describe the technique for application. Excellent photos are included so that the surgeon and therapist know exactly how to fabricate and place the splint. There are also references for videos available on the *Journal of Hand Surgery* website. He then includes a section on pearls and pitfalls that I found most helpful.

This article is equally important for the surgeon and therapist. It presents new and creative ways to use low-profile splinting to encourage early active motion. As we continue to work toward early motion, allowing greater function and compliance with our patient population, additional applications will emerge that will further advance the use of controlled active motion splinting. I have personally had good success using this technique to treat chronic loss of proximal interphalangeal (PIP) extension postfracture or sprain of the PIP joint. We owe a debt of gratitude to Dr Merritt for pioneering the use of relative motion splinting and giving us the tools outlined in this article to use in our practice. This technique has great advantages that serve our patients well.

S. J. Clark, OTR/L, CHT

4 Wrist Arthroscopy

Does Body Mass Index Affect Outcomes of Ambulatory Knee and Shoulder Surgery?

Kluczynski MA, Bisson LJ, Marzo JM (Univ at Buffalo, NY)

Arthroscopy 30:856-865, 2014

Purpose.—Obesity is highly prevalent among patients with knee and shoulder injuries and is associated with greater odds of surgical treatment for these injuries. The purpose of this systematic review was to summarize the literature that has examined the association between body mass index (BMI) and outcomes of ambulatory knee and shoulder surgery.

Methods.—A literature search of PubMed and Medline was conducted up to December 2013. Studies that examined the association between BMI and outcomes after ambulatory knee and shoulder surgery (arthroscopy, repairs, and reconstructions) were included. Outcomes included postoperative functional scores, clinical scores, and complications.

Results.—Eighteen studies were included in this review; 13 involved knee surgery and 5 involved shoulder surgery. Seven knee studies and 2 shoulder studies found increased BMI to be associated with worse postoperative outcomes, whereas the remaining 9 studies did not find an association. Increased BMI was associated with worse clinical scores and less patient satisfaction after arthroscopic meniscectomy or debridement, and with worse clinical scores and lower activity levels after anterior cruciate ligament (ACL) reconstruction. It was also associated with worse clinical scores and a longer hospital stay after rotator cuff repair and with longer time to return to work after subacromial decompression. Six studies examined the association between BMI and complications, but all reported null findings.

Conclusions.—There is a lack of consensus in the literature regarding the association between BMI and ambulatory knee and shoulder surgery. Several factors may have contributed to contradictory findings, including variation in measuring and classifying anthropometry, postoperative outcomes, and follow-up time.

Level of Evidence.—Level IV, systematic review of Level I, III, and IV studies.

► This study is a systematic review of 18 articles looking at the association between body mass index (BMI) and outcomes after ambulatory knee and shoulder surgery. There is substantial evidence in the literature reporting on worse outcomes after total joint replacement surgery. However, this trend became less obvious when ambulatory surgeries were evaluated in this study. In this review, a greater percentage of knee studies documented adverse affects of elevated BMI on postoperative results compared with shoulder studies. This result is expected, as the knee joint is a weight-bearing joint, whereas the shoulder is not, and if a patient has a higher BMI, it may result in higher loads across the knee. Interestingly, neither knee nor shoulder articles reviewed here showed an increased complication risk with an increasing BMI. Part of this surprising finding can be explained by the fact that only 6 of 18 articles looked at the complications, but they all were reporting postoperative outcomes. Obesity has been the most important factor for extended stay after my ambulatory surgeries, as especially morbidly obese patients almost invariably have obstructive sleep apnea requiring longer observation periods in the postoperative period.

A. Cil, MD

Arthroscopy After Locked Plating of Proximal Humeral Fractures: Implant Removal, Capsular Release, and Intra-articular Findings

Katthagen JC, Hennecke D, Jensen G, et al (Diakoniekrankenhaus Friederikenstift gGmbH, Hannover, Germany)

Arthroscopy 30:1061-1067, 2014

Purpose.—The purpose of this study was to determine the outcomes of arthroscopy after proximal humeral plating and the occurrence of concomitant pathology and avascular necrosis.

Methods.—Forty-five patients (28 women; median age, 58.5 years [range, 30 to 82 years]) underwent arthroscopies of 46 shoulders because of unsatisfactory results after locked plating of proximal humeral fractures. They were prospectively followed up for 3, 12, and 24 months postoperatively. Relevant intra-articular lesions were documented. The patients were assigned to 1 of the following groups: (1) articular screw perforation, (2) subacromial plate impingement, or (3) post-traumatic/postoperative shoulder stiffness. Shoulder range of motion and function as measured with the age- and gender-adjusted Constant-Murley score, as well as the Simple Shoulder Test, were compared among the groups.

Results.—Concomitant lesions of the articular cartilage, long head of the biceps tendon, tuberosities, and rotator cuff were found in 34 patients (75%). Two-thirds of patients (n = 31) had a partial or complete 270° capsular release. Of the patients, 84% (n = 38) underwent 3 and 12 months' follow-up and 82% (n = 37) underwent 24 months' follow-up. The active range of abduction (P = .029), flexion (P = .048), and internal rotation (P = .0005) had improved significantly at 24 months' follow-up compared with the preoperative status. The mean adjusted Constant-Murley score of patients with post-traumatic shoulder stiffness (n = 15, 64.2% ± 7.9%) and articular screw perforation (n = 19, 73.3% ± 8.4%) was significantly lower (P = .0089 and P = .042, respectively) than that of patients with subacromial plate impingement (n = 12, 93.4% ± 4.3%).

Conclusions.—High rates of relevant articular pathologies and the necessity of capsular release in a majority of patients with unsatisfactory results after locked plating of proximal humeral fractures make arthroscopy a valuable revision tool with promising results in cases of high plate positioning, screw perforation, and postoperative/post- traumatic shoulder stiffness.

Level of Evidence.—Level IV, therapeutic case series.

▶ This article is important for shoulder surgeons because it presents an alternative procedure to open surgery for complications after locking plates for proximal humerus fractures. The main strength is that authors highlight the benefits of performing arthroscopy for these patients. What is more relevant is the fact that arthroscopy permits the surgeon to diagnose and treat intraarticular findings that might be otherwise missed with standard open procedures. The main weakness is that there is no control or comparative group to fully assess the clinical outcomes after removing implants either by arthroscopy or open surgery, and arthroscopic capsular release compared with rehabilitation for postoperative stiffness. Personally, I favor removing hardware with an open or minimally invasive procedure. After reading this article, I am now willing to perform a diagnostic arthroscopy before hardware removal because the authors have shown a high rate (75%) of concomitant intraarticular pathology. This might result in cost-effective care that could benefit patient outcomes and may become part of the standard procedure for hardware removal in the near future.

J. P. Simone, MD

5 Carpus

Pisiform Excision for Pisotriquetral Instability and Arthritis

Campion H, Goad A, Rayan G, et al (Univ of Oklahoma Med School)

J Hand Surg Am 39:1251-1257.e1, 2014

Purpose.—To evaluate wrist strength and kinematics after pisiform excision and preservation of its soft tissue confluence for pisotriquetral instability and arthritis.

Methods.—We evaluated 12 patients, (14 wrists) subjectively and objectively an average of 7.5 years after pisiform excision. Three additional patients were interviewed by phone. Subjective evaluation included inquiry about pain and satisfaction with the treatment. Objective testing included measuring wrist flexion and extension range of motion, grip strength, and static and dynamic flexion and ulnar deviation strengths of the operative hand compared with the nonsurgical normal hand. Four patients had concomitant ulnar nerve decompression at the wrist.

Results.—All patients were satisfied with the outcome. Wrist flexion averaged 99% and wrist extension averaged 95% of the nonsurgical hand. Mean grip strength of the operative hand was 90% of the nonsurgical hand. Mean static flexion strength of the operative hand was 94% of the nonsurgical hand, whereas mean dynamic flexion strength was 113%. Mean static ulnar deviation strength of the operative hand was 87% of the nonsurgical hand. The mean dynamic ulnar deviation strength of the operative hand was 103% of the nonsurgical hand.

Conclusions.—Soft tissue confluence-preserving pisiform excision relieved pain and retained wrist motion and static and dynamic strength. Associated ulnar nerve compression was a confounding factor that may have affected outcomes.

Type of Study/Level of Evidence.—Therapeutic IV.

▶ Pisotriquetral (PT) joint problems are uncommon yet an important cause of chronic ulnar wrist pain. Diagnosis depends on a high degree of clinical alertness and the ability to elicit appropriate physical signs and to order specific radiologic investigations. There is a paucity of literature on the precise anatomy, biomechanics, and function of this apparently insignificant component of the wrist joint. Nevertheless, the numerous soft-tissue attachments to the pisiform connected directly or indirectly with the forearm bones, carpal bones, and metacarpal bones naturally imply a considerable role of the bone and the joint in contributing stability and possibly proprioceptive function to the ulnar side of wrist, of which the precise role is still poorly understood. Since Caroll and

Coyle advocated excision of the pisiform bone to treat various dysfunctions of the PT joint 30 years ago, the pisiformectomy option seemed to become a standard method of treatment. However, the impact to the ulnar wrist stability had not been formally addressed until recently.

The author of this report attempted to address this issue by emphasizing the preservation of the soft-tissue confluence around the pisiform and a meticulous repair of the flexor carpi ulnaris tendon to the piso-metacarpal ligament after excision of the pisiform. They evaluated the pain, return to work, satisfaction, grip strength, range of motion, static and dynamic flexion, and ulnar deviation strength at an average follow-up of 6.9 years with good outcome compared with the unaffected side. They have mentioned the examination for distal radio-ulnar joint and ulno-carpal joint stability in their evaluation, but no result was reported. The major weakness of this study is, however, the very low follow-up rate of the cohort. Only 39.5% of the patients could be reached, including the 3 patients by phone interview only, which can hardly produce any convincing results for the whole group of patients. Like other studies, they failed to address the time interval to achieve maximal pain relief. In my experience, many patients after pisiformectomy often require extended time of up to a year before the pain and discomfort can resolve. It can be attributed to the disruption of the fine balance between the dynamic and static stabilizing structures such as the force couple of the flexor carpi ulnaris and extensor carpi ulnaris muscles. The prolonged time to attain a clinical resolution is a drawback of this operation. The lengthy recovery time and the potential threat to the ulnar wrist stability prompt me and others to consider pisotriquetral stabilization or fusion as an alternative to treat symptomatic PT instability or arthritis, with the aim to truly preserve the peri-pisiform stability. Fusion can be achieved by a compression headless screw.

P. C. Ho, MD

Surgical management of the wrist in children with cerebral palsy and traumatic brain injury

Koman LA, Smith BP (Wake Forest School of Medicine, Winston-Salem, NC)

Hand 9:471-477, 2014

Background.—Upper extremity disabilities are common in children with hemiplegia/quadriplegia caused by cerebral palsy or traumatic brain injury. Often wrist function is compromised with respect to flexion and hyperextension. Fewer than 20% of children with cerebral palsy and 30% of those with traumatic brain injury are candidates for wrist surgery. The goals of treatment are to improve function, eliminate or diminish pain and/or discomfort, improve appearance, bolster self-esteem, and enhance caregiver activities. The optimal time for surgical treatment is difficult to establish, requiring a balance between performing procedures before growth is completed and intervening only after irreversible joint deformity or contracture has occurred. The treatment options to manage wrist spasticity related to cerebral palsy and traumatic brain injury were outlined.

Evaluation.—A careful history and physical examination are required to identify the time course of the deformity and disability, previous treatment interventions and their outcomes, pain, spasticity, impact on health-related quality of life and function, goals, and feasibility of interventions. Essential aspects include active, gross, and fine motor control, active and passive wrist range of motion, sensibility, proprioception, and presence and extent of movement disorders. Treatment decisions include the patient's input and seek to set realistic goals and address the unique problems involved. Hand and wrist function are closely tied, so wrist procedures cannot be planned in isolation.

Treatment Options.—Nonoperative treatment options include therapy, splinting, oral drugs such as baclofen and tizanidine, and parenteral neuromuscular blocking agents such as botulinum toxins. No pharmacologic agents are specifically labeled for managing spasticity in children, and most have significant side effects.

Surgical options include soft tissue and osseous procedures, with the choice depending on deformity severity. Soft tissue procedures are designed to balance muscle forces across joints and include tendon transfers, tendon lengthening and/or shortening, combinations approaches, serial casting, and the use of a multiplanar, geared external fixator. Osseous procedures include distal radius osteotomy, hemiepiphysiodesis, proximal row carpectomy, radial shortening, and wrist fusion with or without carpal resection. Casting or splinting is required after these surgical procedures. The wrist position chosen should protect tendon transfers and/or plications and maintain joint position after carpectomy or arthrodesis. After a cast is applied for 4 to 5 weeks, splinting is done to prevent finger stiffness and maintain function. Active and passive range of motion and strengthening exercises are initiated after 4 weeks of immobilization. The wrist is splinted in optimal corrected position for at least 8 hours daily. Electrical stimulation can benefit some patients. Botulinium toxin used intraoperatively offers the potential advantages of decreasing pain postoperatively, protecting the repair site, and facilitating rehabilitation efforts.

Conclusions.—Wrist arthrodesis can improve wrist position and facilitate hygiene for children with cerebral palsy or traumatic brain injury who have wrist disabilities. Often, additional surgery is needed to extrinsic finger flexors and extensors to optimize the outcome.

► The authors present a review article discussing the surgical management of the wrist in pediatric patients with cerebral palsy and traumatic brain injuries. Many children with these disease processes have wrist flexion deformity that can interfere with grasp. This deformity can be further compounded by spasticity of the extensor carpi ulnaris and forearm pronation. Surgical treatment should be aimed primarily at improvement in function and secondarily at improvement in cosmesis. Commonly used techniques include arthrodesis, which usually requires a wedge resection to be performed, and tendon transfers. The most commonly utilized tendon transfers are the flexor carpi ulnaris (FCU) to extensor carpi radialis longus or extensor carpi radialis brevis, FCU to extensor digitorum communis, and extensor carpi ulnaris to the 4th metacarpal. Passage of the FCU around the ulnar border of the forearm as opposed to through the interosseous membrane can provide a supination moment, thus, counteracting the pronation forces. Care must be taken when performing wrist procedures in these patient populations because finger flexor and extensor muscle and tendon lengths can be altered, necessitating additional further surgery on these structures.

J. Abzug, MD

Distal Scaphoid Resection for Degenerative Arthritis Secondary to Scaphoid Nonunion: A 20-Year Experience

Malerich MM, Catalano LW III, Weidner ZD, et al (St. Luke's-Roosevelt Hosp, NY)

J Hand Surg Am 39:1669-1676, 2014

Purpose.—To evaluate the long-term results of distal scaphoid excision for degenerative arthritis secondary to scaphoid nonunion and compare them with our original results published in 1999.

Methods.—Nineteen patients who were treated by distal scaphoid resection arthroplasty from 1987 through 2010 were included. The mean follow-up was 15 years (range, 10–25 y) vs 4 years in the previous study. Clinical evaluation included measurement of the visual analog pain scale, wrist range of motion, and grip strength. Radiographs were taken at follow-up to assess for signs of arthritis and wrist collapse.

Results.—The outcomes of this procedure include increased grip strength and total arc of motion, a small decrease in revised carpal height ratio, and a small increase in radiolunate angle. Two patients failed distal scaphoid resection arthroplasty necessitating proximal row carpectomy (1) and wrist arthrodesis (1) for recalcitrant pain. More than half of the remaining patients developed midcarpal arthritis on radiographs that was asymptomatic. No patients developed radiolunate arthritis.

Conclusions.—This study showed that distal scaphoid resection arthroplasty produced favorable, long-term clinical results and did not result in noteworthy wrist collapse. Midcarpal arthritis, which may develop after the procedure, did not cause appreciable deterioration in patient outcomes. This procedure also did not eliminate the option of using additional, more conventional reconstructive procedures if needed.

Type of Study/Level of Evidence.—Therapeutic IV.

▶ Most hand surgeons read several journals regularly amounting to hundreds of articles annually, but it is a rare article that actually changes one's approach to a clinical problem. This article by Malerich et al is one such article for me. The clinical problem of the scaphoid nonunion advanced collapse wrist that does not respond to surgical treatment and develops degenerative changes, but not diffuse osteoarthritis (OA) (midcarpal), has been a problem in my practice without an obvious solution. Bone grafting (conventional or vascularized) combined with styloidectomy in patients with early or stage I OA changes sometimes leads to pain relief, but I have had a number come to union and continue to have pain and limitations. The well-described salvage procedures of 4-bone fusion and *proximal row carpectomy* have limitations, and although typically successful, for a patient population that is typically young (mean age 40 in this series), seem drastic. "Wait, you are going to take out half of the bones in my wrist?" one recent wide-eyed patient remarked. Distal scaphoid excision had been described, but the longevity of the operation and the impact of secondary carpal changes were concerns for me, particularly in younger patients. This study, with a mean follow-up of 15 years and minimum of 10 years, answers the question of longevity and secondary changes. Although most patients had midcarpal OA radiographically in their second decade after surgery, symptomatic OA and need for secondary surgery was around 10%. The authors suggest that capitolunate OA is not a contraindication to this procedure based on the observation that when capitolunate OA developed postoperatively, it was rarely symptomatic. I do not find that their published data completely support this, as the patients in their series who had midcarpal OA preoperatively did poorly compared with those who did not. But this is a topic for further study. I find this report compelling enough to change my practice for this challenging clinical problem.

P. Blazar, MD

Carpal Tunnel Syndrome Impairs Thumb Opposition and Circumduction Motion

Marquardt TL, Nataraj R, Evans PJ, et al (Cleveland Clinic, OH)

Clin Orthop Relat Res 472:2526-2533, 2014

Background.—Carpal tunnel syndrome is associated with sensory and motor impairments resulting from the compressed and malfunctioning median nerve. The thumb is critical to hand function, yet the pathokinematics of the thumb associated with carpal tunnel syndrome are not well understood.

Questions/Purposes.—The purpose of this study was to evaluate thumb motion abnormalities associated with carpal tunnel syndrome. We hypothesized that the ranges of translational and angular motion of the thumb would be reduced as a result of carpal tunnel syndrome.

Methods.—Eleven patients with carpal tunnel syndrome and 11 healthy control subjects voluntarily participated in this study. Translational and angular kinematics of the thumb were obtained using marker-based video motion analysis during thumb opposition and circumduction movements.

Results.—Motion deficits were observed for patients with carpal tunnel syndrome even though maximum pinch strength was similar. The path length, normalized by palm width of the thumb tip for the patients with carpal tunnel syndrome was less than for control participants (opposition:

2.2 palm width [95% CI, 1.8–2.6 palm width] versus 3.1 palm width [95% CI, 2.8–3.4 palm width], $p < 0.001$; circumduction: 2.2 palm width [95% CI, 1.9–2.5 palm width] versus 2.9 palm width [95% CI, 2.7–3.2 palm width], $p < 0.001$). Specifically, patients with carpal tunnel syndrome had a deficit of 0.3 palm width (95% CI, 0.04–0.52 palm width; $p = 0.022$) in the maximum position of their thumb tip ulnarly across the palm during opposition relative to control participants. The angular ROM also was reduced for the patients with carpal tunnel syndrome compared with the control participants in extension/flexion for the metacarpophalangeal (opposition: 34° versus 58°, $p = .004$; circumduction: 33° versus 58°, $p < 0.001$) and interphalangeal (opposition: 37° versus 62°, $p = .028$; circumduction: 41° versus 63°, $p = .025$) joints.

Conclusions.—Carpal tunnel syndrome disrupts kinematics of the thumb during opposition and circumduction despite normal pinch strength.

Clinical Relevance.—Improving understanding of thumb pathokinematics associated with carpal tunnel syndrome may help clarify hand function impairment associated with the syndrome given the critical role of the thumb in dexterous manipulation.

► In this article, the authors investigate the hypothesis that subtle differences in hand range of motion, specifically with regard to the thumb, can be found in patients with carpal tunnel syndrome compared with patients without carpal tunnel syndrome. The study includes 11 patients, all confirmed to be right-handed, with carpal tunnel syndrome and 11 control patients. In this study, the authors measure, with great precision using sensors, the ability of patients to oppose using their thumb and to perform circumduction. Representative data and aggregate data show definitively that patients with the diagnosis of carpal tunnel syndrome seem to have smaller range of motion in both of these tasks compared with others without carpal tunnel syndrome. With relatively few subjects, the authors reveal significant findings, specifically with regard to flexion and extension at the interphalangeal and metacarpophalangeal joints. Patients with carpal tunnel syndrome have a smaller range of motion overall, and these patients are special because they do not have significant differences in pinch strength. The reader is left with the burning question: Could this be yet another entry in the fray of new methods to potentially diagnose carpal tunnel syndrome?

The significance of an approach based on motion to distinguish carpal tunnel syndrome patients cannot be understated. Carpal tunnel syndrome is common, and its functional consequences are of great interest to different populations of care providers, including those involved in occupational medicine, hand surgery, and practitioners simply desiring to diagnose both the presence of carpal tunnel syndrome and the resolution of symptoms. Ever more intricate and perhaps more functionally relevant tests for the existence of carpal tunnel syndrome seem to arise yearly. These tests offer a functional counterweight to the classically accepted electrodiagnostic studies that are used to diagnose carpal tunnel syndrome now. The functional consequences of carpal tunnel syndrome, now discovered in this article to be related to range of motion in the joints of the thumb, should weigh heavier in the final analysis in the diagnosis of a condition that causes functional consequences. Many patients with positive electrodiagnostic studies have few symptoms, and some patients with severe symptoms can have negative electrodiagnostic studies. Purists rely on the electrodiagnostic studies to diagnose carpal tunnel syndrome, rendering those patients with negative studies and obvious symptoms without a clear diagnosis. Most hand surgeons refer to patients who have carpal tunnel syndrome on a symptomatic basis and so the need for a functional measurement that reliably diagnoses and measures the effect of carpal tunnel syndrome and its treatment becomes ever more important.

The results of this study are clear in that range of motion is affected by carpal tunnel syndrome; however, these results must be interpreted with the cautions the authors note in the article. First, the patients with carpal tunnel syndrome did not uniformly have electrodiagnostic studies confirming the presence of slowed conduction across the carpal tunnel. Instead, the authors rely on a 3-out-of-4 diagnosis method that can, in some of the few patients included in this study, allow for the inclusion of a patient with carpal tunnel syndrome symptoms and yet without electrodiagnostic studies confirming slowing. This is acceptable if we believe that patients with carpal tunnel syndrome can have negative electrodiagnostic studies. However, the effect on range of motion should necessarily be related to muscle function, and muscle function is not directly tested in all 11 of these patients. Muscle function by way of electromyography could be coupled with this technique in the future. Second, no assessment is made as to the presence or extent of pain associated with carpal tunnel syndrome. Because range-of-motion deficits could well be related to pain, it should be part of future work using this range of motion–based method to assess carpal tunnel syndrome patients. It would be interesting to know whether the range of motion deficits exhibited in these 11 patients were related to differences in symptoms and differences in effort. One easy way to test this would be to use similar sensors on parts of the hand that are not affected by the median nerve and see whether those ranges of motion are actually affected by the presence or absence of carpal tunnel syndrome. In all cases, electrodiagnostic confirmation of the presence of carpal tunnel syndrome will help these results be more widely accepted by those who do not believe that carpal tunnel syndrome as a diagnosis should be associated with patients who have negative electrodiagnostic studies.

There is no doubt that the approach these authors take is truly novel and interesting. It allows practitioners of hand surgery to consider the possibility that a functional test may, in the end, supersede all the other tests used to diagnose carpal tunnel syndrome. The other tests, both in physical diagnoses and electrodiagnosis, even when grouped together, seem to fall short of predicting who will respond to surgical decompression. This study offers a glimpse into what may be the future in terms of the diagnosis and the outcomes of this common disorder.

J. Elfar, MD

Radiographic Evaluation of the Modified Brunelli Technique Versus a Scapholunotriquetral Transosseous Tenodesis Technique for Scapholunate Dissociation

Hsu JW, Kollitz KM, Jegapragasan M, et al (Univ of Washington Med Ctr, Seattle)

J Hand Surg Am 39:1041-1049, 2014

Purpose.—To compare reduction of the scapholunate articulation using a transosseous tenodesis through the scaphoid, lunate, and triquetrum (SLT) with the modified Brunelli technique (MBT) in a cadaver model, as measured by scapholunate (SL) angle and diastasis on radiographs.

Methods.—Twelve fresh-frozen cadaveric wrists were radiographically examined in a neutral posture, ulnar deviation, and clenched fist position. The SL angle and diastasis were recorded in each position with the SL ligament intact, after sectioning the ligament and secondary restraints, and after reconstruction by either the MBT (6 wrists) or SLT technique (6 wrists). Wrists were cycled through their maximum flexion and extension arc 100 times to simulate wrist motion after ligament sectioning and reconstruction.

Results.—After sectioning and cycling, all wrists demonstrated radiographic evidence of SL diastasis. After ligament reconstruction and cycling, there was no statistically significant difference in diastasis in the MBT reconstructions compared with the SLT reconstructions (3.0 vs 2.4 mm). The SLT group demonstrated better maintenance of the restored SL angle than the MBT reconstructions.

Conclusions.—In this cadaveric model, both MBT and SLT reconstructions restored anatomic parameters in the SL joint, with correction of SL diastasis and SL angle. Future studies to assess the clinical outcomes of SLT tenodesis in patients with chronic SL disruptions are important.

Clinical Relevance.—The SLT tenodesis, with a central biologic tether along the SL axis and dorsal reinforcement, may prove clinically useful.

▶ This is an elegant and well-constructed cadaveric assessment of 2 common techniques to reconstruct the torn and irreparable scapholunate ligament. I do have some concerns, however, as to how accurate intercarpal angles and scapholunate diastasis can be measured by plain radiographs even on cadavers. The modified Brunelli has been the most popular technique in recent years with excellent long-term publications from Wrightington and other institutions in both the general population and also in elite athletes. New techniques will continue to evolve, and the scaphoid, lunate, and triquetrum tenodesis does appear to offer theoretical advantages. In particular, the reconstruction is more likely to reduce the dorsal intercalated segment instability deformity and also support in the midportion of the scaphoid–lunate interval rather than the isolated dorsal reconstruction of the modified Brunelli technique. I share the authors' concerns of iatrogenic fracture using an interference screw in the lunate that has been popularized. The authors accept the limitations of their study being performed in cadavers and not the dynamic multifactorial pathological process that we encounter in our practice. Cadaveric dissection papers such as this allow us to experiment with new techniques that will allow us to further develop reconstruction techniques to help our patients in the long term.

M. Hayton, MD

Vascularized Medial Femoral Trochlea Osteochondral Flap Reconstruction of Advanced Kienböck Disease

Bürger HK, Windhofer C, Gaggl AJ, et al (Privat Hosp Maria Hilf, Klagenfurt; Unfallkrankenhaus, Berlin, Germany; Univ Hosp Salzburg, Austria; et al)

J Hand Surg Am 39:1313-1322, 2014

Purpose.—To describe the operative technique and report the results of 16 consecutive cases of arthroplasty for advanced Kienböck disease using a vascularized osteochondral graft from the medial femoral trochlea (MFT) with a minimum 12-month follow-up.

Methods.—Chart reviews of 16 cases of osteochondral MFT flap transfers for lunate reconstruction were performed in 2 institutions. Mean patient age was 35 years (range, 19–51 y). Preoperative Lichtman staging was 2 in 7 patients, 3a in 8 patients, and 3b in 1. Five of 16 patients had undergone a previous procedure for Kienböck disease (3 radial shortening osteotomies, 1 wrist denervation, and 1 distal radius vascularized bone grafting). Ulnar variance recorded at the time of the MFT reconstruction was negative in 8 patients, positive in 6 patients, and neutral in 2 patients. Follow-up data were recorded at a minimum of 12 months (average, 19 mo). Radiographic parameters recorded included preoperative ulnar variance, preoperative and final follow-up radioscaphoid angle, lunate height, lunate diameter, and the Stahl index and Lichtman stage.

Results.—Healing was confirmed in 15 of 16 reconstructed lunates. Lichtman staging remained unchanged in 10 patients, improved in 4 patients from grade 3a and 3b to 2, and worsened in 2 patients from grade 3a to 3b. All but 1 patient experienced improvement in wrist pain (12/16 complete relief; 3/16 incomplete relief). Wrist motion at follow-up averaged 50° extension and 38° flexion, similar to preoperative measurements. Grip strength at follow-up was 85% of the contralateral side.

Conclusions.—Osteochondral vascularized MFT flaps provided a reliable means of lunate reconstruction in advanced Kienböck disease. This flap allowed resection of the proximal portion of the collapsed lunate and reconstruction with an anatomically analogous convex segment of vascularized cartilage-bearing bone.

Type of Study/Level of Evidence.—Therapeutic IV.

▶ The authors have provided a retrospective study of their patients treated with medial femoral trochlear graft for treatment of Stage 2–3b Kienböck disease. They have demonstrated good results and that their technique can be effectively used to treat patients with this condition.

This is a technically demanding procedure, requiring experience with flap harvest and microsurgical anastomosis. The authors do not report on the operative time or duration of inpatient care. The donor site had pain in some instances for 3 months. These surgeons are proficient microsurgeons, and many hand surgeons may not be able to reproduce these results with this procedure.

Several procedures are described for Kienböck disease, including radial shortening or closing wedge osteotomies, capitate shortening, ulnar lengthening, metaphyseal core decompression of the radius and ulna, and lunate decompression, all with level IV evidence of good outcomes. Local vascularized bone grafting has also been shown to produce good results, but there is currently insufficient evidence to recommend 1 treatment routinely over the others. We also do not know whether the long-term outcomes are better with the proximal articular surface of the lunate being replaced as in their technique when compared with more traditional techniques.

Although the results of this retrospective review are compelling, further data are necessary to recommend its routine use, especially given the increase in technical requirements of the flap harvest, microvascular anastomosis, distant donor site morbidity with variable periods of discomfort, longer operative times, and inpatient hospital care. This should currently be reserved for those surgeons with microsurgical expertise and experience harvesting medial femoral grafts and may be best used as attempted salvage for revision cases.

W. C. Hammert, MD

Comparison of Two Percutaneous Volar Approaches for Screw Fixation of Scaphoid Waist Fractures: Radiographic and Biomechanical Study of an Osteotomy-Simulated Model

Meermans G, Van Glabbeek F, Braem MJ, et al (Lievensberg Hosp, Bergen op Zoom, The Netherlands; Univ of Antwerp, Belgium; et al)

J Bone Joint Surg Am 96:1369-1376, 2014

Background.—When a surgeon uses a percutaneous volar approach to treat scaphoid waist fractures, central screw placement is complicated by the shape of the scaphoid and by obstruction by the trapezium. In this study, we used radiographs and biomechanical tests to compare the standard volar percutaneous approach with the transtrapezial approach, with regard to central screw placement at the distal pole of the scaphoid.

Methods.—Fourteen matched pairs of cadaveric wrists were randomly assigned to two treatment groups. Under fluoroscopic control, a guidewire was drilled into the scaphoid, either through a transtrapezial approach or through a standard volar approach that avoided the trapezium. Guidewire position was measured in the coronal and sagittal planes. A transverse osteotomy was performed along the scaphoid waist, and this was followed by the insertion of the longest possible cannulated headless bone screw. Each specimen was placed into a fixture with a pneumatically driven plunger resting on the surface of the distal pole. Load was applied by using a load-controlled test protocol in a hydraulic testing machine.

Results.—All guidewires were inside the central one-third of the proximal pole. The guidewire positions at the distal pole differed significantly between the transtrapezial and standard volar approach groups ($p < 0.001$). The load to 2 mm of displacement and the load to failure averaged, respectively, 324.4 N (standard error of the mean [SEM] = 73.5 N) and 386.4 N (SEM = 65.6 N) for the transtrapezial approach group compared with 125.7 N (SEM = 22.6 N) ($p = 0.002$) and 191.4 N (SEM = 36.30 N) ($p = 0.005$) for the standard volar approach group.

Conclusions.—The data suggest that, in a cadaveric osteotomy-simulated scaphoid waist fracture model, the transtrapezial approach reliably achieves central positioning of a screw in the proximal and distal poles. This position offers a biomechanical advantage compared with central placement in only the proximal pole.

▶ This study provides evidence that in a cadaver model, with soft tissues removed, a screw can be predictably placed in the central axis of the distal and proximal poles using a transtrapezial approach, which had greater stiffness than a screw placed eccentrically in the volar third of the distal pole and central portion of the proximal pole. This study, although adding to the literature, has the typical limitations of a cadaver study. The placement of the wires was done after removing the soft tissues, and the load applied was in 1 direction and continuous, rather than cyclic, the latter of which occurs clinically.

The clinical relevance is that placement in the central axis on both coronal and sagittal planes will allow for more stiffness of the construct and possibly greater chance of union. Crossing the scaphotrapezial trapezoidal (STT) joint with the screw has been shown to increase the incidence of radiographic arthritis, but it is unclear whether this is clinically relevant. In addition, there may be a disruption of volar blood supply and injury to STT ligament, but the clinical importance of this is yet to be determined.

I find it easier and more predictable to place a percutaneous screw from proximal to distal in the central portion of the scaphoid at proximal, waist, and distal aspects. This does violate the articular surface of the scaphoid at the point of articulation of the radiocarpal joint, but there is no evidence to demonstrate that this creates a higher incidence of radiographic or clinically symptomatic arthritis.

W. C. Hammert, MD

6 Distal Radius Fractures

Biomechanical Comparison of Bicortical Locking Versus Unicortical Far-Cortex–Abutting Locking Screw-Plate Fixation for Comminuted Radial Shaft Fractures

Overturf SJ, Morris RP, Gugala Z, et al (Univ of Texas Med Branch, Galveston)

J Hand Surg Am 39:1907-1913, 2014

Purpose.—To provide comparative biomechanical evaluation of bicortical locking versus unicortical-abutting locking screw-plate fixation in a comminuted radius fracture model.

Methods.—A validated synthetic substitute of the adult human radius with a 1.5-cm-long segmental mid-diaphyseal defect was used in the study to simulate a comminuted fracture. Stabilization was achieved with an 8-hole locking plate and either bicortical screws or unicortical-abutting screws. The specimens were tested using nondestructive cyclical loading in 4-point bending, axial compression, and torsion to determine stiffness and displacement and subsequently in 4-point bending to assess load to failure.

Results.—There were no statistically significant differences between bicortical versus unicortical-abutting locking screw fixation in nondestructive 4-point bending, axial compression, and torsion. Both locking screw constructs also demonstrated comparable 4-point bending loads to failure.

Conclusion.—The biomechanical equivalence between bicortical locking versus unicortical-abutting locking screw-plate fixation suggests that adequate locking plate fixation can be achieved without perforation of the far cortex. The abutment of the screw tip within the far cortex enhances the unicortical screw positional stability and thereby effectively opposes the displacement of the screw when subjected to bending or axial or rotational loads.

Clinical Relevance.—Unicortical-abutting screws potentially offer several clinical advantages. They eliminate the need for drilling through the far cortex and thereby a risk of adjacent neurovascular injury or soft tissue structure compromise. They eliminate the issues associated with symptomatic screw prominence. They can decrease risk of refracture after screw-plate removal. In case of revision plating, they permit conversion to bicortical locking screws through the same near-cortex screw holes, which eliminates the need for a longer or repositioned plate.

▶ This biomechanical study examines the strength of unicortical, far-cortex abutting locking screws compared with traditional bicortical locking screws in a saw bone model. The concept is certainly appealing given the lessened risk of soft tissue irritation from traditional bicortical screws assuming mechanical strength is not compromised by the construct. Similar previous studies have shown unicortical locking screws to be weaker, especially when tested in torsion, although these were not far-cortex abutting.

From a design standpoint, the study used a validated synthetic radius substitute but chose a nonosteoporotic model. This is an important limitation because osteoporotic bone is typically cited as an indication for locking screw technology. The results of this study cannot be generalized to include osteoporotic bone. Also surprising is that nonlocking screws were not used in the comparisons. The final study design abnormality, in my opinion, was the decision to plate all radii along the radial border of the bone. Although 1 cadaver study (no saw bones studies) has shown similar biomechanical properties (anterior plating being stronger but not statistically significant compared with lateral plating), a more traditional surgical plate placement on the volar or dorsal surface of the bone would be more clinically relevant.

The results do support the authors' hypothesis that unicortical abutting screws are equal in strength to traditional bicortical locking screws when tested in 4-point bending, axial compression, torsional loading, and load-to-failure testing. The authors did not report the variation in screw length between specimens, which would be interesting to know considering the known influence of screw length and rotational stability. This also has clinical relevance given that screw sizes come in 2-mm increments; therefore, the diaphyseal cortical thickness variability could significantly affect the ability to perform this technique.

This study adds to our understanding of the biomechanics of locking screw technology. In my practice, I routinely drill into but not through the dorsal cortex when applying a volar plate to the distal radius. This study raises the question as to whether this principle could be applied to a diaphyseal radius fracture. The results certainly suggest from a biomechanical standpoint that this could be done. A major limitation for me with this consideration is that the overwhelming majority of diaphyseal radius fractures in my practice are managed with nonlocking screws. Nonlocking screw constructs from previous biomechanical studies have been found to have similar strength to those reported with locking screws in this study and are more cost-effective.

In summary, unicortical, far-cortex abutting locking screws appear to have similar biomechanical strength to traditional bicortical locking screws in a diaphyseal saw bone radius model. Often nonlocking screws are sufficient in radial shaft fractures. If locking screws are deemed necessary, far-cortex abutting unicortical locking screws could be considered. The reproducibility of placing them in a clinical scenario has not been examined, however.

G. Gaston, MD

The Effect of Brachioradialis Release During Distal Radius Fracture Fixation on Elbow Flexion Strength and Wrist Function

Kim JK, Park JS, Shin SJ, et al (Ewha Woman Univ, Seoul, South Korea)

J Hand Surg Am 39:2246-2250, 2014

Purpose.—To identify whether brachioradialis (BR) release during volar plate fixation for a distal radius fracture affects elbow flexion strength and wrist function.

Methods.—A total of 42 consecutive patients who were treated by open reduction volar plate fixation for unstable distal radius fractures were enrolled in this study. The BR was not released in 20 of 42 patients (BR preserved group) and was released in 22 patients (BR released group). The primary outcome variable was isokinetic strength and endurance testing of elbow flexion measured by the Cybex isokinetic system 3 months after surgery. Measured at the same time, secondary outcome variables were grip strength, a visual analog scale score for wrist pain, Disabilities of the Arm, Shoulder, and Hand score, and radiographic parameters. We used Manne—Whitney *U* tests to compare these variables between groups.

Results.—Neither elbow flexion strength and endurance nor any of the secondary outcome variables differed significantly between groups.

Conclusions.—Release of the BR during a volar approach for a distal radius fracture did not adversely affect elbow flexion strength and wrist function.

Type of Study/Level of Evidence.—Prognostic III.

► This is a well-done cohort study that looks at the effect of releasing brachioradialis (BR) on various parameters of upper extremity function during volar approach to the distal radius. Measurements include elbow flexion strength, elbow flexion endurance, visual analog score, grip strength, and Disabilities of the Arm, Shoulder, and Hand score. The study is well organized with thorough patient evaluation; 42 patients were evaluated at 3 months by a therapist who was blinded to the treatment approach. The patients were not randomly assigned, however, and one could suppose that those who underwent BR release had a more comminuted fracture pattern. Perhaps these differences in function would not translate if the fracture patterns were similar or patients randomly assigned.

The biomechanical background in a cadaveric model notes that loss of elbow flexion torque of the BR was less than 10% if the BR was released at the proximal beak of the distal radius.[1] This is consistent with the authors clinical findings as well.

I routinely assess whether the BR needs to be released to obtain an adequate reduction before releasing. I have found, however, that in most of my cases, I am releasing the BR to obtain radial inclination and restoration of height. Although I am not surprised by the authors' results, I am encouraged that the release of the BR does not seem to be clinically significant. A randomized study would lend further support to these findings.

E. Lawler, MD

Reference

1. Tirrell TF, Franko OI, Bhola S, Hentzen ER, Abrams RA, Lieber RL. Functional consequence of distal brachioradialis tendon release: a biomechanical study. *J Hand Surg Am*. 2013;38:920-926.

The Effects of Ulnar Styloid Fractures on Patients Sustaining Distal Radius Fractures

Daneshvar P, Chan R, MacDermid J, et al (St. Joseph's Health Centre, London, Ontario, Canada)
J Hand Surg Am 39:1915-1920, 2014

Purpose.—To determine if ulnar styloid fractures (USF) affect clinical outcome following distal radius fracture (DRF) in adults under 65 years of age.

Methods.—This study involved 312 patients (aged 18–64) with surgically and nonsurgically treated DRFs. Patients were followed prospectively at baseline and 3, 6, and 12 months. The primary outcome was the Patient-Rated Wrist Evaluation (PRWE), and secondary outcomes were range of motion and grip strength. The USFs were classified by location (tip, middle, and base) and union status.

Results.—There were 170 patients with isolated DRFs and 142 with associated USF (64 tip, 32 middle, and 46 base fractures). The mean age of the entire cohort was 48 years with 218 (70%) women. All USFs were treated nonoperatively. There was a trend of higher PRWE scores in DRFs associated with USFs compared to isolated DRFs throughout the study. Associated ulnar styloid base fractures had higher but clinically insignificant PRWE scores than isolated DRFs at 6 and 12 months. Patients with an associated USF had a slower recovery of wrist flexion and grip strength compared to isolated DRF, but values were comparable at 12 months. United USFs and nonunited USFs had similar PRWE scores at all time points.

Conclusions.—Adults under 65 years old with DRFs and associated USFs initially have greater pain and disability than those with isolated DRFs; however, this difference dissipated over time and was not significant at one year. No long-term differences in measured impairments were observed, but the presence of an associated USF resulted in a slower recovery of grip strength and wrist flexion. Presence of a USF nonunion did not significantly affect outcomes.

Type of Study/Level of Evidence.—Prognostic II.

▶ The authors performed a prospective study to assess whether young (less than 65) distal radius fracture patients with ulnar styloid fractures had a difference in recovery time. The assessment tools used were motion and patient-rated wrist evaluation (PRWE). The study involved 312 patients that were followed up at 3, 6, and 12 months. A statistically significant difference in PRWE was seen at baseline and at 3 and 12 months, although at 12 months the difference was not clinically significant. Recovery of wrist motion was significantly slower in patients with ulnar styloid fractures at 3 months but not after 6 months.

This study shows that young patients with ulnar styloid fractures with distal radius fractures may have more pain and slower return of motion at 3 months, but by 12 months the recovery is similar to that of isolated distal radius fractures. The study was well designed and specifically addresses younger patients who tend to have higher demand and use of their hands compared with previous studies that address all ages.

C. Heinrich, MD

Total Joint Arthroplasty of the Distal Radioulnar Joint for Rheumatoid Arthritis

Galvis EJ, Pessa J, Scheker LR (Kleinert Kutz Hand Care Ctr, Louisville, KY)
J Hand Surg Am 39:1699-1704, 2014

Purpose.—To evaluate the clinical and radiological results of primary total distal radioulnar joint (DRUJ) replacement as well as reconstruction following ulnar head excision in patients with rheumatoid arthritis (RA).

Methods.—Seventeen patients with RA underwent 19 total DRUJ replacement between 2005 and 2011. Mean age at the time of the surgery was 57 years. Mean follow-up was 39 months (range, 12–79 mo). Pain level was evaluated using a visual analog scale (VAS). Pronation and supination were recorded before and after surgery. A patient satisfaction survey was used, as well as postoperative Disabilities of the Arm, Shoulder, and Hand (DASH) and Patient- Related Wrist Evaluation (PRWE) scores. Ulnar translocation of the carpus was assessed radiographically, and the presence or absence of radiolucent zones around the implant were recorded.

Results.—The preoperative average VAS score for the 19 joints was 7.3. Pain decreased after surgery to 2.2. Pronation improved from 56° before surgery to 78° afterward, a 39% improvement. Supination improved from 57° before surgery to 71° afterward, a 27%improvement. Final scores were 24 for the DASH and 24 for the PRWE. Fifteen patients reported substantial pain relief. All patients were satisfied with their surgical result.

Conclusions.—The results of this study suggest that total replacement of the DRUJ is of benefit to the patient with RA. Pronation was significantly increased and supination was increased but did not approach significance. Improvement in VAS score suggests that pain was decreased.

Type of study/level of evidence.—Therapeutic IV.

▶ The management of distal radioulnar joint (DRUJ) arthritis has been a vexing problem in hand surgery. Traditional surgical treatments, including Darrach resection, Sauve-Kapandji, and soft-tissue reconstructions, have been met with mixed results. Nonconstrained arthroplasties exist, but there are concerns using them in patients with rheumatoid arthritis (RA) who typically have poor soft-tissue stability at the DRUJ. Total DRUJ replacement offers a potential solution to these traditional procedures but has not been studied to date in the RA population.

The strengths of the study design include its targeted study population of RA patients, validated outcome instruments (Disabilities of the Arm, Shoulder, and Hand [DASH] and Patient-Related Wrist Evaluation [PRWE]) and detailed radiographic follow-up examining loosening in the midterm. The study is limited by its small sample size (17 patients), lack of preoperative DASH and PRWE scores for comparison, and number of concomitant procedures (although this last point is to be expected in an RA patient cohort).

The results the authors report do parallel my experience with this implant, showing improved range of motion (statistically significant for supination), decreased pain (statistically significant decrease in visual analog scale), improved functional outcome (high PRWE scores although no preoperative comparisons are available), and low disability (as seen in DASH results, but again no preoperative comparisons are available).

My experience with this implant has been positive. The procedure does require strict attention to detail, particularly with placement of the radial plate. There is a natural tendency to have the plate angled in a volar direction, and at times aggressive burring is needed to flatten the sigmoid notch and allow it to sit perpendicular to the radius. Interestingly, in the patient without RA, care is supposed to be taken not to position the component too far distally to avoid abutment with the carpus.

From a radiographic standpoint, preoperative ulnar translocation was unchanged after surgery, and the authors cite a potential advantage as a mechanical buttress for the carpus. This is somewhat interesting in that the surgical technique guide describes positioning the implant more proximal to avoid contact with the carpus. The authors did not elaborate on whether they routinely place the implant more distally to try and serve as a mechanical buttress in all patients with RA. Also, it is common in my practice to see some lysis around the distal aspect of the ulnar stem. The authors noted this as well and found no radiographic progression during the study period.

In an era of cost containment, the cost of this implant must also be considered. My preference in the RA patient is to perform a Darrach or Sauve-Kapandji procedure as an index surgery and reserve this implant for a salvage of a failed index case.

The largest limitation of this study is the conflict of interest. Dr Scheker is the designer of the prosthesis, holds the patent for the prosthesis, and is a co-owner of the Aptis Company. Further evidence is still needed, but this is a promising implant for DRUJ arthritis.

G. Gaston, MD

The Effect of Brachioradialis Release During Distal Radius Fracture Fixation on Elbow Flexion Strength and Wrist Function

Kim JK, Park JS, Shin SJ, et al (Ewha Woman Univ, Seoul, South Korea)

J Hand Surg Am 39:2246-2250, 2014

Purpose.—To identify whether brachioradialis (BR) release during volar plate fixation for a distal radius fracture affects elbow flexion strength and wrist function.

Methods.—A total of 42 consecutive patients who were treated by open reduction volar plate fixation for unstable distal radius fractures were enrolled in this study. The BR was not released in 20 of 42 patients (BR preserved group) and was released in 22 patients (BR released group). The primary outcome variable was isokinetic strength and endurance testing of elbow flexion measured by the Cybex isokinetic system 3 months after surgery. Measured at the same time, secondary outcome variables were grip strength, a visual analog scale score for wrist pain, Disabilities of the Arm, Shoulder, and Hand score, and radiographic parameters. We used Manne—Whitney *U* tests to compare these variables between groups.

Results.—Neither elbow flexion strength and endurance nor any of the secondary outcome variables differed significantly between groups.

Conclusions.—Release of the BR during a volar approach for a distal radius fracture did not adversely affect elbow flexion strength and wrist function.

Type of Study/Level of Evidence.—Prognostic III.

▶ This is a nice study supporting brachioradialis (BR) release during distal radius fracture reduction. The attributes of the study groups were comparable. The authors don't provide information about fracture type, but we can suspect that the BR release group was included for more comminuted fractures because the reduction needed the release of the BR insertion. Elbow force was measured objectively by an isokinetic system, and no differences were found between the groups. Additionally, end point radiographic parameters were checked showing no differences. This finding supports the fact that BR release helped in achieving a successful reduction. It would be much more interesting to compare if BR release really helps in achieving better reduction, but in this case similar fracture type groups must be planned for that study. It is hard to set up this kind of research in the clinic. I think that during the procedure, if the BR insertion is not released completely (the authors give good description about the anatomy of that region), the lack of influence on elbow flexion seems not to be a surprising finding.

I do a BR release more frequent mostly to have better control of the radial styloid fragment, and I do it as far as it is necessary to help achieve the reduction. I perform the release gradually in the cases in which my usual dissection is not enough to reduce the fracture, so it appears to be the same as the approach presented by the authors.

P. Czarnecki, MD, PhD

The Effects of Ulnar Styloid Fractures on Patients Sustaining Distal Radius Fractures

Daneshvar P, Chan R, MacDermid J, et al (St. Joseph's Health Centre, London, Ontario, Canada)

J Hand Surg Am 39:1915-1920, 2014

Purpose.—To determine if ulnar styloid fractures (USF) affect clinical outcome following distal radius fracture (DRF) in adults under 65 years of age.

Methods.—This study involved 312 patients (aged 18–64) with surgically and nonsurgically treated DRFs. Patients were followed prospectively at baseline and 3, 6, and 12 months. The primary outcome was the Patient-Rated Wrist Evaluation (PRWE), and secondary outcomes were range of motion and grip strength. The USFs were classified by location (tip, middle, and base) and union status.

Results.—There were 170 patients with isolated DRFs and 142 with associated USF (64 tip, 32 middle, and 46 base fractures). The mean age of the entire cohort was 48 years with 218 (70%) women. All USFs were treated nonoperatively. There was a trend of higher PRWE scores in DRFs associated with USFs compared to isolated DRFs throughout the study. Associated ulnar styloid base fractures had higher but clinically insignificant PRWE scores than isolated DRFs at 6 and 12 months. Patients with an associated USF had a slower recovery of wrist flexion and grip strength compared to isolated DRF, but values were comparable at 12 months. United USFs and nonunited USFs had similar PRWE scores at all time points.

Conclusions.—Adults under 65 years old with DRFs and associated USFs initially have greater pain and disability than those with isolated DRFs; however, this difference dissipated over time and was not significant at one year. No long-term differences in measured impairments were observed, but the presence of an associated USF resulted in a slower recovery of grip strength and wrist flexion. Presence of a USF nonunion did not significantly affect outcomes.

Type of study/level of evidence.—Prognostic II.

▶ This is a nice study on ulnar styloid fractures and their impact on hand function when a distal radius fracture is treated. As in many studies on distal radius fracture and treatment methods, the results do not differ between the groups at the 1 year end point. But authors showed worse results in the ulnar styloid fracture group in the short term. This information can be used to help explain the prognosis to the patient despite initial difficulties in exercises. In this study, the advantage is a higher number of patients (n = 312) and younger age (mean 48) than in other studies on that problem. A weakness of this study is that the authors only used the Patient-Rated Wrist Evaluation as the assessment tool, which could be expanded, and several scores could be used (Mayo, Michigan). Each of these gives different information and could help further elucidate the potential issues arising from a concomitant ulnar styloid fracture.

From my perspective, it always needs explanation that this fracture is only an indirect symptom of ligamentous (distal radioulnar joint [DRUJ]) injuries, which the authors mention in the introduction. We still don't know how it can influence and why it gives different kinds of symptoms in different patients despite the same radiologic findings. Moreover, the study does not consider any treatment of the ulnar styloid fracture, which could be a good idea for the next step of research. We also don't have information about persistent problems such as DRUJ instability or ulnar pain in both groups.

I rarely stabilize ulnar styloid fractures. This is very challenging and unnecessary, and this opinion is based on this and previous studies. If there is evidence of concomitant DRUJ instability, I then stabilize the DRUJ with an additional K-wire for 6 weeks.

P. Czarnecki, MD, PhD

Factors Delaying Recovery After Volar Plate Fixation of Distal Radius Fractures

Roh YH, Lee BK, Noh JH, et al (Gachon Univ of Medicine, Incheon, South Korea; Kangwon Natl Univ Hosp, Gangwon-do, South Korea; Seoul Natl Univ College of Medicine, South Korea)

J Hand Surg Am 39:1465-1470, 2014

Purpose.—To evaluate the factors influencing delayed functional recovery in patients with a distal radius fracture treated by volar plate fixation.

Methods.—A total of 122 patients with a distal radius fracture treated by volar locking plate were enrolled. The wrist range of motion, grip strength, and functional outcome by the Michigan hand score were assessed 3, 6, and 12 months after surgery. The factors assessed for their influence on delayed functional recovery include age, sex, bone mineral density (BMD), hand dominance, the type of fracture, the energy of trauma, the time to surgery, and the duration of immobilization. A multivariate regression analysis was conducted to identify independent predictors of delayed functional recovery in terms of the Michigan hand score.

Results.—There was a significant decrease in the wrist range of motion in patients with a high-energy trauma, severe type fracture, or increase in duration of immobilization at month 3, whereas only a severe fracture type was associated with a decreased range of motion after 6 and 12 months. An increase in age, a decrease in BMD, and high-energy trauma reduced grip strength at months 3 and 6, whereas only an increase in age and a decrease in BMD reduced grip strength at month 12. According to the multivariate regression analysis, severe type fracture and high-energy trauma reduced functional outcomes at months 3 and 6. Conversely, at month 12, an increase in age and a decrease in BMD reduced functional outcome.

Conclusions.—An increase in age and a decrease in BMD were important risk factors influencing delayed functional recovery up to 12 months after distal radius fracture surgery, whereas fracture severity and high-energy trauma were associated with decreased functional outcomes up to 6 months after surgery.

Type of Study/Level of Evidence.—Prognostic II.

▶ The authors investigate parameters that delay functional recovery after operative treatment of distal radius fractures. This study is thoroughly designed, but the outcomes are not really surprising: Patients with more severe fractures recover more slowly, and old patients (with reduced bone mineral density) do not recover as fast as young patients. Most of the parameters investigated were beyond the surgeons' control and could not be altered to improve outcomes. Because only 2 different surgeons were involved, it would have been interesting to also include more technical details such as the number of reductions or operating time. Therefore, the eternal question, why some patients have good functional results (and quicker recovery) despite suboptimal radiographic studies and vice versa, still remains unanswered. The best strategy is to try to restore the original anatomy as closely as possible.

K. Megerle, MD

Distal Radial Fractures in Older Men: A Missed Opportunity?

Harper CM, Fitzpatrick SK, Zurakowski D, et al (Harvard Combined Orthopaedic Residency, Boston, MA; Harvard Med School, Boston, MA; Children's Hosp Boston, MA)

J Bone Joint Surg Am 96:1820-1827, 2014

Background.—Fractures of the distal aspect of the radius are common, yet little is known about this type of fracture among older men. The purpose of this study was to compare fracture characteristics, treatment, and osteoporosis evaluation among men and women who had sustained a distal radial fracture. We hypothesized that the men would have similar patterns of injury and lower rates of evaluation for osteoporosis.

Methods.—We retrospectively reviewed the medical records of ninety-five men and 344 women over the age of fifty years who were treated for a distal radial fracture at a single institution over a five-year period. We assessed whether the patients had received a dual x-ray absorptiometry (DXA) scan and osteoporosis treatment within six months following the injury. Multivariate analysis identified independent predictors of bone mineral density (BMD) testing and osteoporosis treatment.

Results.—Men had less severe fractures than women (a Type-C fracture rate of 20% for men compared with 40% for women; $p = 0.014$).While 184 (53%) of the women had a DXA scan after injury, only seventeen (18%) of the men were evaluated ($p < 0.001$). Among the patients who underwent DXA scan, nine men (9% of men overall) and sixty-five women (19% of women overall) had a diagnosis of osteoporosis ($p = 0.01$). Male sex was an independent predictor of failure to undergo

BMD testing as well as receive subsequent treatment with calcium and vitamin D or bisphosphonates ($p < 0.001$).

Conclusions.—Significantly fewer men received evaluation for osteoporosis following a distal radial fracture, with rates of evaluation unacceptably low according to published guidelines.

▶ The incidence of osteoporosis and fragility fractures in our aging population is increasing dramatically. Distal radius fractures (DRF) have been well recognized as a "sentinel event" that can predict more serious osteoporotic fractures in the future. This puts surgeons who treat DRFs in the important position of often being the first physician to discuss bone health or osteoporosis with these patients. If diagnosed, intervening with treatments at this early stage can have the potential to have a substantial impact on future fragility fractures. Although the study is retrospective and used subjects from a single center, it is well designed, has a large sample size, and has increased awareness of the higher than expected incidence of osteoporosis in men with DRFs. In my experience, although women often ask about osteoporosis at their first visit after DRF, men rarely do. General awareness of the incidence of osteoporosis in men must increase, both in patients and clinicians, because this study reports that only one-third of men with osteoporosis actually receive treatment.

R. Grewal, MD

Radiographic interpretation of distal radius fractures: visual estimations versus digital measuring techniques

O'Malley MP, Rodner C, Ritting A, et al (Univ of Connecticut Health Ctr, Farmington)

Hand 9:488-493, 2014

Purpose.—Distal radius fractures are a common injury. In the emergency room, trainees regularly assess these fractures using visual estimation. Our hypothesis is that assessment of radiographic parameters has sufficient accuracy for rendering treatment consistent with formal measurements.

Methods.—This study compared visual measurements made by 25 orthopaedic residents and attending physicians to formal measurements made by a single fellowship trained musculoskeletal radiologist in a series of patients with distal radius fractures. A search was performed utilizing the ICD-9 code for distal radius fracture in all patients presenting to a single institution emergency department. Participants used visual estimation to rate 25 radiographs. Parameters estimated included radial inclination, radial height, volar tilt, and the presence of intra-articular displacement. Analysis using Lin concordance coefficients, Bland Altman plots, and the Kappa statistic evaluated the agreement between visual estimation and formal measurements. The proportion of raters whose estimates would have resulted in a course of treatment that conflicted with the formal reading quantified the potential impact of visual estimation on treatment.

Results.—Concordance coefficients were poor for radial inclination ($\rho c = 0.13$), radial height ($\rho c = 0.24$), and volar tilt ($\rho c = 0.46$). The Kappa statistic for intra-articular displacement was 0.4. Analysis performed according to level of training did not result in substantial improvements in these statistics. Treatment based on visual estimates conflicted with formal readings 34 % of the time for radial inclination, 38 % of the time for radial height, 27 % of the time for volar tilt, and 31 % of the time for intra-articular displacement.

Discussion.—Visual estimation is not an adequate form of measurement for evaluation of patients with distal radius fractures. Physicians should be mindful of these results when developing treatment plans based solely upon visual estimation.

▶ The message is clear: Visual estimates of radiographic parameters are inaccurate. This is not at all surprising. The methodology of this study, however, is problematic. The raters were placed at a marked disadvantage by asking them to view a slide show of 25 distal radius fractures (DRF) projected onto a screen under ambient light, which washes out the image and is lower resolution than a PACS (picture archiving and communication system) monitor. The authors intended to simulate how DRFs present in the ER, but orthopedic surgeons are certainly not required to evaluate the fractures from a slide show. Most emergency departments have PACS monitors. Even without using the measurement software, the radiographic landmarks are more easily seen.

A single reading of a radiologist, rather than a computed tomography scan, was taken as the gold standard. There was no interobserver calculation between 2 or 3 additional musculoskeletal radiologists, which is a source of bias. The radiologist should have provided his own visual estimates of the parameters to establish his visual accuracy, and the raters should have provided visual estimates after reviewing the X-rays on a PACS monitor. Despite the detailed statistical analysis, the data is questionable because of the flawed methodology. As Szabo stated, "Application of the best statistical methodology to poor-quality data is analogous to claiming that the operation was a success but the patient died."[1]

Although the authors collected data regarding treatment recommendations based on clinical thresholds for the parameters, the actual fracture management in Table 1 in the original article suggests that they did not follow their own treatment recommendations. Most authors would not recommend nonoperative treatment of a C2 articular fracture (5) or a C3 fracture (1) regardless of the radiographic parameters.

My take-home message from this article is not that visual estimates are inaccurate but rather that resident education should emphasize the importance of measuring the radiographic parameters because pencil and goniometer or PACS software are readily available in any emergency department. Adjuvant imaging techniques are often necessary to define the fracture characteristics. In my own practice, the decision to operate is not based on a clinical guess, the radiologist report, nor blind adherence to radiographic parameters. Myriad other factors must be taken into consideration, including patient age and activity level.

D. J. Slutsky, MD

Reference

1. Szabo RM. Statistical analysis as related to hand surgery. *J Hand Surg Am*. 1997; 22:376-385.

Complications Associated With Operative Versus Nonsurgical Treatment of Distal Radius Fractures in Patients Aged 65 Years and Older

Lutz K, Yeoh KM, MacDermid JC, et al (St. Joseph's Health Care, London, Ontario, Canada; Orthosports Orthopaedic and Sports Medicine Service, Sydney, New South Wales, Australia)

J Hand Surg Am 39:1280-1286, 2014

Purpose.—To compare complication rates for distal radius fractures treated operatively versus nonsurgical in patients older than 65 years. We hypothesized that surgical intervention would improve fracture alignment, but it would be associated with more complications and equivalent functional outcomes when compared with the nonsurgical group.

Methods.—Patients (operative, n = 129) and controls (nonsurgical, n = 129) were identified from a prospective clinical and operating room database. They were matched on fracture severity (AO-A/ B/C1 vs AO-C2/C3), sex, age, and energy of injury. Data on complications were extracted from medical charts using a validated complications checklist, and radiologic data were collected for all patients. Functional outcomes (Patient-Related Wrist Evaluation) at 1 year were available in only a subset of patients. We determined differences in complication and reoperation rates using a chi-square test.

Results.—A significant number of patients experienced complications in the operative group (operative = 37 of 129; nonsurgical = 22 of 129). The most common complication was median neuropathy (n = 8 operative; n = 14 nonsurgical), followed by surgical site infections (n = 16 operative; 12 of 16 were pin site infections) and complex regional pain syndrome (n = 4 operative; 3 nonsurgical). The complication rate in patients treated with volar plate was 22% (16 of 74), for dorsal plate it was 50% (2 of 4), for external fixation it was 42% (16 of 38), and for percutaneous pinning it was 23% (3 of 13). The number of patients requiring reoperations was similar in both groups (11 [9%] operative; 7 [5%] nonsurgical). Our secondary radiologic and functional outcomes demonstrate that despite a higher incidence of malunion in nonsurgical patients (nonsurgical: 69% vs operative: 29%), a subset of patients from both groups (n = 140) had minimal pain and disability at 1 year (Patient-Related Wrist Evaluation operative: 16.9 ± 23.2; nonsurgical: 15.7 ± 17.5).

Conclusions.—In a study matching fracture severity, sex, age, and energy of injury, we found that elderly patients with distal radius fractures who underwent surgery had higher complication rates than those treated nonsurgically.

Type of Study/Level of Evidence.—Therapeutic III.

▶ The focus of this study was to compare complication rates for distal radius fractures treated operatively and nonoperatively in patients over 65 years of age. At issue, in this article and in orthopedics as whole, is whether the complications associated with the operative treatment of distal radius fractures when weighed against the complications of nonoperative treatment render surgery the better option. Historically, nonoperative management of all distal radius fractures was the norm and yet recent data show improved radiographic and perhaps functional outcomes with operative management. This trend has, no doubt, been related to the more advanced hardware and more precise technique that can be used for the reduction and fixation of distal radius fractures. However, even within the realm of operative management, no single, clear answer is available to the question of what treatment approach best fits any given fracture type.

In this study, 129 operative patients were compared to 129 nonoperatively treated distal radius fractures. These patients were obtained from an operating room database. Some patients were evaluated functionally using the Patient-Rated Wrist Evaluation at 1 year, and data on complications were obtained from chart review. Interestingly, the most common complication of operatively and nonoperatively managed patients was median nerve compression neuropathy. This was followed by surgical site infection and complex regional pain syndrome. The complication rate for modes of fixation such as volar plate, dorsal plate, and external fixation as well as percutaneous pinning was also obtained. Interestingly, the complication rates associated with volar plate treatment and percutaneous pinning treatment were nearly the same at 22%. However, the complication rate for dorsal plate treatment was 50% in 2 of 4 patients and 42% of patients undergoing external fixation. Perhaps expectedly, nonsurgical management led to a higher incidence of malunion (69% vs 29% in operatively treated patients), and the Patient-Rated Wrist Evaluation was similar at 1 year between the 2 groups at approximately 16. The authors conclude that when patients matched for fracture severity (sex, age, and the energy of injury) are compared, elderly patients with distal radius fractures who undergo surgery have a higher complication rate than those treated nonsurgically.

In this matched, case-controlled-type study, the authors have been able to answer a fundamental question in hand surgery: Is the complication rate for operative management higher than for nonoperative management of distal radius fractures? Secondarily, is the Patient-Rated Wrist Evaluation significantly different between these 2 groups? The answers to these questions seem to be that operative management is associated with more complications and that outcomes, as measured with the Patient-Rated Wrist Evaluation, seemed to be the same in both groups at 1 year. In these cohorts, 29% of patients treated operatively experienced complications, whereas only 17% of those treated nonoperatively experienced complications. Eight of the combined cohort of patients had transient symptoms of median neuropathy, 6 required no treatment, 6 had moderate symptoms, and an additional 8 required surgical release. Surgical site infections occurred in 6% of the operatively treated patients, only 1 of whom required operative incision, drainage, and early removal of hardware. There was a greater number of moderately severe complications in the operative group, which was significant, and these complications were related primarily to infections. Interestingly, patients requiring an operation after the completion of fracture healing were the same in both operative and nonoperative groups, and the most common operation performed on these patients was a carpal tunnel release.

This study contributes much to our understanding of the best way to treat distal radius fractures. In matching cases to controls for fracture severity, the authors are effective at reducing the treatment bias issue because patients were matched for severity in both the operative and nonoperative cohorts. Selection bias, therefore, is less of an issue in this study than it might be in a study in which patients are allocated prospectively to operative or nonoperative treatment solely on the opinion of the treating surgeon. The caveat here is that 13 of the 130 patients with operative management had open fractures, and open fractures are always treated operatively in the study cohort; therefore, the matching of cases for severity cannot possibly fully eliminate bias.

The authors conclude, and we may as well, that the role of surgery in patients over age 65 is not yet clear. Surgery produces perhaps a more anatomic reduction but does not necessarily improve functional outcome and does definitely result in higher complications. The importance of this study goes beyond these conclusions, however. It seems that these authors are asking a more fundamental question than which method of operative management is best; they are asking whether operative management actually results in a better outcome. With so much work and so much literature in our field dedicated to which operative technique does best, it seems that the "holy grail comparison" between operative and nonoperative management is the void that this article fills. The fact remains that the method of operative management is operator-dependent, and the choice of operative management is related to surgeon skill and experience with the technique; however, whether to even perform an operation is a fundamentally important issue to explore with patients in this elderly age group. With almost 260 patients involved in this study, it seems clear and prescient that an orthopedic surgeon must consider the weight of a higher complication rate and possibly unimproved functional outcome in the decision to recommend surgery for a distal radius fracture in practice.

J. Elfar, MD

Accelerated Rehabilitation Compared with a Standard Protocol After Distal Radial Fractures Treated with Volar Open Reduction and Internal Fixation: A Prospective, Randomized, Controlled Study

Brehmer JL, Husband JB (Univ of Minnesota, MN; TRIA Orthopaedic Ctr, Bloomington, MN)

J Bone Joint Surg Am 96:1621-1630, 2014

Background.—There are relatively few studies in the literature that specifically evaluate accelerated rehabilitation protocols for distal radial fractures treated with open reduction and internal fixation (ORIF). The purpose of this study was to compare the early postoperative outcomes (at zero to twelve weeks postoperatively) of patients enrolled in an accelerated rehabilitation protocol with those of patients enrolled in a standard rehabilitation protocol following ORIF for a distal radial fracture. We hypothesized that patients with accelerated rehabilitation after volar ORIF for a distal radial fracture would have an earlier return to function compared with patients who followed a standard protocol.

Methods.—From November 2007 to November 2010, eighty-one patients with an unstable distal radial fracture were prospectively randomized to follow either an accelerated or a standard rehabilitation protocol after undergoing ORIF with a volar plate for a distal radial fracture. Both groups began with gentle active range of motion at three to five days postoperatively. At two weeks, the accelerated group initiated wrist/forearm passive range of motion and strengthening exercises, whereas the standard group initiated passive range of motion and strengthening at six weeks postoperatively. Patients were assessed at three to five days, two weeks, three weeks, four weeks, six weeks, eight weeks, twelve weeks, and six months postoperatively. Outcomes included Disabilities of the Arm, Shoulder and Hand (DASH) scores (primary outcome) and measurements of wrist flexion/extension, supination, pronation, grip strength, and palmar pinch.

Results.—The patients in the accelerated group had better mobility, strength, and DASH scores at the early postoperative time points (zero to eight weeks postoperatively) compared with the patients in the standard rehabilitation group. The difference between the groups was both clinically relevant and statistically significant.

Conclusions.—Patients who follow an accelerated rehabilitation protocol that emphasizes motion immediately postoperatively and initiates strengthening at two weeks after volar ORIF of a distal radial fracture have an earlier return to function than patients who follow a more standard rehabilitation protocol.

Level of Evidence.—Therapeutic Level I. See Instructions for Authors for a complete description of levels of evidence.

► This level I study is important and adds to our understanding of the optimal rehab protocol for one of the most common upper extremity procedures. Volar plate fixation for distal radius fractures has become many surgeons' procedure of choice, although the evidence still supports dorsal plating and external fixation as equally effective. The optimal timing of active motion, passive motion, and strengthening has not been well researched. This prospective, randomized study of 81 patients helps answer this question.

It is critical to understand the exact protocols used in each group. Both groups began gentle active motion at 3 to 5 days' postsurgery and had identical rehabilitation for the first 2 weeks. At 2 weeks, the accelerated protocol began passive range of motion and at 4 weeks strengthening. The standard protocol began passive motion at 6 weeks and strengthening at 8 weeks. In my practice, a more standard protocol would initiate motion at 1 to 2 weeks rather than 3 to 5 days and an accelerated protocol would be as described by the authors. This leads me to believe that the differences could be even greater than the authors report at the earlier time points in my personal practice.

It is perplexing that the results of the DASH and wrist flexion in the accelerated group were statistically significantly better than the standard group at 2 weeks considering the protocols to that point were identical. The DASH results remained statistically better in the accelerated group until 6 months, although were only clinically relevant at 2 time points.

There was a statistically significant improvement in the range of motion in flexion, extension, and supination from 3 weeks until 2 months. Although this was statistically significant, its clinical significance is questionable considering the majority of the time points had a difference of less than 5 degrees.

For me, the main strength of this article is that it validates the safety of both an accelerated and standard protocol. My preference is an accelerated protocol when fracture stability allows. Any time a more comminuted fracture exists or I have concerns over the stability of the initial construct a standard protocol appears to offer similar midterm outcomes. This article supports the commonly held belief that earlier motion is safe and affords earlier recovery of function. Delaying motion, however, delays functional recovery in the short term but does not impact ultimate recovery.

Probably the biggest limitation of the study is that compliance with protocols was not reported. The ability of either group to do more or less than instructed could have an impact on results.

G. Gaston, MD

The Influence of Vitamin C on the Outcome of Distal Radial Fractures: A Double-Blind, Randomized Controlled Trial

Ekrol I, Duckworth AD, Ralston SH, et al (Royal Infirmary of Edinburgh, UK; Univ of Edinburgh, UK)

J Bone Joint Surg Am 96:1451-1459, 2014

Background.—Vitamin C has been proposed to improve outcomes after a distal radial fracture by promotion of bone and soft-tissue healing and reduction of the prevalence of complex regional pain syndrome (CRPS). Our primary aim was to examine the effect of vitamin C on functional outcome after a distal radial fracture.

Methods.—A total of 336 adult patients with an acute fracture of the distal aspect of the radius were recruited over a one-year period and randomized to receive 500 mg of vitamin C or placebo daily for fifty days after the fracture. The primary outcomes were the DASH (Disabilities of the Arm, Shoulder and Hand) score at six weeks and at one year. Secondary variables included complications, wrist and finger motion, grip and pinch strength, pain, and a CRPS score.

Results.—There were no significant differences in patient or fracture characteristics between the treatment groups. There was no significant effect of vitamin C on the DASH score throughout the study period. At six weeks, patients in the vitamin C group with a nondisplaced fracture had a significantly greater wrist flexion deficit ($p = 0.008$) and pinch strength deficit ($p = 0.020$) and a greater rate of CRPS ($p = 0.022$), but there was no difference in the CRPS rate at any other time point. At twenty-six weeks, there was a higher rate of complications ($p = 0.043$) and greater pain with use ($p = 0.045$) in the patients with a displaced fracture treated with vitamin C. There was no significant difference in the time to fracture-healing.

Conclusions.—This study demonstrated no significant difference at one year in the DASH score, other functional outcomes, the rate of CRPS, or osseous healing of nondisplaced or displaced distal radial fractures treated with vitamin C compared with placebo. We conclude that administration of vitamin C confers no benefit to patients with a displaced or nondisplaced fracture of the distal aspect of the radius.

Level of Evidence.—Therapeutic Level II. See Instructions for Authors for a complete description of levels of evidence.

▶ This is a prospective study of the effect of vitamin C on the outcome of 336 patients with an acute fracture of the distal radius. These patients were given either vitamin C or placebo daily for 50 days after the fracture. The outcomes were measured with the Disabilities of the Arm, Shoulder and Hand (DASH) score. DASH and secondary outcome variables included complications in finger and wrist range of motion, among others. Notably, the authors measured the incidence of complex regional pain syndrome (CRPS) as well. They definitively found that there is no effect of vitamin C treatment on either the DASH score or the rate of complex regional pain syndrome. Patients who were taking vitamin C also had a significantly greater wrist flexion deficit, pinch strength deficit, and rate of CRPS in the short term. There was no significant difference between the groups with regard to fracture healing.

The authors note the limitation that, although no differences were found, there may actually be a small difference in the time to fracture healing that they would be able to ascertain if they had more patients. The caveat to this is that if the study needs so many patients to illustrate a difference in time to fracture healing, the difference is actually probably quite small. What they do note is that the dietary vitamin C scores revealed no vitamin C deficits in their patients and that there was a complete absence of an effect of vitamin C supplementation on fracture healing in their study. They note that this could be related to the fact that vitamin C supplementation may be beneficial only in those who are vitamin C deficient.

The most notable result in this study is the fact that CRPS was not reduced in the vitamin C-treated population; in fact, there was significantly greater prevalence of CRPS at 6 weeks in the vitamin C group, and this in the nondisplaced fracture cohort. Yet all of this seems to evaporate by 1 year, rendering vitamin C a not very convincing adjuvant to the treatment of patients with distal radius fractures. Previous studies that found such a difference were based on telephone interviews and inquiry letters and included patients already on vitamin supplements. The overall importance of this finding may be related to vitamin C alone and yet may also be philosophical.

This study seems to underline the need for direct, well-thought-out, and well-executed studies to answer questions such as vitamin C supplementation. Some years ago when it was suggested that vitamin C might improve outcomes after distal radius fractures and other traumatic injuries, those of us involved with teaching trainees were confronted with results derived from incomplete studies governing how we should teach about and care for patients with distal radius fractures. When a study like this one debunks, or at least destabilizes, a theory previously believed to be fact, the cautions of overdetermining incomplete data in other aspects of our practice must be underlined. This study is therefore clinically relevant and excellently performed, as well as an example of how questions ought to be answered and how unanswered questions ought to be identified.

J. Elfar, MD

Percutaneous Distal Radius–Ulna Pinning of Distal Radius Fractures to Prevent Settling

Kim JY, Tae SK (Dongguk Univ College of Medicine, Ilsan, Goyang, Republic of Korea)

J Hand Surg Am 39:1921-1925, 2014

Purpose.—To evaluate the clinical and radiological outcomes of distal radius fractures treated by percutaneous fixation using distal radius–ulna pinning and to assess its effectiveness especially for preventing fracture settling.

Methods.—We retrospectively reviewed 18 distal radius fractures (15 AO type A2 and 3 AO type C1). Range of motion and Disabilities of the Arm, Shoulder, and Hand scores were evaluated. We measured radiographic parameters at the final follow-up and compared them with those on immediate postoperative x-rays.

Results.—All fractures united and average time to initial healing was 6.9 weeks (range, 6–7 wk). Average follow-up was 29 months (range, 26–43 mo). Average wrist flexion and extension were 70° and 65°, respectively. Average forearm supination and pronation were 82° and 83°, respectively. Average pain score was 1.2 and average Disabilities of the Arm, Shoulder, and Hand score was 13. Mean difference of ulnar variance, volar tilt, and radial inclination between immediate and final follow-up x-rays was 0.7 mm, 1°, and less than 1°, respectively.

Conclusions.—Percutaneous fixation of distal radius fractures using distal radius–ulna pinning had favorable radiologic and functional outcomes and was effective in preventing fracture settling during initial healing in unstable extra-articular fractures and some simple sagittal split intra-articular fractures.

Type of Study/Level of Evidence.—Therapeutic III.

► This article introduces a new twist to percutaneous pinning of extra-articular distal radius fractures that may be more effective in preventing postoperative settling. An advantage of this technique is the low cost of the implants. The construct used in this article appeared to be more rigid than crossed k-wires with orthogonal (dorsoulnar) pinning and more effective at preventing fracture site settling. Pin site infections and pin breakage were potential disadvantages.

The numbers of simple articular fractures (3) were not separated out and were too small to make any separate comparisons. There was no case control. The entrance criteria were not specified other than redisplaced fractures. Analysis of variance testing was not performed to control for effects of age and gender. The amount of preoperative displacement was not specified because treating minimally displaced fractures would introduce bias given that they may have also done well with nonsurgical treatment. There were no ranges or standard deviations for the Disabilities of the Arm, Shoulder, and Hand or pain score. A glaring omission was that there was no measurement of radial height, which is regarded as the most important parameter to restore because there can be significant settling despite maintenance of the radial inclination.[1-3] There was an average ulnar variance of 2.7 mm, which ranged as high as 4.8 mm. This indicates that there was a fair amount of subsidence, but the data on this are not presented. The actual wrist motion is not provided, only the averages. The authors compare their results to volar locking plates, but the cohorts are different. Pinning was likely used on simpler extra-articular fractures than those selected for plate fixation.

I personally reserve percutaneous pinning for fractures with marked displacement on the preinjury film because of the likelihood of late collapse or for redisplaced extra-articular fractures. If the patient is over 55 years and/or has comminution, I have followed the advice of Trumble et al[4] and used a bridging external fixation for 6 weeks in addition to adjuvant pinning to prevent collapse.

D. J. Slutsky, MD

References

1. Aro HT, Koivunen T. Minor axial shortening of the radius affects outcome of Colles' fracture treatment. *J Hand Surg Am.* 1991;16:392-398.
2. Fujii K, Henmi T, Kanematsu Y, Mishiro T, Sakai T, Terai T. Fractures of the distal end of radius in elderly patients: a comparative study of anatomical and functional results. *J Orthop Surg (Hong Kong).* 2002;10:9-15.
3. Goldfarb CA, Rudzki JR, Catalano LW, Hughes M, Borrelli J Jr. Fifteen-year outcome of displaced intra-articular fractures of the distal radius. *J Hand Surg Am.* 2006;31:633-639.
4. Trumble TE, Schmitt SR, Vedder NB. Factors affecting functional outcome of displaced intra-articular distal radius fractures. *J Hand Surg Am.* 1994;19:325-340.

Testing the Validity of Preventing Chronic Regional Pain Syndrome With Vitamin C After Distal Radius Fracture

Malay S, Chung KC (Univ of Michigan Health System, Ann Arbor)
J Hand Surg Am 39:2251-2257, 2014

Purpose.—The American Academy of Orthopaedic Surgeons recommends the use of vitamin C to prevent complex regional pain syndrome

(CRPS) for patients with distal radius fractures (DRFs). We hypothesized that the evidence for supporting this recommendation is weak, based on epidemiological principles of association and causality. The specific aim of this project was to test the validity of this recommendation.

Methods.—We conducted a literature review to retrieve articles reporting on the use of vitamin C to prevent CRPS. Data collected included sample size, study design type, dose of vitamin C used, and outcome measures of association expressed as relative risk (RR) and odds ratio. We then applied Hill criteria to evaluate the relationship between vitamin C and CRPS.

Results.—We obtained 225 articles from the database search. After the exclusion of duplicates, unrelated articles, editorial letters, and commentaries, we found 4 articles and 1 systematic review relevant to our topic. Six of the 9 Hill criteria were met, and an earlier meta-analysis showed a quantified reduction in CRPS risk. However, criteria like biological plausibility, specificity, and coherence were not met.

Conclusions.—The number of causal/association criteria met was adequate to support the scientific premise of the effect of vitamin C in preventing CRPS after DRF. Furthermore, vitamin C administration is of relatively low cost and has few complications unless administered in large doses. Owing to sufficient epidemiological evidence availability, the American Academy of Orthopaedic Surgeons recommendation of vitamin C to prevent CRPS has practical merit.

Type of Study/Level of Evidence.—Therapeutic II.

▶ This article is about systematic pooling of the data on vitamin C as a treatment to prevent complex regional pain syndrome (CRPS) after distal radius fracture. The authors hoped to be able to provide a thorough review of the existing literature using Hill's criteria of the strength of the evidence of the effect of vitamin C on CRPS for distal radius fractures. Hill's criteria are 9 conditions that support a causal effect of an intervention and its outcome. The authors found that the available vitamin C data met many of these criteria with the following 6 of the 9 criteria present: reproducibility in different settings, a dose—response relationship, and animal studies supporting vitamin C. The final recommendation of the authors was that the data supported current American Academy of Orthopaedic Surgeons guidelines. It will be interesting to see a rereview of the data with recent trials published by Ekrol that show no effect of vitamin C on CRPS.[1]

This study's methodology adds important depth to the information not found in a simple pooling of 1 outcome. This global view of how well an intervention works using these various metrics levels helps solidify its efficacy and support implementation.

C. Curtin, MD

Reference

1. Ekrol I, Duckworth AD, Ralston SH, Court-Brown CM, McQueen MM. The influence of vitamin C on the outcome of distal radial fractures a double-blind, randomized controlled trial. *J Bone Joint Surg Am.* 2014;96:1451-1459.

Readmissions after treatment of distal radius fractures

Curtin CM, Hernandez-Boussard T (Palo Alto Veterans Hosp, CA; Stanford Univ, Palo Alto, CA)

J Hand Surg Am 39:1926-1932, 2014

Purpose.—To assess the rates and associated diagnoses of readmissions for patients having received an intervention for treatment of distal radius fracture.

Methods.—We analyzed patient discharges from 2005–2011 for California, Florida, and New York. We used Agency for Healthcare Research and Quality data sets: (1) State Inpatient Database, (2) State Ambulatory Surgery Database, and (3) State Emergency Department Database. We examined inpatient, outpatient, and emergency room treatment locations. We identified patients by diagnosis code for distal radius fracture (813.41). Patients were stratified based on procedure codes for open reduction, closed reduction, and external fixation. The cohort was followed for 30 days to examine all-cause 30-day inpatient admissions and emergency department visits.

Results.—We identified 35,241 discharges with a primary diagnosis of distal radius facture. Of those, 18,388 patients underwent a procedure for their fracture, and 1,679 (9%) were readmitted within 30 days of discharge. Readmission rates varied by procedure type: internal fixation 8%, closed reduction 14%, and external fixation 11%. The most common diagnosis codes associated with readmission were general distal radius fracture codes (11%) and pain diagnoses (10%). Open procedures had higher odds of having a readmission associated with pain compared with closed treatment and external fixation.

Conclusions.—Readmissions after treatment of distal radius fracture care are common. Our results show many distal radius fracture patients return to the health care system for pain-related issues. As more emphasis is placed on quality health care delivery, implementation of better pain management will be important to health care providers and patients.

Clinical Relevance.—This study highlights that improved perioperative pain control may improve patient care and reduce readmissions.

► The authors present an observational study examining readmission rates and associated diagnoses for patients who received treatment for distal radius fractures. The investigators analyzed patient discharges from 2005 to 2011 for California, Florida, and New York. Findings concluded that, overall, 9% of patients were readmitted within 30 days after treatments including closed reduction, external fixation, or open reduction. There is a 20% readmission rate of all Medicare patients within 30 days after an inpatient stay. Pain was the primary reason for readmission after the distal radius fracture interventions in one-third of the patients analyzed and was at least 1 of the reasons for two-thirds of patients readmitted. The authors found that Medicare was the primary insurance for the greatest number of patients readmitted followed by private insurance, Medicaid, and self-pay. Overall, multivariate analysis illustrated that closed reduction and Medicaid insurance were associated with increased odds of any readmission.

In my practice, patients who undergo surgical intervention for their distal radius fractures typically receive regional anesthesia with an axillary nerve block. Patients who receive a closed reduction and splinting typically receive a hematoma block for pain control. I believe that patients do not understand the quality or quantity of pain associated with fracturing a bone to such a degree that would require manipulation or surgical intervention. A key factor in controlling patients' postprocedure or postoperative pain is setting their expectations appropriately and making sure they are aware of potential pain intensity and having a variety of pain control methods available to the patient if and when needed.

M. Kessler, MD

Outcomes and Cost of Care for Patients With Distal Radius Fractures

Farner S, Malkani A, Lau E, et al (Univ of Louisville, KY; Exponent, Inc, Menlo Park, CA; et al)

Orthopedics 37:e866-e878, 2014

This study was designed to evaluate treatment patterns in open treatment and percutaneous fixation of distal radius fractures, compare morbidity rates for the 2 types of treatment, and compare costs associated with the procedure and treatment of complications up to 1 year after surgery. From a 5% sample of nationwide Medicare claims records (1997-2009), patients with distal radius fractures were identified with *International Classification of Diseases, 9th revision, Clinical Modification* (ICD-9-CM), codes. Patients who underwent percutaneous fixation and open treatment were tracked with appropriate Current Procedural Terminology codes. Complications were identified at 3 and 12 months. Medicare charges and payments associated with the treatment groups were compiled from the claims data. The rate of surgical treatment increased from 44.7 to 82.0 surgeries per 100,000 persons (+83.0%) over the study period. A total of 9343 procedures met the inclusion criteria between 1998 and 2008. The proportion of open treatment procedures increased from 25.5% in 1998 to 73.4% in 2008. Percutaneous fixation was associated with lower adjusted risk of carpal tunnel syndrome and release and mononeuritis at 3 and 12 months. The percutaneous fixation group had lower adjusted risk of malunion/nonunion at 3 months and tendon rupture at 12 months. Average charges were lower in the percutaneous fixation group for the index operation as well as for treatment of morbidities at 3 and 12 months. The operative fixation rate for distal radius fractures in the Medicare population continues to rise, with a significant trend toward open fixation. Charges and payments associated with open treatment are significantly higher than those for percutaneous fixation.

► The authors give us a sense of the outcomes (including complications) and costs associated with the operative repair of distal radius fractures in the elderly population. Operative repair consisted of both percutaneous fixation and open procedures in this study. Given the sheer number of distal radius fractures in the elderly population, it was necessary to look at a 5% nationwide sample of this population. This study was retrospective and limited by the accuracy of the data they could obtain from the Medicare database, and specific information regarding the injury and treatment in each case was not available.

It is unclear from the many studies in the literature whether nonoperative vs operative treatment is preferred for distal radius fractures in the elderly, much less which surgical treatment modality (percutaneous fixation vs open treatment) is optimal. This study clearly showed an upswing in the operative and open treatment of distal radius fractures in this population during this period (1997-2009), and therefore an increase in the cost associated with these treatments, given the significant expenses associated with surgery and the hardware used (eg, volar plates). This study also noted an increase in the incidence of new carpal tunnel syndrome in the first postoperative year, the treatment of which has its own associated costs. With the increasingly large number of people in the Medicare population and the increasing trend of operative and open repair of distal radius fractures in this population, it is no surprise that the costs associated with these treatments will continue to rise.

I have also seen an increase in the number of distal radius fractures in this population in my practice, and unless there are significant comorbidities that would steer me toward closed and/or percutaneous fixation, my preference is to treat almost all of these fractures with operative and open fixation using a volar plate. With plate fixation, I have less worry of the fracture losing its initially acceptable alignment over the ensuing weeks postinjury, which might make the fracture more difficult to repair if nonoperative treatment is initially chosen, especially if the fracture is comminuted and/or the bone is osteopenic.

S. S. Shin, MD, MMSc

Early Changes in Bone Density, Microarchitecture, Bone Resorption, and Inflammation Predict the Clinical Outcome 12 Weeks After Conservatively Treated Distal Radius Fractures: An Exploratory Study

Meyer U, de Jong JJ, Bours SGP, et al (Maastricht Univ, The Netherlands; Maastricht Univ Med Ctr, The Netherlands; et al)
J Bone Miner Res 29:2065-2073, 2014

Fracture healing is an active process with early changes in bone and inflammation. We performed an exploratory study evaluating the association between early changes in densitometric, structural, biomechanical, and biochemical bone parameters during the first weeks of fracture healing and wrist-specific pain and disability at 12 weeks in postmenopausal women with a conservatively treated distal radius fracture. Eighteen patients (aged 64 ± 8 years) were evaluated at 1 to 2 and 3 to 4 weeks postfracture, using high-resolution peripheral quantitative computed tomography (HR-pQCT), micro-finite element analysis, serum procollagen type-I N-terminal propeptide (P1NP), carboxy-terminal telopeptide of type I collagen (ICTP), and high-sensitive C-reactive protein (hsCRP). After 12 weeks, patients rated their pain and disability using Patient Rated Wrist Evaluation (PRWE) questionnaire. Additionally, Quick Disability of the Arm Shoulder and Hand (QuickDASH) questionnaire and active wrist range of motion was evaluated. Linear regression models were used to study the relationship between changes in bone parameters and in hsCRP from visit 1 to 2 and PRWE score after 12 weeks. A lower PRWE outcome, indicating better outcome, was significantly related to an early increase in trabecular bone mineral density (BMD) (β −0.96 [95% CI −1.75 to −0.16], $R^2 = 0.37$), in torsional stiffness (−0.14 [−0.28 to −0.004], $R^2 = 0.31$), and to an early decrease in trabecular separation (209 [15 to 402], $R^2 = 0.33$) and in ICTP (12.1 [0.0 to 24.1], $R^2 = 0.34$). Similar results were found for QuickDASH. Higher total dorsal and palmar flexion range of motion was significantly related to early increase in hsCRP (9.62 [3.90 to 15.34], $R^2 = 0.52$). This exploratory study indicates that the assessment of early changes in trabecular BMD, trabecular separation, calculated torsional stiffness, bone resorption marker ICTP, and hsCRP after a distal radius fracture provides valuable information regarding the 12-week clinical outcome in terms of pain, disability, and range of motion and validates its use in studies on the process of early fracture healing.

▶ Finally! Here we have an article that correlates quantitative real-science parameters with patient-generated psychometric instruments. Objective truly meets subjective! This study outlines specific correlations using the highly sensitive (and accurate) high-resolution peripheral quantitative computed tomography (HR-pQCT) means of obtaining bone density and peripheral blood markers compared with common hand instruments of the Patient Rated Wrist Evaluation and QuickDASH. Better bone/bone healing yields better patient-perceived results, and they proved it!

I am excited about this study because not only is it well executed, but the authors also identify future steps to expand their approach into meaningful diagnostic and treatment measures. Although HR-pQCT is expensive, it provides superior quantitative and qualitative information of specific bone targeted areas, compared with the homogenous snapshot that comprises bone densitometry (which is lousy for the distal radius). The authors propose how the effect of vitamin D, calcium therapy, and other pharmacologic agents could be immediately measured to influence bone density and quality in fracture treatment. The expansion of this modality is promising for fractures throughout the body and for a variety of musculoskeletal conditions. I truly hope similar studies are in progress because our exhaustive foray into psychometric testing has begged for this type of robust evidence to make it all worthwhile.

A. Ladd, MD

The Impact of Coronal Alignment on Distal Radioulnar Joint Stability Following Distal Radius Fracture

Dy CJ, Jang E, Taylor SA, et al (Hosp for Special Surgery, NY)

J Hand Surg Am 39:1264-1272, 2014

Purpose.—Shift of the distal fragment of a distal radius fracture (DRF) in the coronal plane (coronal shift) may compromise the contributions of the distal oblique bundle (DOB) of the interosseous membrane to distal radioulnar joint (DRUJ) stability. The purpose of the study was to test our hypothesis that coronal shift of the distal fragment would increase dorsal-volar DRUJ displacement in response to applied load.

Methods.—A distal radius osteotomy was performed proximal to the sigmoid notch base and the ulnar styloid was cut (to simulate triangular fibrocartilage complex detachment) in 10 cadaveric specimens. A volarly placed plate was used to shift the distal radius fragment radially in 2-mm increments. A mechanical testing apparatus applied a 20 N load to the distal fragment perpendicular to the volar cortex with the forearm in neutral, 60° pronation, and 60° supination. Dorsal-volar displacement of the radius relative to the fixed ulna was measured in the control state (DRF and ulnar styloid anatomically fixed) and in 3 positions (anatomical reduction, 2-mm coronal shift, 4-mm coronal shift) with ulnar styloid displacement. The specimens were dissected post hoc to evaluate for a distinct DOB (thickness, > 0.5 mm). Dorsal-volar DRUJ displacement was compared among testing and control states using analysis of variance.

Results.—In specimens with a distinct DOB, 2-mm coronal shift significantly increased dorsal-volar DRUJ displacement. However, there was no difference in DRUJ displacement between 4-mm coronal shift and control state. Coronal shift did not affect dorsal-volar DRUJ displacement in specimens without a distinct DOB.

Conclusions.—In the setting of an ulnar styloid fracture, a 2-mm (but not a 4-mm) coronal shift of the DRF is associated with increased dorsal-volar DRUJ displacement in specimens with a distinct DOB, but not in specimens without a distinct DOB.

Clinical Relevance.—Awareness of the importance of coronal shift may aid in prevention of DRUJ instability associated with DRF, especially in patients with a DOB.

▶ The triangular fibrocartilage, complex along with the deep radioulnar ligament (RUL), is the primary stabilizer of the distal radioulnar joint (DRUJ).[1] The distal interosseous membrane (DIOM) is a secondary stabilizer of the DRUJ.[2] Ulnar translation of the proximal radial shaft has the potential to cause DRUJ instability if the deep RUL is also injured by detensioning of the DIOM.[3] The dorsal oblique bundle (DOB) is an inconstant thick fiber bundle within the DIOM that may provide additional DRUJ stability.[4]

The authors' data indicate that a slight coronal shift should alert the surgeon to the risk of DRUJ instability and the benefit of correcting this when a DOB is present.

There is no reliable, noninvasive method to determine which patients have a DOB. The deep RUL was not directly visualized to determine whether it was actually detached by the ulnar styloid osteotomy and did not directly verify that tensioning the DOB occurred. If the DOB is detensioned at 2 mm, this effect should be even more pronounced with 4 mm of coronal shift, but this was not seen. Conversely, others have demonstrated that a 5-mm coronal shift resulted in a bidirectional DRUJ instability when the deep RUL was disrupted.[2]

With distal radius fractures, DRUJ instability with an associated disruption of the deep RUL can be stabilized by anatomic fixation of the DRF fracture without directly repairing the deep RUL. Correction of ulnar translation of the radial shaft restores the DIOM tension, which subsequently holds the ulnar head firmly in the concavity of the sigmoid notch.[5] It is important to recognize the function of the DIOM with injuries in which DRUJ instability accompanies distal radius fractures.

In my experience, DRUJ instability from the disruption of the deep RUL may be the primary cause that leads to a coronal shift, rather than vice versa. I have treated a patient with a DRF in which the radial translation could not be corrected until the deep RUL was reattached by internal fixation of a basilar ulnar styloid fracture. This concept has been verified by Nakamura et al.[6]

D. J. Slutsky, MD

References

1. Watanabe H, Berger RA, Berglund LJ, Zobitz ME, An KN. Contribution of the interosseous membrane to distal radioulnar joint constraint. *J Hand Surg Am.* 2005;30:1164-1171.
2. Moritomo H, Noda K, Goto A, Murase T, Yoshikawa H, Sugamoto K. Interosseous membrane of the forearm: length change of ligaments during forearm rotation. *J Hand Surg Am.* 2009;34:685-691.
3. Ross M. Volar angle stable plating for distal radius fractures. In: Slutsky DJ, ed. *Principles and Practice of Wrist Surgery.* Philadelphia, PA: Saunders; 2010:133-136.
4. Kitamura T, Moritomo H, Arimitsu S, et al. The biomechanical effect of the distal interosseous membrane on distal radioulnar joint stability: a preliminary anatomic study. *J Hand Surg Am.* 2011;36:1626-1630.
5. Moritomo H, Omori S. Influence of ulnar translation of the radial shaft in distal radius fracture on distal radioulnar joint instability. *J Wrist Surg.* 2014;3:18-21.
6. Nakamura T, Iwamoto T, Matsumura N, Sato K, Toyama Y. Radiographic and arthroscopic assessment of DRUJ instability due to foveal avulsion of the radioulnar ligament in distal radius fractures. *J Wrist Surg.* 2014;3:12-17.

Therapist supervised clinic-based therapy versus instruction in a home program following distal radius fracture: A systematic review

Valdes K, Naughton N, Michlovitz S (Rocky Mountain Univ of Health Professions, Provo, UT; Professional Orthopedics Associates, Scranton, PA; Cayuga Hand Therapy PT, Ithaca, NY; et al)

J Hand Ther 27:165-174, 2014

Purpose.—The primary purpose of this systematic review is to determine the effectiveness of a home program or a structured therapy program for patients following distal radius fracture.

Methods.—A search was performed using terms wrist fracture, supervised therapy, occupational therapy, physical therapy, splint, orthosis, distal radius fracture, exercise, and home program. Studies that met the inclusion criteria were evaluated for research quality using The Structured Effectiveness for Quality Evaluation of Study (SEQES).

Results.—Five of the seven trials found no difference between outcomes for their subjects that had uncomplicated distal radius fractures. The population that has complications following distal radius fractures was not represented in the studies reviewed.

Conclusion.—The available evidence from randomized controlled trials is insufficient to support a home program or therapist supervised clinic-based program as a superior method of treatment for adults following a distal radius fracture without complications or the presence of comorbidities.

▶ This systematic review tackles one of the current hot topics in hand therapy and hand surgery. How effective is a structured therapy program vs a home program in post–distal radius fracture management? From a pool of 383 articles, the authors worked to identify 7 articles that met their criteria for review. Of these, 4 studies compared supervised therapy in a clinic, including a home program to a therapist instructed home exercise program (HEP). Three studies compared supervised therapy in the clinic with a HEP to a HEP with instruction provided by the physician.

It is not surprising that all the subjects included in these studies made significant clinical gains in all outcomes measured. The authors listed all variances noted in outcomes in the studies, with no clear advantage to one program over the other. They also noted design flaws in the reviewed studies that may change the clinical significance of these outcomes.

The secondary purpose of this article was to access whether the studies reviewed accurately represented the patient population post–distal radius fracture. Because the inclusion criteria often excludes those patients with comorbidities and complexities that require more care, the need for supervised therapy may not be fully accounted for. Indeed, the current studies do not reflect the complete patient population, so the conclusion that supervised therapy and a well-instructed HEP provide the same results should be questioned. The authors do an excellent job outlining the complications that warrant therapy in the clinic as well as the need for further studies.

It is my bias that all patients post–distal radius fracture should be referred to hand therapy. The hand therapist can then provide both supervised therapy and a well-designed home program. If the patient progresses well, he or she can be discharged to home management. If complications are present, the patient is already enrolled in an established therapy program that can be continued until the best possible outcomes are met.

S. J. Clark, OTR/L, CHT

Intraoperative evaluation of dorsal screw prominence after polyaxial volar plate fixation of distal radius fractures utilizing the Hoya view: a cadaveric study

Dolce D, Goodwin D, Ludwig M, et al (Georgetown Univ Hosp, Washington, DC; et al)
Hand 9:511-515, 2014

Background.—The irregular nature of the dorsal surface of the distal radius makes it difficult to detect prominent screws with volar plate fixation for distal radius fractures using standard fluoroscopic images. This study evaluates the accuracy of a new radiographic method, the Hoya view, for the assessment of dorsal cortical screw penetration with volar plate fixation.

Methods.—Eight cadaveric upper extremities underwent application of a volar distal radius plate with polyaxial locking screws placed distally. Utilizing a mini C-arm, lateral and Hoya views were obtained with notation of any dorsal cortical screw prominence. Dissection of the cadavers was then performed for direct visualization of screw prominence. The screws were then exchanged sequentially for screws 2-mm longer than their initial measurements with repeated imaging and direct visualization.

Results.—The Hoya view revealed that 9.4% of the screws penetrated the dorsal cortex with an average screw prominence of 1.08 mm (range 0.5–2 mm). None of the six prominent screws were detected with lateral views. With the Hoya view, six of six prominent screws were identified. With locking screws exchanged for screws 2-mm longer, 76.6% of the screws had violated the dorsal cortex; of these, 24.5% were detected with lateral imaging versus 100% with the Hoya view.

Conclusions.—This study supports the intraoperative use of the Hoya view to evaluate screw length and dorsal cortical screw penetration in volar plate fixation of distal radius fractures. However, this view may be difficult to obtain in patients with limitations in elbow or shoulder range of motion.

▶ This article describes a novel radiographic view of the distal radius that can assess for dorsal cortical screw penetration with volar plate fixation. This was a well-performed cadaveric study; however, one weakness is that the authors drilled bicortically yet used only locking screws for their fixation. It is well known that bicortical drilling is not necessary for locking screw fixation, and this is indeed one of the benefits of using unicortical-abutting locking screws. Surgeons who repair distal radius fractures with a volar plate are always concerned about dorsal screw penetration, with its inherent risks (eg, tendon irritation/rupture, intraarticular screw penetration, and nerve injury). With this additional view, these risks can be decreased.

Like many other surgeons, volar plate fixation is an important part of my armamentarium in the treatment of distal radius fractures. I try to be as diligent as I can to avoid dorsal cortical screw penetration. To this end, once I have achieved satisfactory reduction of the fracture (ie, apposition of the plate with the volar cortex of the distal radius using the minimum number of cortical screws), I proceed to use unicortical locking screws for the remaining distal holes. Although I was unfamiliar with the Hoya view and am unsure of its practical utility, it is at least another tool for the surgeon who is concerned about the distal screws being too long.

S. S. Shin, MD, MMSc

Ultrasound-Assisted Closed Reduction of Distal Radius Fractures

Kodama N, Takemura Y, Ueba H, et al (Shiga Univ of Med Science, Otsu, Japan)

J Hand Surg Am 39:1287-1294, 2014

Purpose.—To assess the accuracy and ability of ultrasound for monitoring closed reduction for distal radius fractures.

Methods.—Consecutive patients undergoing ultrasound-guided closed reduction of acute, displaced distal radius fractures between January 2003 and December 2006 at our department were enrolled. The control group was extracted from patients who underwent a closed reduction for similar fractures under fluoroscopy or without any imaging assistance. To confirm the accuracy of the ultrasonography measurements, displacement distance values were compared with those on radiographic imaging before and after reduction. X-ray parameters for pre- and postreduction, reduction time, total cost, and success rate were compared between the ultrasound-guided and the control groups.

Results.—The ultrasound-guided group consisted of 43 patients (mean age, 68 y) and the control group consisted of 57 patients, which included 35 patients (mean age, 74 y) with fluoroscopic reduction and of 22 patients (mean age, 72 y) with reduction unaided by imaging. There were no significant displacement differences between radiographic and ultrasound measurements. In x-ray parameters for pre- and postreduction, there were no significant differences between the 2 groups. Ultrasound-guided reduction took longer than the other 2 methods. The success rate of the ultrasound and the fluoroscopic groups were similar (95% and 94%, respectively).

Conclusions.—Our data suggest that ultrasound assistance can aid reduction of distal radius fractures as well as fluoroscopy.

Type of Study/Level of Evidence.—Therapeutic II.

▶ The authors present a well-designed study comparing a prospective cohort of patients who underwent closed reduction of distal radius fractures using ultrasound guidance with a retrospective cohort of patients who underwent closed reduction of distal radius fractures using fluoroscopic guidance or blind manipulation. Currently, fluoroscopically assisted reduction or blind manipulation are the most common methods of reducing distal radius fractures around the world. The authors suggest that because ultrasound uses no radiation and is less expensive to purchase than a fluoroscopy machine, there may be a utility for this technique where access to fluoroscopic technology is limited. The authors note that interpreting the ultrasound images before, during, and after reduction requires training and experience. Also, ultrasound is limited in visualizing the articular surface and may sometimes show good alignment of the bony cortices when the distal and proximal cortices overlap. The authors were unable to show a significant difference in adequacy of reduction comparing the 3 methods of reduction.

In my practice, with limited experience using ultrasound, I perform closed reductions of distal radius fractures with fluoroscopic guidance. The mini-fluoroscopy units have been shown not to require lead aprons for protection and provide clear visualization of the cortices and articular surface. This also limits reduction attempts and pain experienced by the patient. Ultrasound guided reduction of distal radius fractures may become a more frequently used technique in the future if orthopedists and emergency room physicians are appropriately trained in the procedure and feel that they can obtain an equal reduction to that achieved with fluoroscopic guidance or blind manipulation.

M. Kessler, MD

Malpractice in Distal Radius Fracture Management: An Analysis of Closed Claims

DeNoble PH, Marshall AC, Barron OA, et al (St. Luke's-Roosevelt Hosp, NY)
J Hand Surg Am 39:1480-1488, 2014

Purpose.—Distal radius fractures comprise the majority of hand- and wrist-related malpractice claims. We hypothesized that a majority of lawsuits would be for malunions resulting from nonsurgical treatment. Additional goals of this study were to quantify costs associated with claims, determine independent risk factors for making an indemnity payment, and illustrate trends over time.

Methods.—Seventy closed malpractice claims filed for alleged negligent treatment of distal radius fractures by orthopedic surgeons insured by the largest medical professional liability insurer in New York State (NYS) from 1981 to 2005 were reviewed. We separately reviewed defendants' personal closed malpractice claim histories from 1975 to 2011. Overall incidence of malpractice claims among distal radius fractures treated in NYS was calculated using the NYS Statewide Planning and Research Cooperative System database and the 2008 American Academy of Orthopedic Surgeons census data.

Results.—The overall incidence of malpractice claims for distal radius fracture management was low. Malunion was the most common complaint across claims regardless of treatment type. Claims for surgically treated fractures increased over time. A majority of claims documented poor doctor-patient relationships. Male plaintiffs in this group were significantly older than males treated for distal radius fractures in NYS. Most defendants had a history of multiple malpractice suits, all were male, and only a small percentage were fellowship-trained in hand surgery.

Defendants lacking American Board of Orthopedic Surgery certification were significantly more likely to make indemnity payments. Thirty-eight of 70 cases resulted in an indemnity payment.

Conclusions.—Malunion and poor doctor-patient relationships are the major features of malpractice litigation involving distal radius fracture management. Older defendant age and lack of American Board of Orthopedic Surgery certification increase the likelihood of making an indemnity payment.

Type of Study/Level of Evidence.—Economic and decision analyses II.

▶ This study analyzed 70 closed malpractice claims for alleged negligent treatment of distal radius fractures by orthopedic surgeons in New York State insured by the largest medical professional liability insurer. Malunion was the most common complaint, with 80% of the claims noted in those treated nonoperatively. In those treated surgically, claims resulted from either a loss of reduction or failure to restore alignment during the initial procedure. Of the 70 claims, 38 resulted in indemnity payments with 35 claims "settled" and 3 guilty verdicts. Thirty-two claims were dismissed, discontinued, successfully defended, or the defendant was separated from the suit. Absence of American Board of Orthopaedic Surgery certification was a significant factor in the likelihood of making an indemnity payment. The authors also report that "strained doctor-patient relationships" were a common feature and were identified in 51 of 70 (73%).

The study is interesting, and of note is that of the 70 claims, only 4 were against hand surgeons, whereas the remaining 66 were against general orthopedic surgeons. A breakdown in the doctor-patient relationship continues to be identified as a significant factor in those individuals that file malpractice suits. For me, at times it continues to be challenging when considering operative vs nonoperative treatment, particularly in the elderly with a displaced and comminuted distal radius fracture. Deciding who is truly "low demand" and will tolerate a malunion remains problematic. This often requires a lengthy conversation, including family members, if possible. Accurate documentation, particularly if one opts for nonoperative treatment in the setting of significant displacement, is critical. Frequent follow-up in this setting is also vital and often identifies a patient who has a change of heart and subsequently opts for surgical treatment in the setting of a nascent malunion.

D. Zelouf, MD

Radiographic Scoring System to Evaluate Union of Distal Radius Fractures

Patel SP, Anthony SG, Zurakowski D, et al (Harvard Med School, Boston, MA; Boston Children's Hosp, Boston, MA)

J Hand Surg Am 39:1471-1479, 2014

Purpose.—To evaluate the intra- and interobserver reliability of a scoring system for distal radius fracture union based on specific radiographic parameters obtainable from x-rays.

Methods.—Two sets of 35 anteroposterior and lateral x-rays were obtained by retrospective review of consecutive patients with distal radius fractures (AO types A and C) treated by a single surgeon in 2009. One set was assembled for those patients treated nonsurgically and 1 set for those treated with open reduction and internal fixation (ORIF) with volar plating. Radius union scoring system (RUSS) scores were compiled from a 5-person review panel consisting of hand surgeons and musculoskeletal radiologists. Union of each of the 4 cortices was graded on a 3-point scale (0, fracture line visible with no callus; 1, callus formation but fracture line present; 2, cortical bridging without clear fracture line). Reviewers also recorded their overall impression of fracture union (united or not united). Each set of radiographs was reviewed twice by the 5 reviewers, 2 weeks apart. Inter- and intraobserver reliability were determined using intraclass correlation coefficients.

Results.—For nonsurgically treated fractures, substantial agreement in union scores was found with regard to both intra- and interobserver reliability. For fractures treated with ORIF, substantial agreement was found in union scores with regard to intraobserver reliability and moderate agreement with regard to interobserver reliability. In addition, when using the reviewers' overall assessment of union as a reference standard, RUSS had a statistically significant predictive value in being able to differentiate between united and not united fractures.

Conclusions.—This radiographic union tool demonstrated substantial intra- and interobserver reliability for the determination of fracture union in the distal radius. The RUSS is a simple method for a standardized assessment of radiographic union of DRF treated nonsurgically or with ORIF.

Type of Study/Level of Evidence.—Economic/decision analysis IV.

▶ The authors propose a radiographic scoring system to assess union of distal radius fractures and demonstrated substantial intra- and interobserver reliability for both nonsurgically and surgically treated fractures. Like other scoring systems widely used to assess union in the tibia and hip, the Radius Union Scoring System (RUSS) has the advantage of focusing on cortical bridging with callus as demonstrated on standard x-rays, thus being less expensive and readily available for routine use in the clinic.

However, because it only takes into account radiographic criteria, further studies are required to correlate RUSS scores to clinically relevant information such as bone strength and possibility of load bearing, which would represent the most interesting field of application for such an easy and reliable tool.

A. Atzei, MD

7 Elbow: Trauma

Surgical Treatment of Posterolateral Rotatory Instability of the Elbow

Anakwenze OA, Kwon D, O'Donnell E, et al (Kaiser Permanente, San Diego, CA; Columbia Univ, NY)

Arthroscopy 30:866-871, 2014

Purpose.—The purpose of this systematic review was to critically examine the outcomes of lateral ulnar collateral ligament reconstruction for posterolateral rotatory instability (PLRI) of the elbow.

Methods.—A systematic review of the literature was performed. Two reviewers assessed and confirmed the methodologic and patient data from the included studies. Frequency-weighted means were calculated for outcomes that were present in multiple studies.

Results.—Eight studies fulfilled our criteria, and they included 130 patients. The mean age was 38.1 years, and the mean follow-up period was 44.5 months. Traumatic dislocation was the most common cause of PLRI. Of the studies that reported the Mayo Elbow Performance Score, 91% of patients had good or excellent results, with a frequency-weighted mean of 91. Improvement in elbow range of motion was noted (133° to 138° of flexion [$P < .0001$] and 6.6° to 3.9° of extension [$P = .005$]). A complication rate of 11% was noted, with recurrent instability noted to occur in 8% of patients.

Conclusions.—PLRI of the elbow remains to be fully understood. Treatment strategies vary and should be performed based on surgeon experience and evidence available. Most patients will have good or excellent results after surgery; however, up to 11% of patients may have complications.

Level of Evidence.—Level IV, systematic review of Level II through IV studies.

► A review of more than 2000 studies yielded 130 patients with surgically treated posterolateral rotatory instability from 8 usable publications. The reviewed group did not include patients that had concomitant surgery or fractures, such that it was relatively homogeneous.

Multiple different reconstructions of the lateral collateral ligament were performed. Half of the patients in whom graft selection could be determined had a triceps fascial graft, which was surprising to this reviewer.

Only 3 of the studies used outcome scoring. Of those 47 patients, scores of more than 90% were good and excellent, with less than 10% fair, and no poor ratings in the Mayo Elbow Performance Score. The overall failure rate of 8% was not broken down by graft type. Seven of the 8 studies listed complication data and 6 patients had recurrent instability. The overall failure rate of 8% was not broken down by graft type.

R. Papandrea, MD

Reduction of Pulled Elbow

Aylor M, Anderson JM, Vanderford P, et al (Oregon Health and Science Univ, Portland)
N Engl J Med 371:e32.1-e32.3, 2014

Background.—Annular ligament displacement or radial-head subluxation (pulled elbow) occurs often in children, with 2.7 per 1000 emergency room visits by persons under age 18 years in the United States involving this injury. Median age when it occurs is 2 years, reflecting the anatomy of the radial head at this age that allows it to become displaced. Diagnosis and treatment of pulled elbow were discussed.

Diagnosis.—A careful history may reveal the forceful traction often associated with this injury. Pulled elbow occurs when the child is pulled or lifted by the arm, which pulls the radial head under the annular ligament and traps the ligament at the level of the radiocapitellar joint. On physical examination the child will hold the elbow in a slightly flexed position with the hand pronated. Pseudoparalysis is common, as are pain with movement (usually pronation and supination), tenderness to palpation on the lateral side of the elbow, and a normal-appearing elbow with no effusion, bruising, or obvious deformity. Radiographs are usually normal and should be reserved for patients with equivocal signs. Often positioning the elbow for radiographs can be therapeutic in reducing the displacement. If the history or examination indicates fracture, radiographs should be obtained and any attempt at reduction postponed until the results are available. Reduction is not attempted if other abnormalities are present; further evaluation should be conducted.

Treatment Options and Follow-up.—Reduction is the treatment for pulled elbow and it requires no equipment other than clean hands. Caregivers should be advised that the child will experience some discomfort for several minutes after the reduction is performed.

The two techniques for reduction are supination and hyperpronation. For the supination technique, the child is seated on the caregiver's lap facing the examiner. Both the hand and elbow of the arm are grasped, with the fingers or thumb overlying the radial head, although these positions are not critical to the procedure's success. The forearm is supinated and flexed until the ligament moves into position, which is often accompanied by a click. Children are generally pain free and able to move normally in 5 to 30 minutes. For the hyperpronation technique, the child is again positioned on the caregiver's lap and facing the examiner. The child's hand is clasped as for a handshake, with the examiner's other hand supporting the patient's elbow. The wrist is hyperpronated until the ligament returns to position, often accompanied by a click. The child's pain and movement should be normal in 5 to 30 minutes.

Usually a single attempt is successful, but if it is not, the technique can be repeated or the alternate method used. If three or four attempts are made without success, a radiograph is indicated. The elbow is then splinted at an angle of about 90 degrees and the child referred to an orthopedic surgeon. The period of immobilization may resolve the problem.

Caregivers should be cautioned that the pulled elbow may recur and advised about how to minimize recurrence by avoiding pulling, lifting, or swinging the child by the arms. Family members may also be instructed in how to reduce the pulled elbow at home.

Conclusions.—Reducing a pulled elbow is simple and relatively uncomplicated.

▶ This video provides a nice overview of the common orthopedic condition known as nursemaid's elbow. The diagrams and explanations are simple and well presented. Although this information is unlikely to affect orthopedic practices, this is an excellent way to educate our colleagues in pediatrics and the emergency department. Videos such as these will assist in providing timely and appropriate care to patients in a more cost-effective manner. I think this is an example of how the hand and upper extremity community could work to educate our medical colleagues and improve patient care.

E. Lawler, MD

Hinged external fixation for complex fracture-dislocation of the elbow in elderly people

Maniscalco P, Pizzoli AL, Renzi Brivio L, et al (Guglielmo da Saliceto Hosp, Piacenza, Italy; C. Poma Hosp, Mantua, Italy)

Injury 45:S53-S57, 2014

The authors report their experience of treating complex elbow fracture-dislocations in elderly people, using a minimally-invasive approach with a new articulated external fixator that is associated with minimal internal fixation. The clinical results for 19 patients are presented according to outcome factors, such as range of motion, pain and function, rate and type of complications, and reoperation rate. The results indicate that this treatment strategy should be considered as a good alternative to other treatment options reported in the literature, including conservative treatment, ORIF with angular stable plates and total elbow arthroplasty.

▶ Complex elbow fracture dislocations can be difficult to treat in the best of circumstances, let alone in the elderly. Current treatment options include open reduction internal fixation, total elbow arthroplasty, ligament reconstruction, or a combination thereof. The current study is a case series of 19 patients treated with a hinged elbow external fixator with combined minimal fixation for complex elbow fracture dislocations. As with any case series, the main weaknesses of the study include the small number of patients, lack of a control group, lack of patient-reported outcomes, and relatively short follow-up period. This last factor is especially important because of the need to evaluate these patients for possible conversion to total elbow arthroplasty.

However, the study presents an intriguing option to conventional methods for treatment of a difficult problem. Although a generalization, most physicians choose not to use a hinged elbow external fixator secondary to the difficulty of application when trying to find the elbow axis of rotation. The authors of the article do not address how the axis of the elbow was decided in patients with comminuted fractures. For the commentator, this is the most important step in the use of any hinged external fixator, and one would have expected a detailed explanation in the article. For the fixation method to become mainstream, it must be easily reproducible for the average orthopedic surgeon.

The results were impressive, with the average time of fixation being 7 weeks (range 6–12 weeks), the average range of motion obtained with the fixator ranged between 20 and 118 degrees and was improved at follow-up (3–120 degrees); the average prono-supination ranged from 72 degrees to 73 degrees. Although interesting, the article also does not discuss the options of using a static fixator to stabilize these elbows.

M. B. Gottschalk, MD
J. T. Capo, MD

Long-Term Outcomes of Isolated Stable Radial Head Fractures

Duckworth AD, Wickramasinghe NR, Clement ND, et al (Royal Infirmary of Edinburgh, Scotland)

J Bone Joint Surg Am 96:1716-1723, 2014

Background.—There is evidence to support primary nonoperative management of isolated stable fractures of the radial head, although minimal data exist regarding long-term outcomes. The aim of this study was to report subjective long-term outcomes of isolated stable fractures of the radial head and neck following primary nonoperative management.

Methods.—From a prospective database of proximal radial fractures, we identified all skeletally mature patients who sustained an isolated stable Mason type-1 or type-2 fracture of the radial head or neck during an eighteen-month period. Inclusion criteria were a confirmed isolated stable fracture of the proximal aspect of the radius, primarily managed nonoperatively. The primary long-term outcome measure was the Disabilities of the Arm, Shoulder and Hand (DASH) score.

Results.—The study cohort comprised 100 patients with a mean age of forty-six years (range, seventeen to seventy-nine years). A fall from a standing height accounted for 69% of all injuries. Thirty-five percent of the patients had one or more comorbidities. There were fifty-seven Mason type-1 fractures and forty-three Mason type-2 fractures. At a mean of ten years post injury (range, 8.8 to 10.2 years), the mean DASH score was 5.8 (range, 0 to 67.2) and the mean Oxford Elbow Score (OES) was 46 (range, 14 to

48). Fourteen (14%) of the patients reported stiffness and twenty-four (24%) reported some degree of pain. A worse DASH score was associated with older age ($p = 0.002$), one or more comorbidities ($p = 0.008$), increasing socioeconomic deprivation by Index of Multiple Deprivation quintile ($p = 0.026$), increasing amount of fracture displacement ($p = 0.041$), and involvement in compensation proceedings ($p = 0.006$).

Conclusions.—Long-term patient-reported outcomes were excellent following the nonoperative management of isolated stable fractures of the radial head or neck. We suggest that routine primary nonoperative management of these fractures provides a satisfactory outcome for the majority of patients, with few patients in our study requiring further intervention for persisting complaints.

Level of Evidence.—Therapeutic Level IV. See Instructions for Authors for a complete description of levels of evidence.

► This is the largest series in the literature documenting subjective, long-term patient outcomes after primary nonoperative intervention for an isolated stable fracture (Mason Type 1 and 2) of the radial head. Their data further confirm what has been previously published in other studies: that conservative management of this injury is a reliable treatment option, yielding an excellent or good long-term result in the majority of cases. Despite a small number of patients reporting persistent pain and stiffness, patient satisfaction was high (92% were satisfied with their long-term outcome). Two percent of patients in this series required additional surgery. Persistent elbow stiffness was found in 14% of patients. Median time to return to work was 2 weeks, and median time for return to sports was 6 weeks. Exceptions to nonoperative management of Mason Type 2 fractures are fractures with a clinically relevant associated injury pattern and/or elbow or forearm instability and high-energy injuries, which may be part of a complex injury pattern. Increasing fracture displacement was the only injury characteristic that was predictive of long-term outcome, potentially suggesting that above a certain degree of displacement, surgery might be indicated. However, no firm conclusions could be drawn from these findings because of the small sample size and the inevitable degree of intraobserver and interobserver variability associated with measuring fracture displacement. The authors reiterate that the absolute indications for operative intervention is crepitus on forearm rotation or an established block to forearm rotation.

E. Cheung, MD

Is ORIF Superior to Nonoperative Treatment in Isolated Displaced Partial Articular Fractures of the Radial Head?

Yoon A, King GJW, Grewal R (North Shore Hosp, Auckland, New Zealand; St Joseph's Health Care London, Ontario, Canada)
Clin Orthop Relat Res 472:2105-2112, 2014

Background.—While good results have been reported with both nonoperative and operative treatment of isolated displaced partial radial head fractures, there remains considerable disagreement about the role of surgery in the management of these injuries.

Questions/Purposes.—We (1) compared isolated displaced partial articular radial head fractures treated nonoperatively with open reduction internal fixation (ORIF) in terms of validated outcomes scores, ROM, and strength; (2) assessed whether there were any predictor variables for outcomes; and (3) compared complications between groups.

Methods.—We retrospectively compared patients with isolated partial articular radial head fractures displaced greater than 2 mm but less than 5 mm who received either nonoperative treatment (30 patients) or ORIF (30 patients). We reviewed the nonoperative and ORIF groups at a mean of 3 and 4.5 years, respectively. The nonoperative and ORIF groups were similar except for age (51 ± 17 years versus 39 ± 10 years, respectively) and fracture displacement (2.3 ± 0.3 mm versus 2.8 ± 0.6 mm, respectively). As there were no definitive guidelines on which treatment represented best management, treatment type was decided by the attending surgeon in conjunction with the patient on a case-by-case basis. Patients were evaluated using the Patient-rated Elbow Evaluation (PREE) (primary outcome measure), Mayo Elbow Performance Score (MEPS), QuickDASH, SF-12, clinical examination, and radiographic evaluation (14 and 28 in the nonoperative and ORIF groups, respectively). Elbow ROM was assessed with a goniometer and hand grip strength with calibrated strength testing. We assessed possible predictive variables (age, displacement, energy of injury) for clinical outcome scores and recorded complications.

Results.—PREE scores were not different between groups, but the MEPS favored the nonoperative group (93 versus 86; $p = 0.012$). ROM and grip strength were similar between groups. Younger age was associated with worse outcome, but displacement and energy were not. More complications occurred in the ORIF group (eight cases of mild heterotopic ossification, two cases of hardware failure) than in the nonoperative group (one case of mild heterotopic ossification, one case of complex regional pain syndrome).

Conclusions.—No clinical benefit with ORIF could be found compared to nonoperative management of isolated partial articular radial head fractures with displacement of greater than 2 mm but less than 5 mm at short-term followup. A well-designed randomized trial and followup at longer term are required to provide better information about how to treat these common fractures.

Level of Evidence.—Level III, therapeutic study. See Instructions for Authors for a complete description of levels of evidence.

▶ There is paucity in the literature directly comparing open reduction internal fixation (ORIF) vs conservative treatment for isolated Mason type II radial head fractures. This study contains a relatively large number of cases. Patient age of 60 years or more was found to be an independent predictor of better outcome. Fracture displacement and the amount of energy involved in the injury were not found to be independent predictors. Weaknesses of the study include the fact that it is a nonrandomized review with inherent selection bias and that the 2 groups had significant differences in terms of age, fracture displacement, and length of follow-up. Lower patient age or a larger displacement of fracture would influence management toward operative intervention, and we accept that these variables could affect outcomes. The longer-term follow-up in the ORIF group may be a confounder because time may reveal problems that are not obvious early on. Additionally, there were insufficient numbers of long-term follow-up radiographs for a meaningful comparative analysis of radial head morphology and presence of arthritis between the 2 groups, and the more significant limitation of long-term radiographic follow-up in the nonoperative group compared with the ORIF group means the rate of heterotopic ossification in the nonoperative group may be relatively underreported. In conclusion, there was no clinically significant difference in outcomes, range of motion, or strength between patients treated nonoperatively and those treated with ORIF for isolated displaced partial articular radial head fractures. Younger patients fared worse, and the ORIF group had more complications. Although no benefit to ORIF over nonoperative treatment could be found in this study, it should be well noted that the 2 groups were different with respect to age, and this was found to be an independent predictor of outcome. The authors suggest that a randomized controlled trial with long-term follow-up will reduce the bias encountered in this study and may provide further guidelines as to the optimal management of these fractures. Because this was a retrospective comparison, the presence or absence of a mechanical block to rotation influencing the choice of treatment was not considered in this study, and it should be noted that, in treating an isolated displaced partial articular radial head fracture, the presence of a mechanical block to rotation remains an absolute indication for surgical intervention.

E. Cheung, MD

The treatment of the acute Essex-Lopresti injury

Grassmann JP, Hakimi M, Gehrmann SV, et al (Univ Hosp Duesseldorf, Germany)
Bone Joint J 96-B:1385-1391, 2014

The Essex-Lopresti injury (ELI) of the forearm is a rare and serious condition which is often overlooked, leading to a poor outcome.

The purpose of this retrospective case study was to establish whether early surgery can give good medium-term results.

From a group of 295 patients with a fracture of the radial head, 12 patients were diagnosed with ELI on MRI which confirmed injury to the interosseous membrane (IOM) and ligament (IOL). They were treated by reduction and temporary Kirschner (K)-wire stabilisation of the distal radioulnar joint (DRUJ). In addition, eight patients had a radial head replacement, and two a radial head reconstruction.

All patients were examined clinically and radiologically 59 months (25 to 90) after surgery when the mean Mayo Modified Wrist Score (MMWS) was 88.4 (78 to 94), the mean Mayo Elbow Performance Scores (MEPS) 86.7 (77 to 95) and the mean disabilities of arm, shoulder and hand (DASH) score 20.5 (16 to 31): all of these indicate a good outcome.

In case of a high index of suspicion for ELI in patients with a radial head fracture, we recommend the following: confirmation of IOM and IOL injury with an early MRI scan; early surgery with reduction and temporary K-wire stabilisation of the DRUJ; preservation of the radial head if at all possible or replacement if not, and functional bracing in supination. This will increase the prospect of a good result, and avoid the complications of a missed diagnosis and the difficulties of late treatment.

▶ The authors present a retrospective case series of 12 patients diagnosed with Essex-Lopresti injury (ELI) of the forearm and treated surgically after a mean of 5 days from injury. The study achieves its aim to demonstrate that early surgical treatment of ELI can provide good midterm results, especially when compared with the results of treatment of chronic ELI, thus supporting the crucial importance of early diagnosis and treatment. According to the authors' experience, careful examination and comparative radiographs of the wrist are advocated with any elbow injury. In the current study, 1.5-Tesla magnetic resonance imaging assessment of interosseous membrane integrity was undertaken, regardless of the severity of radial head fracture or presence of radial shortening exceeding 1.9 mm. Despite its costs, this approach shows that improved diagnostic accuracy (especially compared with ultrasound investigation) may help reduce the number of underestimated cases that come to consultation once they have become chronic, thus deemed to have a poor prognosis and subject to increased overall costs. We agree that the most important step in the early treatment is restoration of normal radioulnar variance and distal radioulnar joint (DRUJ) reduction and stabilization. Use of simple percutaneous pinning and prolonged immobilization confirms that triangular fibrocartilage complex (TFCC) and DRUJ ligaments may heal spontaneously when treated in the acute setting. My personal preference is to perform an arthroscopic foveal repair of the TFCC because restoration of the DRUJ alignment is facilitated by wrist tower distraction, and early arthroscopic fixation reduces postoperative immobilization up to 3 weeks.

A. Atzei, MD

Anconeus pedicle olecranon flip osteotomy: an approach for the fixation of complex intra-articular distal humeral fractures

Habib M, Tanwar YS, Jaiswal A, et al (RML Hosp and PGIMER, New Delhi, India; Bokaro General Hosp, Jharkhand, India)

Bone Joint J 96-B:1252-1257, 2014

In order to achieve satisfactory reduction of complex distal humeral fractures, adequate exposure of the fracture fragments and the joint surface is required. Several surgical exposures have been described for distal humeral fractures. We report our experience using the anconeus pedicle olecranon flip osteotomy approach. This involves detachment of the triceps along with a sliver of olecranon, which retains the anconeus pedicle. We report the use of this approach in ten patients (six male, four female) with a mean age of 38.4 years (28 to 51). The mean follow-up was 15 months (12 to 18) with no loss to follow-up. Elbow function was graded using the Mayo Score. The results were excellent in four patients, good in five and fair in one patient. The mean time to both fracture and osteotomy union was 10.6 weeks (8 to 12) and 7.1 weeks (6 to 8), respectively. We found this approach gave reliably good exposure for these difficult fractures enabling anatomical reduction and bicondylar plating without complications.

▶ Several surgical methods for intra-articular elbow injuries have been described in the literature. This case series of 10 patients adds to the evolving literature on elbow fracture fixation exposure but for the commentator does not change his current clinical practice. The article is well written with sound methods, patient-reported outcomes, and clinically relevant follow-up time. Unfortunately, there are several weaknesses, which degrade the merit of the article. First, the case series nature of the article and small number of patients does not allow for direct comparison against other relevant elbow exposures, for example, olecranon osteotomy. For instance, the article's results show that patients with an AO 13-C3 fracture did "Fair to Good." It is hard to draw conclusions as to whether this was owing to inadequate exposure to allow anatomic reduction, which may have been possible with an olecranon osteotomy, or whether it is the inherent nature of the injury itself. Second, certain elbow injuries within the AO type C fracture class, such as AO 13-C1, can be treated with less extensive exposures. In addition, including elbow strength measurements of flexion and extension, compared with the contralateral arm, would have strengthened the study.

Although the authors state a risk of proximal ulna fracture in the elderly, for the commentator, the clinical merit of this technique would be in this specific subset given the potential need for a conversion to a total elbow arthroplasty, which may be technically difficult after an olecranon osteotomy.

Some of the proposed merits of the exposure include decreased hardware irritation and nonunion rates when compared with an olecranon osteotomy. However, using this anconeus flip osteotomy carries the risk of triceps attachment problems and inadequate exposure of the articular surface in complex articular fractures. This article shows in a small case series that this approach is a reasonable alternative for these injuries.

M. B. Gottschalk, MD
J. T. Capo, MD

Distribution of Coronoid Fracture Lines by Specific Patterns of Traumatic Elbow Instability

Mellema JJ, Doornberg JN, Dyer GSM, et al (Massachusetts General Hosp, Boston; Brigham and Women's Hosp, Boston, MA; Academic Med Ctr, Amsterdam, The Netherlands)
J Hand Surg Am 39:2041-2046, 2014

Purpose.—To determine if specific coronoid fractures relate to specific overall traumatic elbow instability injury patterns and to depict any relationship on fracture maps and heat maps.

Methods.—We collected 110 computed tomography (CT) studies from patients with coronoid fractures. Fracture types and pattern of injury were characterized based on anteroposterior and lateral radiographs, 2- and 3-dimensional CT scans, and intraoperative findings as described in operative reports. Using quantitative 3-dimensional CT techniques we were able to reconstruct the coronoid and reduce fracture fragments. Based on these reconstructions, fracture lines were identified and graphically superimposed onto a standard template in order to create 2-dimensional fracture maps. To further emphasize the fracture maps, the initial diagrams were converted into fracture heat maps following arbitrary units of measure. The Fisher exact test was used to evaluate the association between coronoid fracture types and elbow fracture-dislocation patterns.

Results.—Forty-seven coronoid fractures were associated with a terrible triad fracture dislocation, 30 with a varus posteromedial rotational injury, 1 with a anterior olecranon fracture dislocation, 22 with a posterior olecranon fracture dislocation, and 7 with a posterior Monteggia injury associated with terrible triad fracture dislocation of the elbow. The association between coronoid fracture types and elbow fracture-dislocation patterns, as shown on 2-dimensional fracture and heat maps, was strongly significant.

Conclusions.—Our fracture maps and heat maps support the observation that specific patterns of traumatic elbow instability have correspondingly specific coronoid fracture patterns. Knowledge of these patterns is useful for planning management because it directs exposure and fixation and helps identify associated ligament injuries and fractures that might benefit from treatment.

Clinical Relevance.—Two-dimensional fracture and heat mapping techniques may help surgeons to predict the distribution of coronoid fracture lines associated with specific injury patterns.

▶ Mellema et al studied fracture patterns of the coronoid by grouping them in terms of injury pattern. They were able to harness new quantitative CT data to reconstruct an image of the coronoid fracture in 2 dimensions including the fracture line. They found a high level of correlation between injury pattern and pattern of the coronoid fracture. The coronoid fracture patterns correlated well with the work of Doornberg and Ring, giving clinical validation to the previously reported classification system they described.

Although the fracture patterns do help us understand the mechanism of injury, I have not found this system to clinically alter my approach to these injuries. It is without question important to recognize the presence of a coronoid fracture; however, the fixation of the fracture itself is unaltered by this information. Small fragments can be excised or fixed using a suture lasso technique, and operative fixation of larger fragments necessitates a medial exposure of the coronoid for fixation with plates or screws. It seems the article is just an attempt to highlight the impressive pictures associated with fracture and heat maps; however, the information gleaned from it is largely academic.

L. T. Kroonen, MD

Radial Head Reconstruction in Elbow Fracture-Dislocation: Monopolar or Bipolar Prosthesis?

Hartzler RU, Morrey BF, Steinmann SP, et al (San Antonio Orthopaedic Group, TX; Mayo Clinic Rochester, MN; et al)

Clin Orthop Relat Res 472:2144-2150, 2014

Background.—Monopolar and bipolar radial head prosthetic arthroplasties have been used successfully to treat elbow fracture-dislocation with unsalvageable radial head fractures. The relative stability of these two designs in different clinical situations is a topic of ongoing investigation.

Questions/Purposes.—We tested the effects of monopolar and bipolar fixed-neck prosthetic radial head implants on improvement in elbow coronal and axial plane laxity in a terrible triad biomechanical model that accounted for lateral collateral ligament integrity and the presence of a transverse coronoid fracture.

Methods.—Kinematic data were collected on six fresh-frozen cadaveric upper extremities tested with passive motion throughout the flexion arc. Varus and valgus gravity stress were applied with the wrist in neutral position. A lateral collateral ligament reconstruction was simulated. We assessed instability after radial head resection and reconstruction with either a monopolar or bipolar implant in the presence of a transversely fractured (Regan and Morrey Type 2) or fixed coronoid process.

Results.—With collateral ligament integrity, no difference was detected, with the numbers available, in valgus laxity between implants under valgus stress ($p = 1.0$). Laxity improvement with each prosthesis was higher when the coronoid was fractured (mean ± SD: monopolar: 7.4° ± 1.6°, $p < 0.001$; bipolar: 6.4° ± 1.6°, $p = 0.003$) than when it was fixed (monopolar: 4.0° ± 1.6°, $p = 0.02$; bipolar: 4.2° ± 1.6°, $p = 0.01$). With the numbers available, there was no difference in external rotation laxity between implants under valgus stress ($p = 1.0$). The greatest stabilizing effect of the prostheses occurred when the coronoid was fractured (monopolar: 3.3° ± 1.2°, $p = 0.15$; bipolar: 3.3° ± 1.2°, $p = 0.17$). Radial head arthroplasty offered no substantial stability under varus stress for varus or internal rotation laxity.

Conclusions.—In our terrible triad cadaveric model, coronoid fixation was effective in improving varus laxity with a monopolar or bipolar prosthesis in place. Also, both types of prostheses were effective in improving valgus and external rotation laxity to the elbow, regardless of coronoid status. With collateral ligaments reconstructed, no large kinematic differences were noted between implants regardless of the varus-valgus position or whether the coronoid was fractured or fixed.

Clinical Relevance.—The data from our cadaveric model support the use of either implant type in terrible triad injuries if the collateral ligaments are intact or reconstructed.

▶ When treating an elbow fracture-dislocation, the unsalvageable radial head fractures are treated with arthroplasty. The authors acknowledge the proposed advantage of the bipolar design to improve tracking and decrease contact pressures. However, the authors review several problems and disadvantages, including concerns regarding less resistance to radiocapitellar joint subluxation.

This study uses a terrible-triad model in 6 cadavers to compare a monopolar with a bipolar radial head prosthetic design using a fixed stem and repaired lateral collateral ligament. The use of passive motion with gravity stress and the forearm in neutral may not show the full spectrum of instability that occurs with these injuries. Additionally, this study only evaluates fixed stem prosthesis and does not evaluate other designs.

The authors should be commended, however, in their evaluation of the 2 prostheses in a terrible-triad model that is commonly encountered in clinical practice, although there are some differences. The contribution of the radial head to stability to valgus and external rotation laxity is clearly seen, with no difference shown between prosthetic designs.

In the terrible-triad injury, there is not a significant advantage to the use of a bipolar prosthesis, and it is more costly. The authors show that the bipolar and monopolar radial head arthroplasty designs successfully restore stability to the elbow.

J. Geissler, MD

The Management of Elbow Instability Using an Internal Joint Stabilizer: Preliminary Results

Orbay JL, Mijares MR (The Miami Hand and Upper Extremity Inst, FL)

Clin Orthop Relat Res 472:2049-2060, 2014

Background.—Nonsurgical and surgical treatments such as immobilization, transarticular pinning, and hinged or nonhinged external fixation have been used to treat unstable elbows. These methods all have drawbacks. We thought that a bent Steinmann pin introduced through the axis of ulnohumeral rotation and attached to the ulna could provide an improved method of treatment and that this could result in the development of a proper internal joint fixator that may have widespread application.

Questions/Purposes.—Does a fully internal hinged fixator crafted intraoperatively by the surgeon from a Steinmann pin for patients undergoing surgery for severe elbow instability result in restoration of range of motion and elbow stability? Does it result in new complications?

Methods.—We reviewed the first 10 patients treated with the method for elbow instability. Diagnoses included fracture-dislocations of the elbow that remain unstable after fracture repair and unstable elbows that result from release of contracture or ulnohumeral synostosis. During that time, all patients meeting these criteria who underwent surgery by this surgeon (JLO) were treated with this approach. Charts, radiographs, and therapy notes were assessed at a minimum of 14 months (mean, 32 months; range, 14–59 months); no patients were lost to followup. Data recorded included age, sex, and elbow and forearm range of motion as well as any complications and reoperations that occurred. The absence of elbow instability was determined initially by radiographically observing concentric reduction of the ulnohumeral and radiocapitellar joints and later by radiography plus the absence of clinical signs and symptoms of elbow instability.

Results.—Mean range of motion at latest followup was flexion 134°, extension −19°, pronation 75°, and supination 64°. All elbows were clinically and radiographically stable. Complications resulting in additional procedures occurred in four patients, including one recurrent deep infection in a patient with a remote history of sepsis, one wound hematoma that resolved after a drainage procedure performed in the office, one prominent implant treated by partial removal, and one patient with heterotopic ossification treated with excision of the heterotopic bone.

Conclusions.—This technique restores elbow stability and permits motion without the use of transcutaneous pins. It seems promising for the treatment of patients with severe elbow instability but requires a second procedure for removal. Further investigation is needed to understand its place in the surgeon's toolbox and what drawbacks it may have.

Level of Evidence.—Level IV, therapeutic study. See Guidelines for Authors for a complete description of levels of evidence.

▶ In this report, the authors describe their series of patients treated with a novel internal elbow fixator fabricated from two 3.5-mm screws and a contoured 2.5-mm Steinmann pin. Ten patients with different primary reasons for elbow instability were reviewed. Their results were shown and compared with reported results using other techniques such as an external fixator. All of the patients achieved a stable elbow with an acceptable range of motion. There was a 40% complication rate, which seems reasonable given the difficult pathology. Two of the 10 patients elected to not have the device removed and showed no problem at 5-year follow-up.

I found this article and technique very intriguing. Although in my practice I rarely use external fixation to achieve elbow stability, the concept of a simple, buried construct is interesting and shows great promise. Posttraumatic and postsurgical elbow instability is a complex problem that deserves continued innovation. I imagine I'll use this technique in the future.

There was one obvious omission in the article. It seems that the authors almost intentionally hold back the details of the device. There was only a hint about the technique for bending and implanting the wire. I expect that we will see a commercial version available in the near future.

N. A. Hoekzema, MD

Comparison of lateral and posterior surgical approach in management of extra-articular distal humeral shaft fractures

Yin P, Zhang L, Mao Z, et al (Chinese PLA General Hosp, Beijing, PR China)
Injury 45:1121-1125, 2014

Objective.—The objective of this study was to compare treatment results and complication rates between lateral and posterior approaches in surgical treatment of extra-articular distal humeral shaft fractures.

Material and Methods.—Between June 2008 and May 2012, a total of 68 patients with extra-articular distal humeral shaft fractures were treated by lateral and posterior approaches. Of the patients, 30 were operated by a lateral approach (group I) and 26 patients were operated by a posterior approach (group II). There was no statistical significance between the two groups in sex distribution, age, the mechanism of the injury, injured arms, AO/ASIF (Arbeitsgemeinschaft für Osteosynthesefragen/ Association for the Study of Internal Fixation) classification, and the time from injury to surgery ($P > 0.05$). Operation time, intraoperative bleeding volume, hospitalisation, clinical outcomes, and complications were compared between the two groups. The elbow functional results were evaluated by the Mayo Elbow Performance Score (MEPS).

Results.—All patients were followed up. The average of follow-up in group I was 15.53 ± 2.636 months (range, 12–22 months), and was 16.12 ± 2.889 months (range, 12–22 months) in group II. There was no significant difference in the operation time, intraoperative bleeding time, and hospitalisation between the two groups ($P > 0.05$). In group I, the mean time of bone union was 12.87 ± 1.852 weeks (range, 10–16 weeks), the mean degrees of elbow flexion was 139.20° ± 3.274° (range, 134–146°), the mean degrees of elbow extension was 4.77° ± 1.906° (range, 0–8°), and the mean points of MEPS was 87.00 ± 7.724 (range, 70–100 points). In group II, the mean time of bone union was 12.96 ± 2.218 weeks (range, 10–16 weeks), the mean degrees of elbow flexion was 137.85° ± 4.076° (range, 130–145°), the mean degrees of elbow extension was 5.15° ± 2.327° (range, 0–9°), and the mean points of MEPS was 86.15 ± 7.656 (range, 70–100 points). There was no significant difference in the bone union, range of elbow flexion, range of elbow extension and MEPS between the two groups ($P > 0.05$). The overall complication rate in group I was lower than that in group II ($P = 0.041$).

Conclusions.—Both lateral and posterior surgical approaches acquired satisfied treatment results in the management of extra-articular distal humeral shaft fractures, and there was a lower complication rate using the lateral approach.

► Yin and colleagues present a retrospective comparison of lateral and posterior approaches to distal humeral shaft fractures. Their description of their approaches indicates that their lateral approach is paratricipital, and their posterior approach splits the triceps. Although they found no significant differences with respect to time to union, operating time, blood loss, and clinical outcomes, they noted a higher complication rate with the posterior triceps-splitting approach. Their complications were iatrogenic radial nerve palsy in 3 patients and prominent hardware in 2 patients.

The study does not clearly define their indication for surgery. However, many of these humeral shaft fractures can be treated nonoperatively in a coaptation splint followed by a fracture brace. In the rare case in which operative intervention is warranted, either because of open injury or significant displacement that cannot be adequately controlled nonoperatively, either approach can be used. My preference has been using a posterior paratricipital approach. Working on either side of the triceps allows for easy mobilization of the radial nerve, as opposed to the triceps-splitting approach. The posterior incision is often noted to be more cosmetically appealing than a lateral incision.

The retrospective nature of this study, with follow-up at only set intervals, does not allow for accurate determination of time to union, but it is comforting to know that either approach will result in comparable Mayo Elbow Performance Score and range of motion. Ultimately, as noted in the report, the decision as to which approach to use should be dictated by fracture characteristics and surgeon preference. There does not seem to be a clear benefit of one approach vs the other.

L. T. Kroonen, MD

CORR Insights®: Long-term Outcome of Displaced, Transverse, Noncomminuted Olecranon Fractures

Zelle BA (UT Health Science Ctr at San Antonio)

Clin Orthop Relat Res 472:1962-1963, 2014

This CORR Insights® is a commentary on the article "Long-term Outcome of Displaced, Transverse, Noncomminuted Olecranon Fractures" by Flinterman and colleagues available at http://dx.doi.org/10.1007/s11999-014-3481-5.

► The author of this editorial aptly credits the authors for a long-term follow-up study (20 years) on the treatment of olecranon fractures. The results of the study suggest the use of tension band fixation for fixation of noncomminuted, transverse olecranon fractures. This is not to say that reoperation is infrequent, as the data in this study resulted in a 7% reoperation rate, presumably for failure of fixation or hardware removal. Further, there was a recorded ulnar nerve compression rate of 13%.

I continue to use tension band fixation in my practice in the above-noted fracture pattern. In the setting of higher degrees of comminution, fractures proximal to the coronoid process, or evidence of elbow instability, my preference remains rigid plate fixation. Regardless of the chosen surgical technique, painful hardware, surgical site infection, decreased range of motion, posttraumatic arthritis, and ulnar neuropathy are some of the commonly reported complications of which the patient should be made aware.

S. M. Jacoby, MD

Determining the Efficacy of Screw and Washer Fixation as a Method for Securing Olecranon Osteotomies Used in the Surgical Management of Intraarticular Distal Humerus Fractures

Woods BI, Rosario BL, Siska PA, et al (Univ of Pittsburgh Med Ctr, PA; Univ of Pittsburgh, PA)

J Orthop Trauma 29:44-49, 2015

Objectives.—The purpose of this study was to critically evaluate the efficacy of single screw and washer fixation in comparison with other methods for securing olecranon osteotomies. The hypothesis is that screw and washer fixation is a safe and effective means of olecranon osteotomy fixation with fusion and complication rates similar to other methods of fixation.

Design.—Retrospective review.

Setting.—Two Level I Urban Trauma Centers.

Patients/Participants.—Patients were treated within the last 20 years and received 1 of 4 types of fixation (screw and washer alone, screw and washer augmented with tension band, tension band alone, or plate and screws) after osteotomy.

Intervention.—Open reduction and internal fixation of OTA/AO 13B/C distal humerus fractures with an olecranon osteotomy.

Main Outcome Measurements.—The primary outcome measure was the presence of osteotomy union. Secondary outcome measures were olecranon nonunion, loss of articular reduction, and removal of hardware. Logistic regression was used to determine the associations between method of osteotomy fixation and removal of hardware or nonunion rates. Comorbidities were stratified using the Charlson comorbidity index.

Results.—One hundred sixty patients met the inclusion criteria. Thirty-nine patients underwent screw fixation alone, 47 had tension band fixation, 16 had plate fixation, and 58 had tension band and screw fixation. Screw fixation demonstrated equal or better rates of union, maintenance of reduction, absence of infection, and implant removal compared with alternative fixation techniques. Higher Charlson scores were associated with higher rates of nonunion.

Conclusions.—Screw and washer fixation is a safe and effective means of securing an olecranon osteotomy. Charlson comorbidity score is one factor that may influence the development of nonunion after osteotomy.

Level of Evidence.—Therapeutic Level III. See Instructions for Authors for a complete description of levels of evidence.

▶ An olecranon osteotomy affords improved visualization for surgical fixation of a distal humeral articular fracture. However, the known complications of the osteotomy, including infection, loss of reduction, and nonunion, are troublesome for the treating surgeon. Various fixation strategies have been proposed, including tension band (TB), plating, and intramedullary screw fixation with or without TB. This study retrospectively evaluated 160 patients with an intra-articular distal humerus fracture treated operatively over a 20-year period. An olecranon osteotomy was used for exposure in all cases, and 4 subsequent fixation techniques were used. The authors' hypothesis was that screw and washer fixation was an efficacious fixation technique and was set as the reference standard for comparison of the other fixation strategies.

The odds of a nonunion developing were 10.06 times higher with TB fixation alone versus screw and washer fixation. There were no significant differences among the other techniques (plating, TB/screw, screw). Similarly, TB removal was 3.68 times more likely than screw and washer removal. The screw and washer fixation method had the lowest rate of infection of the various techniques, at 5.1%, but statistical significance was not provided.

Perhaps the most clinically relevant learning point from this article is the relationship between the Charlson comorbidity index[1] and subsequent risk for postoperative nonunion. The average Charlson score was significantly higher in those patients with a nonunion than those without (1.32 vs 0.56, $P = .04$). This finding held true for the other complications (infection, removal of hardware, and loss of reduction) but was not statistically significant. In addition to the increased risk of nonunion, the risk for loss of reduction was more apparent in the older patient population. In the unhealthy, older patient population, thoughtful surgical planning is imperative when considering the exposure of a distal humerus fracture. Perhaps a nonanatomic articular reduction is more acceptable than an olecranon nonunion. A thorough preoperative surgical discussion will best define the goals of surgical treatment.

This is the largest known series evaluating surgical outcomes of olecranon osteotomies. However, its retrospective nature and lack of clinical outcome measures limit the conclusions. I agree with the authors that a prospective study is necessary to further verify the findings of an otherwise well-done retrospective review.

A. Moeller, MD

Reference

1. Charlson ME, Pompei P, Ales KL, MacKenzie CR. A new method of classifying prognostic comorbidity in longitudinal studies: development and validation. *J Chronic Dis.* 1987;40:373-383.

A Preliminary Report of Acute and Subacute Arthroscopic Repair of the Radial Ulnohumeral Ligament After Elbow Dislocation in the High-Demand Patient

O'Brien MJ, Lee Murphy R, Savoie FH III (Tulane Univ School of Medicine, New Orleans, LA; Mississippi Sports Medicine and Orthopaedic Clinic, Jackson)

Arthroscopy 30:679-687, 2014

Purpose.—The purpose of this study was to evaluate functional outcomes, range of motion (ROM), elbow stability, and time to return to full activities after acute and subacute arthroscopic repair of a simple elbow dislocation in high-demand patients.

Methods.—"High-demand patients" were defined as in-season athletes and individuals who required use of both hands for their profession and believed that they could not miss the 6 weeks of work that may be required with conservative treatment in an elbow brace. We retrospectively reviewed 14 consecutive patients with a simple elbow dislocation who underwent arthroscopic repair of the radial ulnohumeral ligament from 2008-2012. Outcomes measures included the Mayo Elbow Performance Score (MEPS), elbow ROM, elbow stability, and time to return to full activities. Each patient was contacted once by telephone to determine the current activity level and presence of any pain or functional limitations.

Results.—The mean patient age was 25 years, with telephone follow-up at a mean of 30 months and clinical examination after a minimum of 6 months. The postoperative MEPS was excellent (mean, 99.6; range, 95 to 100) for all 14 patients, and all returned to their preinjury level of function with no restrictions or instability. Final ROM averaged −3° of full extension to greater than 130° of flexion. The mean time to return to full activities in and out of a brace was 2.7 weeks and 6.6 weeks, respectively, in the acute group and 4.6 weeks and 8.9 weeks, respectively, in the subacute group. All patients were satisfied with their outcome.

Conclusions.—Conservative management remains the gold standard for most simple elbow dislocations. We believe that certain high-demand patients may be candidates for acute arthroscopic ligamentous repair. Our preliminary data show that acute arthroscopic repair of the radial ulnohumeral ligament is a safe, effective procedure that restores stability to the elbow and allows patients to quickly return to full activities.

Level of Evidence.—Level IV, therapeutic case series.

▶ Nonoperative treatment of simple elbow dislocations is commonly considered to yield satisfactory outcomes[1]. The authors present their results of arthroscopically assisted primary repair of the avulsed lateral collateral ligament complex with the goal to provide a faster return to preinjury elbow function. Return to full activities in the brace occurred between 2 and 6 weeks after surgery and being out of the brace occurred between 6 to 12 weeks after surgery. Although these results appear promising, the study is unable to answer whether primary repair performed in the acute or subacute phase positively affects the natural history of simple elbow dislocations. Furthermore, the potential benefits of arthroscopic over open primary repair cannot be established. Although no intraoperative complications occurred, the reader should be mindful that these procedures were done by a highly experienced arthroscopic surgeon. The presented results may, therefore, not be universally applicable. Arthroscopy in a recently dislocated elbow may have an increased risk for compartment syndrome. Furthermore, anatomic landmarks may be altered, thereby potentially affecting safe placement of arthroscopic portals.

P. Streubel, MD

Reference

1. Anakwe RE, Middleton SD, Jenkins PJ, McQueen MM, Court-Brown CM. Patient-reported outcomes after simple dislocation of the elbow. *J Bone Joint Surg Am.* 2011;93:1220-1226.

Can We Treat Select Terrible Triad Injuries Nonoperatively?

Chan K, MacDermid JC, Faber KJ, et al (McMaster Univ, Hamilton, Ontario, Canada; Univ of Western Ontario, London, Canada)
Clin Orthop Relat Res 472:2092-2099, 2014

Background.—While the majority of terrible triad elbow injuries (ulnohumeral dislocation with radial head and coronoid fractures) are managed surgically, nonoperative treatment may be appropriate in selected patients, but results with this approach have been limited by very small studies.

Questions/Purposes.—We assessed (1) functional outcomes using two validated questionnaires, (2) elbow ROM, strength, and stability, (3) the presence of union and arthritis on radiographs, and (4) complications among a group of patients managed nonoperatively for terrible triad injuries.

Methods.—Between 2006 and 2012, we retrospectively identified 12 patients with terrible triad elbow injuries who were treated nonoperatively and met the following criteria: (1) a concentric joint reduction, (2) a radial head fracture that did not cause a mechanical block to rotation, (3) a smaller coronoid fracture (Regan-Morrey Type 1 or 2), and (4) a stable arc of motion to a minimum of 30° of extension to allow active motion within the first 10 days. Eleven patients were available for followup of at least 12 months after the injury (mean, 36 months; range, 12–90 months). Outcome measures included two patient-reported functional outcome measures (DASH, Mayo Elbow Performance Index [MEPI]), a standardized physical examination to record elbow ROM and stability, isometric strength measurements, and radiographic evidence of bony union and elbow arthrosis. Complications were also recorded.

Results.—At latest followup, mean ± SD DASH score was 8.0 ± 11.0 and mean MEPI score was 94 ± 9. Mean ROM of the affected elbow was 134° ± 5° flexion, 6° ± 8° extension, 87° ± 4° pronation, and 82° ± 10° supination. No instability was detected. Strength assessments demonstrated the following mean percentages of the contralateral, unaffected elbow: flexion 100%, extension 89%, pronation 79%, and supination 89%. Four patients had arthritic changes on radiographs that did not call for treatment as of latest followup. Complications included one patient who underwent surgical stabilization for early recurrent instability and another who underwent arthroscopic débridement for heterotopic bone.

Conclusions.—In selected patients, nonoperative treatment of terrible triad injuries is an option that can provide good function and restore stable elbow ROM. However, nonoperative management requires close clinical and radiographic followup to monitor for any delayed elbow subluxation or fracture displacement.

Level of Evidence.—Level IV, therapeutic study. See Instructions for Authors for a complete description of levels of evidence.

► In this report, the authors retrospectively reviewed 11 cases of elbow terrible-triad fracture dislocations, which were treated without surgical stabilization. This report has a larger number of patients (11) and also longer follow-up (mean, 36 months; range, 12-90) than the prior 2010 report by Guitton and Ring (4 patients).[1]

In this article, the patients underwent initial reduction of the elbow under anesthesia. To be included in the study, the elbow then had to be well reduced on 2 radiographic views, have no block to motion from the radial head fracture, a smaller coronoid fracture, and a stable arc of motion to 30° of extension. The patients were followed carefully and underwent early therapy for range of motion. One patient had to be surgically stabilized 3 weeks after injury, and one patient had heterotopic ossification, which was arthroscopically resected.

Overall, I felt that this was a clinically helpful report. However, the reader must understand both the strict inclusion criteria that was in place and that this cohort was a very small percentage of the patients presenting to their institution with terrible-triad injuries. I can think of one patient that I treated in a similar nonoperative fashion, but these patients are few and far between.

I was slightly surprised by their use of the Regan-Morrey coronoid fracture classification even though injury CT scans were available. It might have been helpful to know a little more detail about the smaller coronoid fractures for considering future patients for nonoperative treatment.

These injuries are devastating. Even in the best-case presentation, there will be permanent changes in the injured elbow and most require surgical treatment.

N. A. Hoekzema, MD

Reference

1. Guitton TG, Ring D. Nonsurgically treated terrible triad injuries of the elbow: report of four cases. *J Hand Surg Am.* 2010;35:464-467.

Transverse Coronoid Fracture: When Does It Have to Be Fixed?

Hartzler RU, Llusa-Perez M, Steinmann SP, et al (San Antonio Orthopaedic Group, TX; Universitat de Barcelona, Spain; Mayo Clinic Rochester, MN)

Clin Orthop Relat Res 472:2068-2074, 2014

Background.—After elbow fracture-dislocation, surgeons confront numerous treatment options in pursuing a stable joint for early motion. The relative contributions of the radial head and coronoid, in combination, to elbow stability have not been defined fully.

Questions/Purposes.—The purpose of this study was to evaluate the effect of an approximately 50% transverse coronoid fracture and fixation in the setting of an intact or resected radial head on coronal (varus/valgus) and axial (internal and external rotational) laxity in (1) gravity varus stress; and (2) gravity valgus stress models.

Methods.—Kinematic data were collected on six fresh-frozen cadaveric upper extremities tested with passive motion throughout the flexion arc under varus and valgus gravity stress with lateral collateral ligaments reconstructed. Testing included coronoid fracture and osteosynthesis with and without a radial head.

Results.—In the varus gravity stress model, fixation of the coronoid improved varus stability (fixed: 1.6° [95% confidence interval, 1.0–2.2], fractured: 5.6° [4.2–7.0], $p < 0.001$) and internal rotational stability (fixed: 1.8° [0.9–2.7], fractured: 5.4° [4.0–6.8], $p < 0.001$), but radial head fixation did not contribute to varus stability (intact head: 2.7° [1.3–4.1], resected head: 3.8° [2.3–5.3], $p = 0.4$) or rotational stability (intact: 2.7° [0.9–4.5], resected head: 3.9° [1.5–6.3], $p = 0.4$). With valgus stress, coronoid fixation improved valgus stability (fixed: 2.1° [1.0–3.1], fractured: 3.8° [1.8–5.8], $p < 0.04$) and external rotation stability (fixed: 0.8° [0.1–1.5], fractured: 2.1° [0.9–3.4], $p < 0.04$), but the radial head played a more important role in providing valgus stability (intact: 1.4° [0.8–2.0], resected head: 7.1° [3.5–10.7], $p < 0.001$).

Conclusions.—Fixation of a 50% transverse coronoid fracture improves varus and internal rotatory laxity but is unlikely to meaningfully improve valgus or external rotation laxity. The radial head, on the other hand, is a stabilizer to resist valgus stress regardless of the status of the coronoid.

Clinical Relevance.—Determination as to whether it is necessary to fix a coronoid fracture should be based on the stability of the elbow when tested with a varus load. The elbow may potentially be stable with fractures involving less than 50% of the coronoid. Under all circumstances, the radial head should be fixed or replaced to ensure valgus external rotatory stability.

▶ This purpose of this report "was to evaluate the effect of an approximately 50% transverse coronoid fracture and fixation in the setting of an intact or resected radial head on coronal (varus/valgus) and axial (internal and external rotational) laxity in (1) gravity varus stress; and (2) gravity valgus stress models." A cadaveric testing apparatus was designed to evaluate elbow stability with a combination of native radial head presence versus excision and type II coronoid fractured versus type II coronoid *open reduction and internal fixation*.

The results of the study were that fixation of a "50% coronoid fracture" added to varus and internal rotatory stability but were unlikely to improve valgus or external rotatory stability.

Strengths of the study include a meticulous design and execution. The methods were well described as were the numerical data. Limitations of the study include the small number of cadaveric specimens and the repetitive stressing of the cadaveric elbow.

My concern with the study design was more with the simulated coronoid fracture. The osteotomy was made carefully at 50% coronoid height in a straight transverse pattern reproducing a Regan-Morrey type II fracture. Although the original Regan-Morrey classification is useful and quoted clinically,[1] it likely underestimates the complexities of these fractures—which has been seen in several studies on coronoid fracture patterns by CT scans.[2]

I feel that the authors achieved their goal as quoted above from the report, but I do not feel that they answered the question proposed by their title. Complete understanding of native, posttraumatic, and postsurgical elbow stability is a complex, dynamic topic that is elusive and still being hunted. This report gives us a little more ammunition.

N. A. Hoekzema, MD

References

1. Regan W, Morrey BF. Classification and treatment of coronoid process fractures. *Orthopedics*. 1992;15:845-848.
2. O'Driscoll SW, Jupiter JB, Cohen MS, Ring D, McKee MD. Difficult elbow fractures; pearls and pitfalls. *Instr Course Lect*. 2003;52:113-134.

Injury Patterns and Outcomes of Open Fractures of the Proximal Ulna Do Not Differ From Closed Fractures

Yi PH, Weening AA, Shin SR, et al (Boston Univ Med Ctr, MA; Massachusetts General Hosp, Boston)

Clin Orthop Relat Res 472:2100-2104, 2014

Background.—The incidence and injury patterns of open fractures of the proximal ulna are poorly elucidated and little evidence exists to guide management.

Questions/Purposes.—The purpose of this study was to compare the (1) bony injury patterns; (2) range of motion (ROM) and frequency of union; and (3) postoperative complications between open and closed fractures of the proximal ulna.

Methods.—Seventy-nine consecutive open fractures of the proximal ulna were identified. After excluding fracture-dislocations, penetrating injuries, and pediatric injuries, 60 were compared in a retrospective case-control study with an age- and sex-matched group of 91 closed fractures to compare the bony injury patterns based on radiographic review.

In a subset of 39 open and 39 closed fractures with sufficient followup, chart and radiographic review was performed by someone other than the operating surgeon to compare differences in final ROM, union, and postoperative complication rates at a minimum followup of 3 months (mean, 22 and 15 months; range, 3–86 months and 3–51 months for open and closed fractures, respectively). A total of 12% of the fractures were open (79 of 671) at the three study centers, and the majority of fractures were intraarticular (45 of 60 [75%]) with Gustilo-Anderson Type I and II wounds (54 of 60 [90%]).

Results.—Overall, open fractures of the proximal ulna overall did not have more complex bony injury patterns, but there were more anterior olecranon fracture-dislocations among the open fracture group (nine of 60 [15%] versus two of 91 [2%]; $p = 0.004$) and more posterior olecranon fracture-dislocations in the closed fracture group (31 of 91 [34%] versus seven of 60 [12%]; $p = 0.002$). Final ROM was not different in both groups and all fractures healed. There was no difference in wound infection rate but a higher secondary procedure rate among open fractures of the proximal ulna (39% versus 23%, $p = 0.014$).

Conclusions.—In contrast to open fractures of the distal humerus, open fractures of the proximal ulna present with mild soft tissue injuries and do not have more complex bony injury patterns than closed fractures. Our findings suggest that open fractures of the proximal ulna are the result of tension failure of the skin secondary to the limited soft tissue envelope around the proximal ulna. Open fractures of the proximal ulna should be regarded as relatively mild injuries that are not different in severity and prognosis compared with closed fractures.

Level of Evidence.—Level III, therapeutic study. See Guidelines for Authors for a complete description of levels of evidence.

► The authors of this retrospective, case-control study of open proximal ulna fractures present a convincing argument that most of these injuries are associated with mild soft tissue trauma and that the outcomes after treatment of these injuries are similar to those of closed proximal ulna fractures.

It is interesting to note that the time to debridement of the open fractures in this study was variable, ranging from within 6 hours to 96 hours. Despite this variability, most fractures underwent immediate open reduction and internal fixation, and the wound infection rate did not differ significantly from that of closed fractures. Therefore, it would seem that the treating surgeon has some discretion in operative timing based on the degree of soft tissue injury in open proximal ulna fractures.

A concern is raised in the discussion section that all of the trauma centers in this study were located in the same city. However, the fact that there were 21 attending surgeons involved in the care of the patients in this study would seem to make the outcomes reported more applicable to surgeons located in other cities.

This report is a nice review of an injury that has received little attention in the literature, and the data presented will benefit future surgeons treating open proximal ulna fractures.

E. Kinnucan, MD

Surgical Techniques of Olecranon Fractures

Wilkerson JA, Rosenwasser MP (New York Orthopaedic Hosp)

J Hand Surg Am 39:1606-1614, 2014

Olecranon fractures are common upper extremity injuries. The vast majority are treated with operative fixation. Many treatment techniques have been described including tension band and plating. This review covers the most commonly used fixation techniques in detail, including pearls and pitfalls with case examples of both successful treatments and potential complications.

▶ Several surgical treatment methods for olecranon fractures have been described. This article is a nice review of some of the current available techniques for fracture fixation. The report is well written with the only limitation being that it is expert opinion. It is important to re-emphasize the main goals of olecranon fracture treatment. The first is to provide good stabilization with anatomic articular reduction and to allow fracture healing regardless of surgical construct. The second is to allow a painless arc of functional motion. How these activities are accomplished is up to the treating surgeon, and the surgeon's experience with different surgical techniques should dictate what should be performed. For the commentator, if the fracture is transverse with minimal comminution, a tension band technique should be used. The commentator's preferred technique includes the use of prefabricated k-wires with distal engagement into the anterior cortex of the ulna. Eighteen-gauge wire or braided reinforced suture can be used with newer articles indicating less hardware irritation with reinforced braided suture. In the case of complex fractures or severe comminution, a plate construct should be used. It is important to discuss with the patient that there may be a need for hardware removal should the plate be symptomatic. It is equally important to recognize if there is inadequate purchase in the proximal fragment. Should this be the case, several techniques can be used. The first is to pick a plate with more additional proximal screw holes. The second is to add suture fixation to the triceps tendon to neutralize the deforming force. As with any case, the patient's preference and specific injury pattern, combined with the treating surgeon's experience, should help dictate the appropriate management.

M. B. Gottschalk, MD

J. T. Capo, MD

Terrible Triad Injuries of the Elbow: Does the Coronoid Always Need to Be Fixed?

Papatheodorou LK, Rubright JH, Heim KA, et al (Univ of Pittsburgh School of Medicine, PA)

Clin Orthop Relat Res 472:2084-2091, 2014

Background.—The "terrible triad" of the elbow is a complex injury that can lead to pain, stiffness, and posttraumatic arthritis if not appropriately treated. The primary goal of surgery for these injuries is to restore stability of the joint sufficient to permit early motion. Although most reports recommend repair and/or replacement of all coronoid and radial head fractures when possible, a recent cadaveric study demonstrated that type II coronoid fractures are stable unless the radial head is removed and not replaced.

Questions/purposes.—The purposes of this study were to determine the (1) range of motion; (2) clinical scores using the Disabilities of the Arm, Shoulder and Hand (DASH) and the Broberg-Morrey questionnaires; and (3) rate of arthritic changes, heterotopic ossification (HO), or elbow instability postoperatively in patients whose terrible triad injuries of the elbow included Reagan-Morrey type I or II coronoid fractures that were treated without fixation.

Methods.—Between April 2008 and December 2010, 14 consecutive patients were treated for acute terrible triad injuries that included two Regan-Morrey type I and 12 Regan-Morrey type II coronoid fractures. Based on the senior author's (DGS) clinical experience that coronoid fractures classified as such do not require fixation to restore intraoperative stability to the posterolaterally dislocated elbow, all injuries were treated by the senior author with a surgical protocol that included radial head repair or prosthetic replacement and repair of the lateral ulnar collateral ligament (LUCL) followed by intraoperative fluoroscopic examination through a range of 20° to 130° of elbow flexion to confirm concentric reduction of the ulnohumeral joint. Using this protocol, intraoperative stability was confirmed in all cases without any attempt at coronoid or anterior capsular repair. Repair of the medial collateral ligament or application of external fixation was not performed in any case. All patients were available for followup at a minimum of 24 months (mean, 41 months; range, 24–56 months). The mean patient age was 52 years (range, 32–58 years). At the followup all patients were evaluated clinically and radiographically by the senior author. Outcome measures included elbow range of motion, forearm rotation, elbow stability, and radiographic evidence of HO or arthritic changes using the Broberg and Morrey scale. Elbow instability was defined as clinical or radiographic evidence of recurrent ulnohumeral dislocation or subluxation at final followup. Clinical outcomes were assessed with the patient-reported DASH questionnaire and the physician-administered Broberg-Morrey elbow rating system.

Results.—The mean arc of ulnohumeral motion at final followup was 123° (range, 75°–140°) and mean forearm rotation was 145° (range, 70°–170°). The mean Broberg and Morrey score was 90 of 100 (range, 70–100, higher scores reflecting better results) and the average DASH score was 14 of 100 (range, 0–38, higher scores reflecting poorer results). Radiographs revealed mild arthritic changes in one patient. One patient developed radiographically apparent but asymptomatic HO. None of the patients demonstrated instability postoperatively.

Conclusions.—These findings demonstrate that terrible triad injuries with type I and II coronoid process fractures can be effectively treated without fixation of coronoid fractures when repair or replacement of the radial head fracture and reconstruction of the LUCL complex sufficiently restores intraoperative stability of the elbow through a functional range of motion.

Level of Evidence.—Level IV, therapeutic study. See Guidelines to Authors for a complete description of levels of evidence.

▶ Terrible-triad injuries of the elbow represent a complex injury to the supporting structures of the elbow. Most authors advocate repair or replacement of the radial head and the lateral ulnar collateral ligament (LUCL). It is often debated if the medial ulnar collateral ligament (MUCL) and at times the coronoid need to be repaired. This article aims to answer the question, do all coronoid fractures need to be fixed? The article is well written and has the usual limitations of a case series, including lack of a control group, small sample size, and the inability to compare this series of patients with other potentially biased case series. One of the more difficult limitations is to ascertain where on the spectrum of terrible-triad injury patterns did most of these patients present, as not all injuries are equal. It appears that these injuries were diagnosed with plain radiographs and that CT scans were not utilized. This fact limits the authors' ability to detect what type of coronoid fracture existed. It is often difficult to tell the difference between a type II and III fractures on plain films alone.

When these limitations are taken into account, the question is clearly answered that not all coronoid fractures need fixation. Unfortunately, the report does not address how to determine which fractures do need to be surgically repaired. For the commentator, the goals for terrible-triad injuries are simple and include a painless stable elbow with a functional range of motion. It is the commentator's expert opinion that the treating surgeon needs to be ready to treat all aspects of the injury, which may include repair vs replacement of the radial head, repair of the LUCL or MUCL, repair of the coronoid, and, when necessary, an external fixator. The commentator uses a similar approach as the senior author of the article and will test the elbow through a functional arc of motion under fluoroscopy to see if the coronoid needs to be addressed. This is normally done prior to tightening the sutures for the LUCL repair. As more studies are performed and the surgeon's understanding of such fractures is improved, treatment methods will continue to evolve.

M. B. Gottschalk, MD

J. T. Capo, MD

Comparative Study of Simple and Complex Open Elbow Dislocations

Boretto JG, Rodriguez Sammartino M, Gallucci G, et al (Hosp Italiano de Buenos Aires, Argentina; Clínica de Fracturas y Ortopedia, Mar del Plata, Argentina; et al)

Clin Orthop Relat Res 472:2037-2043, 2014

Background.—Open elbow dislocations are rare injuries. Most of the evidence related to these dislocations is found in case reports or in series with closed injuries. We reviewed the experiences of three centers in the treatment of open elbow dislocations.

Question/Purposes.—We compared the results after operative treatment of simple and complex open dislocations in terms of (1) ROM, (2) functional score, and (3) complications.

Methods.—Eighteen patients were retrospectively included in this study: 11 with simple open elbow dislocations and seven with complex open elbow dislocations. Mean age was 40 years. Thirteen were men. Eight patients presented neurovascular injuries. Evaluation included ROM of the elbow and forearm as measured by hand-held goniometer. We then classified the results using the 100-point Broberg and Morrey functional rating index based on ROM, grip strength, elbow stability, and pain. Scores of 95 to 100 were considered excellent, 80 to 94 good, 60 to 79 fair, and less than 60 poor. Complications were recorded. Minimum followup was 6 months (mean, 25 months; range, 6-72 months).

Results.—We found no differences between simple and complex open elbow dislocations related to ROM (median flexion/extension: 117° versus 110°, $p = 0.12$; forearm rotation: 160° versus 170°, $p = 0.67$). According to the Broberg and Morrey score, four patients had excellent results, five good, and one fair in the simple dislocation group, whereas in the complex dislocation group, four patients had excellent results, two good, and one fair ($p = 0.8$). No difference in complication rate was found between groups ($p = 0.63$). All complications in the simple dislocation group were neurovascular. In the complex dislocation group, there was one case of brachial artery occlusion, two cases of heterotopic ossification, one case of infection and nonunion, and one case of infection. No patients had recurrent elbow instability.

Conclusions.—No differences between simple and complex open elbow dislocations were found in terms of ROM, functional results, and rate of complications. Complications in the simple dislocation group were related to neurovascular injuries in contrast to the complex dislocation group where complications were associated with the bony injury.

Level of Evidence.—Level IV, prognostic study. See Instructions for Authors for a complete description of levels of evidence (Fig 2).

▶ Boretto and colleagues provide a retrospective review of 18 patients from 3 centers with open elbow dislocations and fracture dislocations. Their series represents the largest series of such open injuries, indicating the relative paucity of literature addressing these rare injuries. Their functional outcomes in both

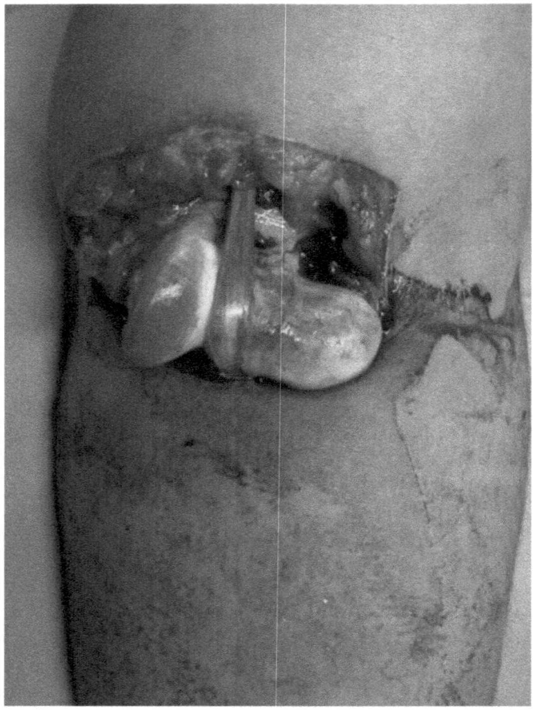

FIGURE 2.—A photograph shows a simple open elbow dislocation with the distal humerus extremity fully exposed. Note the median nerve pulled in the trochlear notch. (With kind permission from Springer Science+Business Media: Boretto JG, Rodriguez Sammartino M, Gallucci G, et al. Comparative study of simple and complex open elbow dislocations. *Clin Orthop Relat Res.* 2014;472:2037-2043, with permission from The Association of Bone and Joint Surgeons.)

groups showed overall good to excellent results in most patients. This review will assist us in appropriately counseling patients that it is reasonable to expect good outcomes despite these severe open injuries.

The major difference they found was related to the types of complications. Interestingly, the open simple dislocations were associated more commonly with neurovascular injuries, whereas the open fracture dislocations were associated with other complications including brachial artery occlusion, infection, heterotypic ossification, and nonunion. This difference is intuitive. If the bony structures stay intact, but are imparted with enough force to cause an open injury, they will pull any neuromuscular structures out of the body with them, as was seen in Fig 2. However, if the bony structures give way, less tension will be seen by the neuromuscular structures.

This study is limited by the small sample size, which cannot be faulted given the rarity of these injuries. However, the sample provides us with the comfort of knowing that outcomes with these open injuries are comparable to the equivalent closed injuries.

Of note is the mechanism of injury in this series. All injuries were from blunt trauma, either fall from a height or motor vehicle-related trauma. However, similar injuries can be seen as a result of penetrating projectile trauma. It is important to recognize the difference with such injuries, as their results would not be expected to be comparable with the results reported in this series.

L. T. Kroonen, MD

Radiographic Loss of Contact Between Radial Head Fracture Fragments Is Moderately Reliable

Bruinsma WE, Science of Variation Group (Academic Med Ctr, Amsterdam, The Netherlands; et al)

Clin Orthop Relat Res 472:2113-2119, 2014

Background.—Loss of contact between radial head fracture fragments is strongly associated with other elbow or forearm injuries. If this finding has adequate interobserver reliability, it could help examiners identify and treat associated ligament injuries and fractures (eg, forearm interosseous ligament injury or elbow dislocation).

Questions/Purposes.—(1) What is the interobserver agreement on radiographic loss of contact between radial head fracture fragments? (2) Are there factors associated with the observer such as location of practice or subspecialization that increase interobserver reliability?

Methods.—Fully trained practicing orthopaedic and trauma surgeons from around the world evaluated 27 anteroposterior and lateral radiographs of radial head fractures on a web-based platform for the following characteristics: (1) loss of contact between at least one radial head fracture fragment and the remaining radial head and neck; (2) a gap between fragments of 2 mm or greater; (3) anticipated fracture instability (mobility) on operative exposure; (4) anticipated associated ligament injuries; and (5) recommendation for treatment. Agreement among observers was measured using the multirater kappa measure. Kappas for various observer characteristics were compared using 95% confidence intervals.

Results.—The overall interobserver agreement was moderate (range, 0.49—0.55) for each question except associated ligament injury, which was fair (0.33). Shoulder and elbow surgeons had substantial agreement (range, 0.51—0.61) in many areas, but kappas were generally in the moderate range (0.41—0.59) based on number of years in practice, radial head fractures treated per year, and trainee supervision.

Conclusions.—Radiographic signs of radial head fracture instability such as loss of contact have moderate reliability. This characteristic seems clinically useful, because loss of contact between at least one radial head fracture fragment and the remaining radial head and neck is strongly associated with associated ligament injury or other fractures.

Level of Evidence.—Level III, diagnostic study. See Guidelines for Authors for a complete description of levels of evidence.

▶ This is an article written by the Science of Variation Group, and it investigates the interobserver agreement for questions posed to orthopedic surgeons of different levels of experience regarding fractures of the radial head. The overall aim is to see whether surgeons can simply look at images and know or believe that there are associated other injuries to the elbow and forearm that may indicate instability. The current classification systems used to grade radial head fractures focus on fragments, both number and displacement, toward the end of defining whether the fragment is going to produce a block to motion. The authors were curious as to whether radiologic fracture parameters, such as a gap between the fracture fragments or loss of contact, indicate which fractures would be mobile on operative exposure and, more important, which would be associated with other fractures or ligament injuries. It has previously been reported that partial articular radial head fractures with at least 1 bony fragment not in contact are more than 20 times more likely to be associated with a complex, unstable injury pattern in the elbow. This study aims to directly test whether there is interobserver reliability on this assessment. Simply put: Do observers agree on the implications of the displacement of a radial head fracture, and is this agreement related to observer experience or practice subspecialization?

The study involves 27 sets of elbow radiographs from patients treated with radial head fractures. The images were selected based on image quality and provided a spectrum of displacement and injury patterns. Fourteen of the 27 sets had displaced radial head fractures according to criteria previously reported as being significant for more unstable injury patterns. One hundred sixty-eight surgeons completed the online survey. Almost 80% of the surgeons had greater than 5 years of experience and some form of subspecialty practice, either in hand and wrist surgery or orthopedic traumatology, and approximately 80% were involved in the training of less experienced surgeons.

The results were somewhat intriguing. First, the interobserver reliability for diagnosing a gap of 2 mm in radial head fragments was only moderate. This was also true for diagnosing a complete loss of bony contact between the fragments and classifying the fracture of a radial head as indicating elbow instability of the radial head fracture as well as recommending operative treatment. There was, however, moderate to fair interobserver reliability for diagnosing an anticipated ligament injury. Notably, shoulder and elbow surgeons seemed to have a greater interobserver reliability for diagnosing a fracture gap greater than 2 mm and anticipating fracture instability and recommending operative treatment. Those specializing in hand and wrist surgery and orthopedic traumatology did not agree as substantially.

In light of the fact that loss of contact of fragments of the radial head is probably important in predicting instability in the elbow, it would seem as if this important factor would garner more interobserver reliability between the surgeons most likely to treat these fractures, and yet this study shows, perhaps definitively, that interobserver reliability and likely the prediction of operative management differs significantly, even based on these agreed-on criteria.

It is hard to interpret whether patients managed operatively will differ in outcome based on the results of this study. This is because an operative surgeon independent of experience and his or her interpretation of the radiographs may act in a more uniform manner relative to other surgeons when confronted with a greater injury at the time of surgery than he or she may have expected. As such, the issue of interobserver reliability, simply based on radiographs, may not be the most important factor in predicting outcome after operative management. Although some information is known about the outcomes of nonoperative management with severe injuries in the elbow, little can be said about the relationship between this step-off and the overall outcome of both of these methods of treatment for these injuries are not so common as to allow large series to compare operative and nonoperative management. This notwithstanding, it seems pretty clear that fractures with no contact between the radial head fragment and the rest of the radius involve a more severe blow to the elbow and more likely instability, which should respond to operative management in the acute or subacute setting. As such, the diagnosis of this instability, as evaluated by this study, is both important and not standard. This study goes a long way to underline the differences in opinions regarding the diagnostic features of proximal radius fractures and, therefore, deserves recognition for its novel approach, its large sample size, and its definitive conclusion that interobserver agreement on the diagnosis of an unstable elbow based on radiographs alone is only fair. It contributes to our understanding of just how far we are from definitively setting down a treatment algorithm for these injuries. It would be interesting to see the results of the study repeated with the presence of critical CT and/or MRI information in the future.

J. Elfar, MD

Open Reduction and Internal Fixation of Radial Head Fractures: Do Outcomes Differ Between Simple and Complex Injuries?

Pike JM, Grewal R, Athwal GS, et al (Univ of British Columbia, Vancouver, Canada; Univ of Western Ontario, London, Canada)

Clin Orthop Relat Res 472:2120-2127, 2014

Background.—Radial head fractures can occur in isolation or in association with elbow and forearm injuries. Treatment options include nonoperative management, fragment or whole-head excision, open reduction and internal fixation (ORIF), and radial head arthroplasty. However, the evidence supporting ORIF for repairable radial head fractures is inconclusive.

Questions/Purposes.—We compared patients undergoing ORIF for isolated radial head fractures or for radial head fractures associated with other fractures or elbow dislocations in terms of patient-related disability, presence of posttraumatic arthritis, complications, and rate of reoperation for capsular release.

Methods.—Between 1997 and 2008, 52 patients underwent ORIF of the radial head for isolated radial head fractures (simple group) and 29 underwent ORIF for radial head fracture with an associated fracture or dislocation (complex group). General indications for ORIF included displaced radial fractures, large articular surface fragments, and greater than 2 mm of displacement and/or a mechanical block to forearm rotation or associated fractures or ligament injuries requiring surgery. Thirty-one patients (60%) in the simple group and 20 (69%) in the complex group were available for followup at a mean of 4 years (range, 1.0–9.5 years). We evaluated the patients using a validated self-reported pain and disability questionnaire (Patient-rated Elbow Evaluation [PREE]). Records review included radiographic examination and assessment of major complications and secondary surgery rates for capsular release.

Results.—With the numbers available, the groups were not different in terms of the mean PREE scores (8 versus 15 for the simple and complex groups, respectively; $p = 0.13$, lower values indicate lower pain and disability). The simple and complex groups were also not different with the numbers available in terms of major complications (13% versus 25%, respectively; $p = 0.29$) or secondary capsular release (3% versus 20%, respectively; $p = 0.07$).

Conclusions.—At short term, we found no differences between patients treated with ORIF for isolated radial head fractures and those treated for radial head fractures in association with other elbow injuries with regard to pain and disability scores; loss to followup in this series precludes making statements with great confidence about function after these injuries. However, the substantial capsular release and complication rates should weigh into the preoperative discussion with patients before selecting ORIF for radial head fractures.

Level of Evidence.—Level III, therapeutic study. See Instructions for Authors for a complete description of levels of evidence Table 2

▶ The authors present a retrospective review of outcomes of open reduction and internal fixation (ORIF) of radial head fractures, comparing simple isolated injuries and complex fracture patterns associated with other fractures or elbow dislocations. During the study period, there were 52 patients for simple fractures with 31 available for follow-up and 29 with complex injury patterns with 20 available for follow-up (minimum 1 year). With the numbers available, the authors conclude that there were no significant differences in Patient-Rated Elbow Evaluation scores, complication rate, or need for secondary capsular release. However, there was a trend toward worse outcomes with the complex injuries, suggesting a type 2 error in the authors' reporting of no differences between the 2 cohorts, which the authors acknowledged in the Discussion section. Overall, the radial head fractures were more comminuted with more fragments in the complex group. The main limitation was that there was no comparison group of nonoperative radial head fractures or those undergoing radial head arthroplasty. However, based on the data presented, patients must be counseled on the high rate of major complications (hardware failure, disabling stiffness, etc) when discussing nonoperative vs surgical treatment of these injuries. Moreover, even at short term, there was a high rate of radiocapitellar arthritis and capitellar abnormalities in the 2 groups. Currently, I treat the majority of isolated radial head fractures nonoperatively even with an articular stepoff, unless there is a mechanical block to elbow motion or forearm rotation. Younger patients with more than 2 to 3 mm articular stepoff are counseled on the increased risk of future radiocapitellar arthritis. With complex radial head

TABLE 2.—Outcomes (by Group)

Variable	Simple Group (Isolated Radial Head Fractures) (n = 31)	Complex Group (Complex Fracture Patterns with Radial Head Fractures) (n = 20)	*p* Value
PREE (points)*	8 (13)	15 (20)	0.13#
Major complications (%)†	13	25	0.29**
Secondary capsular release (%)‡	3	20	0.07**
Prevalence of ulnotrochlear arthritis (%)	13	25	0.29**
Prevalence of radiocapitellar arthritis (%)§	32	40	0.76**
Prevalence of any capitellar abnormality (%)‖	61	60	1.0**
Crepitus detected with motion (%)¶	29	47	0.23**

*Values are expressed as mean, with SD in parentheses.
†Collapse with prominent hardware, disabling elbow stiffness (concomitant complex regional pain syndrome [n = 1; simple group], ulnar neuritis [n = 1; complex group]), or posterolateral joint subluxation requiring external fixation revision (n = 1; complex group).
‡One patient underwent concomitant ulnar nerve transposition.
§At least mild joint space narrowing and mild osteophyte formation (Broberg-Morrey Grade 1 posttraumatic arthritis of the elbow) compared to radiographs of the contralateral elbow.
‖Including subtle irregularity of the subchondral bone, osteopenia, or cysts not sufficient to warrant the diagnosis of mild radiographic arthritis (any joint space narrowing, osteophyte formation compared bilaterally).
¶Crepitus noted in the radiocapitellar joint and/or the ulnohumeral joint.
#Unpaired t-test.
**Fisher's exact test; PREE = Patient-rated Elbow Evaluation.
With kind permission from Springer Science+Business Media: Pike JM, Grewal R, Athwal GS, et al. Open Reduction and Internal Fixation of Radial Head Fractures: Do Outcomes Differ Between Simple and Complex Injuries? Clin Orthop Relat Res. 2014;472:2120-2127.

fracture patterns including Monteggia variants and terrible triads, ORIF is recommended for 2-part fractures. Three-part fractures, as shown by Ring et al and others, have a high risk of failure with ORIF. In those cases, radial head arthroplasty is recommended because there are no concerns of loss of fixation, and early range of motion protocols can be initiated.

J. I. Huang, MD

8 Elbow: Miscellaneous

Stress Ultrasound Evaluation of Medial Elbow Instability in a Cadaveric Model

Ciccotti MC, Hammoud S, Dodson CC, et al (Thomas Jefferson Univ Hosp, Philadelphia, PA)
Am J Sports Med 42:2463-2469, 2014

Background.—An injury of the ulnar collateral ligament (UCL) is potentially career threatening for elite overhead-throwing athletes. Stress ultrasonography (SUS) allows for a rapid, cost-effective, and noninvasive evaluation of the UCL and elbow joint both at rest and with applied stress.

Purpose/Hypothesis.—To determine the amount of cadaveric elbow valgus gapping with sequential sectioning of medial elbow structures as measured by SUS. It was hypothesized that the greatest increase in ulnohumeral joint gapping would be noted with release of the anterior bundle of the UCL.

Study Design.—Descriptive laboratory study.

Methods.—Twelve cadaveric elbows were divided into 2 groups and dissected in reverse sequences under the direct supervision of an experienced orthopaedic surgeon. Baseline ultrasound and SUS with applied valgus loads were performed by an experienced radiologist. A valgus load was applied at each sectioning interval using a standardized device. Ulnohumeral joint gapping in millimeters was measured by SUS for each step as the width of the medial joint from the trochlea to the sublime tubercle. The mean increases in joint gapping (Δ) between each step were calculated to quantify the additional gapping achieved with release of each sequential stabilizer.

Results.—Release of the anterior band of the anterior bundle resulted in a mean Δ of 2.0 mm (95% CI, 1.1-2.8 mm). Release of the posterior band of the anterior bundle resulted in a mean Δ of 1.4 mm (95% CI, 0.6-2.2 mm). Release of the entire anterior bundle caused a mean increase in ulnohumeral valgus joint gapping of 3.4 mm (95% CI, 2.4-4.3 mm). Release of the remaining individual structures each resulted in a mean increase in valgus joint gapping of ≤0.8 mm.

Conclusion.—The results of the current cadaveric study suggest that different amounts of gapping are seen on SUS with sectioning of the medial elbow stabilizers. The hypothesis was confirmed with release of the anterior bundle of the UCL resulting in the greatest increase in joint gapping as measured by SUS.

Clinical Relevance.—This study illustrates that SUS can identify the contributions of each anatomic portion of the UCL and the flexor-pronator mass to ulnohumeral joint stability in a cadaveric model.

▶ Overhead-throwing athletes may experience ulnar collateral ligament (UCL) injuries that produce pain and instability with valgus stress.

This is the first study using stress ultrasound to quantify the relative amounts of ulnohumeral gapping that occurs with sequential sectioning of the medial elbow structures in cadavers at 30 degrees. The structures sectioned were the transverse bundle of the UCL, posterior bundle of UCL, anterior band of the anterior bundle of the UCL, posterior band of the anterior bundle of the UCL, and the flexor-pronator mass.

The authors demonstrated that sectioning of portions anterior bundle showed the greatest change in joint gapping with stress. This correlates to other reported findings and current treatment for elbow valgus instability with reconstruction of both bands of the anterior bundle of the UCL.

The authors were thoughtful in designing their study to section the structures in 2 orders to try to distinguish each structure's contribution rather than the additive effect; however, isolated sectioning may have more directly answered their question. Additionally, the use of cadaveric specimen carries the usual limitations. The small number of specimens, the presumed advanced age, and stress testing at only 30 degrees of valgus limits this study in its ability to mimic the clinical scenario experienced by the relatively young overhead-throwing athlete with dynamic stabilizers. This is certainly a step forward in understanding each structure's role, however.

Their use of a single experienced radiologist may limit the application and extrapolation of these data. Fortunately, ultrasound experience and standardization of techniques are becoming more available.

The authors are commended for their excellent literature review on this pathology, which is most commonly symptomatic in elite athletes, as well as for planning further research of commonly identified injury patterns.

J. Geissler, MD

Anconeus Interposition Arthroplasty: Mid- to Long-term Results

Baghdadi YMK, Morrey BF, Sanchez-Sotelo J (Mayo Clinic, Rochester, MN)

Clin Orthop Relat Res 472:2151-2161, 2014

Background.—Radiocapitellar arthritis and/or proximal radioulnar impingement can be difficult to treat. Interposition of the anconeus muscle has been described in the past as an alternative option in managing arthritis, but there are little published data about relief of pain and restoration of function over the long term in patients treated with this approach.

Questions/Purposes.—We sought (1) to determine whether interposition of the anconeus muscle in the radiocapitellar and/or proximal radioulnar joint relieves pain and restores elbow function; and (2) to identify complications and reoperations after anconeus interposition arthroplasty.

Methods.—Between 1992 and 2012, we surgically treated 39 patients having radiocapitellar arthritis and/or proximal radioulnar impingement with an anconeus interposition arthroplasty. These were performed for situations in which capitellar and/or radial head pathology was deemed not amenable to implant replacement. We had complete followup on 29 of them (74%) at a minimum of 1 year (mean, 10 years; range, 1–20 years). These 29 patients (21 males, eight females) had interposition of the anconeus muscle at the radiocapitellar joint (10 elbows), the proximal radioulnar joint (two elbows), or both (17 elbows). Their mean age at the time of surgery was 39 years (range, 14–58 years). The reasons for the previous determination or the indications included lateral-side elbow symptoms after radial head resection (eight elbows), failed internal fixation of radial head fracture (two elbows), failed radial head replacement with or without capitellar replacement (four elbows), osteoarthritis and Essex-Lopresti injury (six elbows), failed internal fixation of distal humeral fracture involving the capitellum (two elbows), posttraumatic osteoarthritis involving the lateral compartment (one elbow), lateral compartment osteoarthritis associated with chondropathies (three elbows), and primary osteoarthritis affecting the lateral compartment (three elbows). Patient-reported outcome tools included the quick-Disabilities of the Arm, Shoulder and Hand (quick-DASH) and the Mayo Elbow Performance Score (MEPS); we also performed a chart review for complications and reoperations.

Results.—During the followup duration, the mean MEPS was significantly improved from (mean ± SD) 64 ± 17 points before surgery to 82 ± 14 points after surgery ($p < 0.001$) with 21 elbows (72%) graded as excellent or good at most recent followup. The mean quick-DASH score was 24 ± 17 points (n = 25) at latest evaluation. Two patients (7%) had perioperative complications, including wound dehiscence (one elbow) and transient posterior interosseous nerve palsy (one elbow). Seven patients (24%) underwent additional surgery.

Conclusions.—Anconeus arthroplasty provides a reasonable surgical alternative in the armamentarium of procedures to address pathology at the radiocapitellar and/or proximal radioulnar joint. This procedure is especially attractive when other alternatives such as radial head replacement may be problematic secondary to capitellar erosion or marked proximal radius bone loss.

Level of Evidence.—Level IV, therapeutic study. See Guidelines for Authors for a complete description of levels of evidence.

► Anconeus interposition arthroplasty can alleviate pain and improve function in patients with conditions affecting the radiocapitellar and/or proximal radioulnar joint, but there is little reported in the literature on this procedure. This is an interesting article reporting on a rather large retrospective review of a cohort of 29 patients who received an anconeus interposition at the Mayo Clinic with minimum follow-up of 1 year (mean, 10 years; range, 1-20 years). The anconeus muscle was interposed in 3 ways, between the radius and ulna (type III, surrounding the proximal radius stump) in 2 elbows, between the radius and capitellum (type I) in 10 elbows, and at both locations (type II) in 17 elbows. For the interposition at both locations, the anconeus muscle was passed under the lateral collateral ligament complex after being released distally. Then the flap substance was interposed between the radius and capitellum and between the radius and ulna. The proximal portion of the anconeus was fixed to the capitellum, and the distal portion was fixed with sutures passing drill holes through the proximal radius. Additional procedures were also performed at the time of the interposition to address an undergoing pathologic process causing patient symptoms and disability. This interposition procedure was thought to provide a viable treatment option for these difficult patients in whom capitellar and/or radial head pathology was deemed not amenable to prosthetic replacement. Although the interposed anconeus did not provide much stability against valgus stress or proximal migration of the radius radiographically, it was thought to tighten the lateral collateral ligament complex. This procedure is particularly attractive for those patients with a resected or damaged radial head when replacement with a prosthesis would be problematic as a result of marked proximal radius bone loss or capitellar damage.

The mechanism by which the anconeus interposition arthroplasty provides pain relief in these complex cases is unclear. For example, if the muscle itself is still innervated, would it become a pain generator as it offsets some load bearing at the radiocapitellar and proximal radioulnar joint, and how might the muscle belly atrophy over time? Nonetheless, this is another tool the surgeon may employ in certain salvage situations.

E. Cheung, MD

Fixation Versus Replacement of Radial Head in Terrible Triad: Is There a Difference in Elbow Stability and Prognosis?

Watters TS, Garrigues GE, Ring D, et al (Duke Univ Med Ctr, Durham, NC; Massachusetts General Hosp, Boston)

Clin Orthop Relat Res 472:2128-2135, 2014

Background.—Surgical treatment for terrible triad injuries of the elbow (defined as elbow dislocations with concomitant fractures of the radial head and coronoid) remains a challenging clinical problem. Specifically, the question of whether to repair or replace the radial head remains controversial.

Questions/Purposes.—We compared patients with terrible triad injuries of the elbow whose radial head fracture was treated with either internal fixation and internal fixation (ORIF) or radial head arthroplasty in terms of (1) clinical outcome measures (DASH and Broberg-Morrey scores, ROM), (2) elbow stability and radiographic signs of arthrosis, and (3) complications and reoperation rates.

Methods.—Retrospective review identified 39 patients with terrible triad injuries and minimum 18-month complete clinical and radiographic followup (mean, 24 months; range, 18–53 months). Patients were managed with a standard algorithm consisting of (1) repair (n = 9) or replacement (n = 30) of the radial head, (2) repair of the lateral ulnar collateral ligament, and (3) repair of the coronoid fracture. During the study period, the radial head generally was internally fixed when there were fewer than four articular fragments; otherwise, it was replaced. Evaluation included the DASH score, the Broberg-Morrey index, measurements of elbow stability and motion, and radiographic assessment for signs of arthrosis; chart review was performed for complications and reoperations. Complete followup was available on 87% (39 of 45 patients).

Results.—There were no differences between groups in terms of ROM or elbow scores. All patients who underwent radial head arthroplasty at the index procedure had a stable elbow at final followup whereas three of nine patients who underwent ORIF were unstable ($p = 0.009$). However, 11 patients who underwent arthroplasty demonstrated radiographic signs of arthrosis compared to none in the ORIF group ($p = 0.04$). Eleven patients (28%) underwent reoperation (seven arthroplasty, four ORIF) for various reasons. With the numbers available, there was no difference in reoperation rate between groups ($p = 0.45$).

Conclusions.—For terrible triad injuries, radial head arthroplasty afforded the ability to obtain elbow stability with comparable overall outcomes when compared to ORIF. As these injuries commonly occur in younger patients, longer-term studies will be required to ascertain whether the apparent benefits of radial head arthroplasty are offset by late complications of arthroplasty, such as loosening.

Level of Evidence.—Level III, therapeutic study. See the Instructions for Authors for a complete description of levels of evidence.

▶ The authors performed a retrospective review of 39 patients with terrible-triad injuries of the elbow and compared the results of patients treated with open reduction and internal fixation (ORIF) of the radial head (n = 9) vs those that were treated with arthroplasty (n = 30). All patients were also treated with repair of the coronoid and repair of the lateral ulnar collateral ligament. For patients in whom the radial head was not excised, coronoid repair was approached medially. Some patients also required an additional medial approach for medial lateral ulnar collateral ligament repair (n = 2), and some required external fixation for persistent instability (n = 3). The results were reported with a minimum follow-up of 18 months, and the chart review included a comparative analysis of elbow range of motion (ROM), Disabilities of the Arm, Shoulder and Hand (DASH) score, the Broberg-Morrey index, clinical assessment of elbow stability, radiographic assessment of arthrosis, and reoperation rates.

The authors reported no difference between radial head ORIF versus arthroplasty with regard to ROM and DASH scores. However, they reported significant differences in elbow stability and radiographic signs of arthrosis. Three of 9 patients who were treated with ORIF developed instability that required reoperation, and 11 of 30 patients treated with arthroplasty demonstrated radiographic signs of arthrosis, 7 of which required reoperation. Although radial head preservation makes coronoid exposure much more difficult in most cases, I always take great care to preserve and repair the radial head whenever possible. This study provides some confirmation of my personal bias that while radial head arthroplasty can improve elbow stability in high-energy injuries, it can also contribute to potentially higher rates of posttraumatic arthrosis.

J. Tueting, MD

Terrible Triad Injuries of the Elbow: Does the Coronoid Always Need to Be Fixed?

Papatheodorou LK, Rubright JH, Heim KA, et al (Univ of Pittsburgh School of Medicine, PA)

Clin Orthop Relat Res 472:2084-2091, 2014

Background.—The "terrible triad" of the elbow is a complex injury that can lead to pain, stiffness, and posttraumatic arthritis if not appropriately treated. The primary goal of surgery for these injuries is to restore stability of the joint sufficient to permit early motion. Although most reports recommend repair and/or replacement of all coronoid and radial head fractures when possible, a recent cadaveric study demonstrated that type II coronoid fractures are stable unless the radial head is removed and not replaced.

Questions/Purposes.—The purposes of this study were to determine the (1) range of motion; (2) clinical scores using the Disabilities of the Arm, Shoulder and Hand (DASH) and the Broberg-Morrey questionnaires; and (3) rate of arthritic changes, heterotopic ossification (HO), or elbow instability postoperatively in patients whose terrible triad injuries of the elbow included Reagan-Morrey type I or II coronoid fractures that were treated without fixation.

Methods.—Between April 2008 and December 2010, 14 consecutive patients were treated for acute terrible triad injuries that included two Regan-Morrey type I and 12 Regan-Morrey type II coronoid fractures. Based on the senior author's (DGS) clinical experience that coronoid fractures classified as such do not require fixation to restore intraoperative stability to the posterolaterally dislocated elbow, all injuries were treated by the senior author with a surgical protocol that included radial head repair or prosthetic replacement and repair of the lateral ulnar collateral ligament (LUCL) followed by intraoperative fluoroscopic examination through a range of 20° to 130° of elbow flexion to confirm concentric reduction of the ulnohumeral joint. Using this protocol, intraoperative stability was confirmed in all cases without any attempt at coronoid or anterior capsular repair. Repair of the medial collateral ligament or application of external fixation was not performed in any case. All patients were available for followup at a minimum of 24 months (mean, 41 months; range, 24–56 months). The mean patient age was 52 years (range, 32–58 years). At the followup all patients were evaluated clinically and radiographically by the senior author. Outcome measures included elbow range of motion, forearm rotation, elbow stability, and radiographic evidence of HO or arthritic changes using the Broberg and Morrey scale. Elbow instability was defined as clinical or radiographic evidence of recurrent ulnohumeral dislocation or subluxation at final followup. Clinical outcomes were assessed with the patient-reported DASH questionnaire and the physician-administered Broberg-Morrey elbow rating system.

Results.—The mean arc of ulnohumeral motion at final followup was 123° (range, 75°–140°) and mean forearm rotation was 145° (range, 70°–170°). The mean Broberg and Morrey score was 90 of 100 (range, 70–100, higher scores reflecting better results) and the average DASH score was 14 of 100 (range, 0–38, higher scores reflecting poorer results). Radiographs revealed mild arthritic changes in one patient. One patient developed radiographically apparent but asymptomatic HO. None of the patients demonstrated instability postoperatively.

Conclusions.—These findings demonstrate that terrible triad injuries with type I and II coronoid process fractures can be effectively treated without fixation of coronoid fractures when repair or replacement of the radial head fracture and reconstruction of the LUCL complex sufficiently restores intraoperative stability of the elbow through a functional range of motion.

Level of Evidence.—Level IV, therapeutic study. See Guidelines to Authors for a complete description of levels of evidence.

▶ The authors presented data from a retrospective cohort study without controls based on the senior author's operative treatment of 14 consecutive patients with acute terrible-triad elbow fracture dislocations (April 2008–December 2010) with either Reagan-Morrey type I (n = 2) or type II (n = 12) coronoid fractures. This study provided the results of the surgical treatment of these injuries using radial head open reduction and internal fixation or replacement with lateral ulnar collateral ligament (LUCL) repair without coronoid fixation or anterior capsular repair. The results are reported in terms of Disabilities of the Arm, Shoulder and Hand (DASH), Broberg and Morrey score, range of motion (ROM), radiographic interpretation of instability, heterotopic ossification, and posttraumatic arthritis. At a minimum follow-up of 24 months, the authors found a good to excellent result in 13 of 14 patients, a restoration of functional ROM in all cases, no cases of late instability, and only 1 case of heterotopic ossification.

The authors challenged the concept of mandatory coronoid fixation in acute terrible-triad injuries and concluded that coronoid fixation is not always required if the radial head is fixed or replaced and the LUCL is repaired. Limitations of this study include retrospective design, no comparison group, and a relatively small number of patients. The authors admit that this study was not meant to provide therapeutic recommendations and was open to selection bias that includes a select population that may represent lower-energy injuries.

In my practice, I always proceed cautiously when treating terrible-triad injuries and have a low threshold for coronoid fixation as a means to manage even the subtlest instability. Although this study was limited to only lateral (Kaplan) approaches to the elbow, I almost always approach these injuries through a direct posterior incision to easily access both the lateral and medial stabilizing structures when necessary. Going forward, I may consider avoiding the extra soft tissue dissection that is required for coronoid fixation with the hope that this may perhaps decrease the chances for heterotopic ossification and posttraumatic arthrosis. I would only apply this type of treatment in cases of low-energy terrible-triad injuries and those without tendency toward instability and will proceed cautiously with incorporating this methodology into my current treatment algorithm.

J. Tueting, MD

Three-Tesla MR imaging of the elbow in non-symptomatic professional baseball pitchers

Del Grande F, Aro M, Farahani SJ, et al (Johns Hopkins Univ School of Medicine, Baltimore, MD; et al)

Skelet Radiol 44:115-123, 2015

Objectives.—To retrospectively evaluate the qualitative and quantitative 3-T MR imaging features of the elbow in non-symptomatic professional baseball pitchers presenting as major league draft picks or trades.

Materials and Methods.—The Institutional Review Board (IRB) approved the HIPPA-compliant study. Informed consent was waived. Twenty-one professional non-symptomatic baseball pitchers (mean age 23, range 18 to 34 years old) underwent 3-T MR imaging of the pitching elbow. Two experienced readers independently performed qualitative (collateral ligaments, tendons, cartilage, bones, ulnar nerve, olecranon fossa, and joint fluid) and quantitative (collateral ligaments and posteromedial plica) evaluation. Descriptive statistics were calculated.

Results.—Collateral ligament thickening was seen in a high proportion, nearly half, however, without features of full thickness tearing. Tendinosis without tearing was seen in 19% (4/21) of common extensors. Cartilage abnormalities were infrequent. Bone abnormalities manifested as edema in 24% (5/21) and humeroulnar osteophytosis. Ulnar nerve signal and/or morphologic abnormalities were seen in a very high proportion, up to 81% (17/21). The olceranon fat pad showed scarring features in about one third. The median ligament thicknesses in mm measured: 4.6 UCL anterior bundle, 1.8 UCL posterior bundle, 1.9 RCL, 2.5 LUCL, and 0.7 mm anular. The median plica dimensions were 5.3 by 2.2 by 2.7 mm.

Conclusion.—High-resolution 3-T MR imaging frequently shows abnormalities involving the ligaments, tendons, nerves, olecranon fat pad, and bones in non-symptomatic baseball pitchers.

▶ Magnetic resonance imaging (MRI) is one of the most important inventions in the modern medical era. As MRI has become less expensive and more available, the indications for MRI have expanded. This article presents the MRI findings in a case series of asymptomatic professional baseball players. The article reported a defined incidence of apparent pathology in these asymptomatic athletes. The findings included collateral ligament thickening in nearly half, tendinosis without tearing in 19% (4 of 21) of common extensors, bone abnormalities manifested as edema in 24% (5 of 21), and humeroulnar osteophytosis. Ulnar nerve signal or morphologic abnormalities were seen in a very high proportion, up to 81% (17 of 21). The olecranon fat pad showed scarring features in about one-third.

The article gives us a baseline value for asymptomatic findings in this high-performance group of athletes, which is useful information. Although these findings are interesting, the clinical implications remain to be seen. Because these MRIs were ordered as part of a screening physical, all potential trades and draft players would have a tendency to claim to be asymptomatic. As is commonly seen in overhead athletes, the shoulder and elbow are prone to repetitive stresses. The article does a good job of presenting the pathologic findings that one can expect to find secondary to these stresses. Unfortunately, the article fails to answer the question of why some patients are symptomatic with these identical findings while others are not. For the commentator, the article does not add important clinical information for the average physician, but it is relevant for those few physicians that treat professional sports players. The finding of frequent collateral ligament thickening may now be regarded as adaptive rather than pathologic in these high-performance athletes.

M. B. Gottschalk, MD
J. T. Capo, MD

Prevalence and Clinical Characteristics of Osteochondritis Dissecans of the Humeral Capitellum Among Adolescent Baseball Players

Kida Y, Morihara T, Kotoura Y, et al (Kyoto Prefectural Univ of Medicine, Japan; et al)

Am J Sports Med 42:1963-1971, 2014

Background.—The prevalence and clinical characteristics of osteochondritis dissecans (OCD) of the humeral capitellum among adolescent baseball players are unknown.

Purpose.—To determine the OCD prevalence in adolescent competitive baseball players and to investigate the clinical characteristics of these patients.

Study Design.—Cross-sectional and case-control study; Level of evidence, 3.

Methods.—A total of 2433 baseball players (mean age, 14.5 ± 1.5 years) belonging to junior high school and high school baseball clubs were enrolled. Players completed a questionnaire, and the elbow of each player's throwing arm was assessed by ultrasonography. Participants with abnormal results on ultrasonography were further examined through radiographic study. The OCD lesions were classified into stages based on radiographic results, and demographic data were compared between players with and without OCD lesions.

Results.—Osteochondritis dissecans of the humeral capitellum was found in 82 (3.4%) elbows by ultrasonography. Players with an OCD lesion began playing baseball at an earlier age ($P = .016$), had a longer duration of competitive play ($P = .0013$), and had experienced more present ($P = .0025$) and past ($P < .0001$) elbow pain compared with players without a lesion. There were no differences between the 2 groups in the position played ($P = .26$). Sixty-eight patients underwent further radiographic examination for OCD (radiography, computed tomography, magnetic resonance imaging). Of these players, 10 (14.7%) were classified as having stage I OCD (radiolucent stage); 26 (38.2%), stage II (fragmentation stage); 9 (13.2%), stage III (loose body stage); 9 (13.2%), stage IV (residual stage); and 14 (23.5%), stage V (postoperative stage).

Conclusion.—The prevalence of OCD of the humeral capitellum, including latent cases, was 3.4% among adolescent baseball players. Players with OCD lesions began playing baseball at earlier ages, had played for longer periods, and had experienced more elbow pain. The player's current baseball position may not be related to the existence of OCD lesions in adolescents.

► This is an insightful report regarding the prevalence of a relatively uncommon condition in a population of younger baseball players.

The report is reflective of my clinical experience in that students with the greater exposure have a higher prevalence of the condition. So intuitively, beginning at an earlier age or having a longer duration of competitive play would result in greater exposure and, thus, a higher prevalence.

Although the findings are valid, one must note that these students were selected from baseball camps. This is a select population of players who may have logged more throwing hours than the average junior high or high school baseball player. Thus, the prevalence may not be reflective of the average youth baseball player.

One key point illustrated by this report is that this condition is not exclusive to pitchers and should be considered in all players, irrespective of position.

There were some limitations of the study, which were well acknowledged by the authors. Despite this, the information is clinically useful.

J. Ortiz, Jr, MD

Risk Factors for Shoulder and Elbow Injuries in High School Baseball Pitchers: The Role of Preseason Strength and Range of Motion

Tyler TF, Mullaney MJ, Mirabella MR, et al (Pro Sports Physical Therapy, Scarsdale, NY; Lenox Hill Hosp, NY)

Am J Sports Med 42:1993-1999, 2014

Background.—Shoulder strength and motion deficits in high school baseball pitchers have been implicated in injury risk.

Purpose/Hypothesis.—To prospectively determine if preseason strength and range of motion (ROM) are predictive of injury in high school baseball pitchers. It was hypothesized that ROM asymmetries and weakness would be predictive of injury.

Study Design.—Case-control study; Level of evidence, 3.

Methods.—Preseason strength and ROM measurements were made on 101 pitchers from 4 different high schools over 4 seasons (total 166 pitcher-seasons: 25 freshman, 46 junior varsity, and 95 varsity player-seasons). Glenohumeral internal rotation (IR), glenohumeral external rotation, and posterior shoulder ROM were measured bilaterally. Strength in IR, external rotation, supraspinatus (empty-can test), and scapular retraction was measured bilaterally (handheld dynamometer). Injury incidence (injuries per 1000 pitches) was computed for players categorized as above normal (≥1 SD above the mean), normal (within 1 standard deviation of the mean), and below normal (≤1 SD below the mean) for each potential risk factor. Injury was defined as a missed game or practice because of shoulder or elbow problem.

Results.—There were 28 upper extremity injuries (19 shoulder, 9 elbow; incidence, 0.58 injuries/1000 pitches). There was a trend for supraspinatus weakness to be associated with increased injury risk (relative risk [RR], 3.60; 95% CI, 0.75-17.32; $P = .09$). When analyzing major injuries only (>3 missed games), preseason supraspinatus weakness was significantly associated with increased injury risk (RR, 4.58; 95% CI, 1.40-15.01; $P = .02$). Paradoxically, pitchers with no IR loss were at increased risk compared with pitchers with ≥20° loss (RR, 4.85; 95% CI, 1.01-23.29; $P = .04$). Other ROM and strength measures were unrelated to injury risk.

Conclusion.—Although excessive loss of IR ROM is thought to be a risk factor for injury, the opposite was the case in this study. The absence of IR ROM loss in high school pitchers may indicate inadequate prior exposure to pitching, resulting in increased injury risk. Preseason supraspinatus weakness was associated with increased risk for a major injury, and preventative supraspinatus strengthening may be beneficial.

▶ This report provides us with some insight to the relative risk of injury to the shoulder or elbow in a select population of pitchers.

The results presented are contrary to prior research that noted loss of internal rotation motion to be associated with increased injury risk. Here, the authors paradoxically find that injuries were seen more frequently in pitchers with no loss of internal rotation motion. This may be because of the younger age of the population studied compared with other studies. This can also be a consequence of the pitchers being studied earlier on the pitching curve experience than in prior studies. They may not have yet developed the adaptive change in range of motion.

In this population of pitchers, there was a trend for pitchers with supraspinatus weakness to have an increased injury risk compared with their normal-strength counterparts. This provides for an opportunity to direct preseason training to strengthen this muscle and thus minimize this risk.

J. Ortiz, Jr, MD

Transcutaneous electrical nerve stimulation as adjunct to primary care management for tennis elbow: pragmatic randomised controlled trial (TATE trial)

Chesterton LS, Lewis AM, Sim J, et al (Keele Univ, UK)

Br J Sports Med 48:1458, 2014

Study Question.—Can transcutaneous electrical nerve stimulation (TENS), as a patient controlled adjunct to primary care management for tennis elbow, provide superior pain relief to primary care management alone.

Summary Answer.—TENS conferred no additional clinical benefit over primary care management consisting of information and advice on analgesia and exercise for patients with tennis elbow, probably partly owing to poor adherence to treatment recommendations.

What is Known and What this Paper Adds.—A need exists for safe, self administered interventions to provide pain relief for patients with tennis elbow. TENS as an adjunct to primary care management failed to show any additional pain relief compared with primary care management alone.

▶ This report is a summary of a study report published in 2013 in the *British Medical Journal*. The original pragmatic, randomized, controlled trial sought to find whether primary care plus patient-controlled transcutaneous electrical nerve stimulation (TENS), as an adjunct to home therapy, is superior to only primary care management of the enigmatic condition, tennis elbow (TE). At the date of original publication, it was the largest study to investigate primary care of TE. A total of 241 adults from 38 practices in one region of Great Britain participated in the study.

The study methods are outlined in the report of the study protocol and in the original article.[1,2] The intervention described is carried out by a general practitioner. All persons were given a 2-week daily diary to record pain intensity, use of analgesics, and use of TENS (if randomly assigned to that group). Persons were randomly assigned at the first visit with the general practitioner, then measured at 6 weeks and 6 and 12 months. Both groups received primary care with instruction. Primary care is described as: (1) dissemination of publicly available written leaflet information on TE; (2) advice and education on TE and its pain; (3) avoidance of pain-producing activities, repetitive elbow extension, forceful elbow activities; (4) council on ergonomic factors of work and recreation, with advice on rest and avoidance techniques, although absolute rest was not advocated; and (5) advice regarding progressing activities and exercises once acute pain subsided.

The primary care plus TENS group received a TENS machine for use at least once a day for a preprogrammed 45-minute session for at least 6 weeks. Multiple sessions per day were allowed.

Primary outcome was pain at 6 weeks. The secondary outcomes were multiple at all time points: pain, participation in work and usual activities, illness perceptions, use of analgesics, functional limitations, symptom recurrence at 6 and

12 months, cost analysis between the groups, patient adherence, and satisfaction of treatment.

Although both groups reported a significant reduction in pain at 6 weeks and other within-group measures were significant at other time points, adherence was low in both groups. Intention-to-treat (ITT) analysis found no significant differences between the groups in relation to pain or other measures by the 12 months, with the exception of satisfaction of care and information received in the TENS group. A limitation in the study, which is reported by the authors, was the low rate of adherence for both groups. This may have contributed strongly to the lack of significant effect for both groups in the primary and secondary outcomes.

The authors note the results represent the challenges of effecting change in behavior and self-management for this diagnosis in primary care. Although the authors did not find significant result between the groups, it may have been owing to more factors than only the division between instruction and instruction plus TENS. No therapy was involved in this primary care model. From this therapist's viewpoint, one clinic visit may not be enough to effect a change. Other research questions to ask of this study: what was the follow through on effective placement of the TENS or other portions of the instruction and advice? These factors may have been larger than expected.

V. H. O'Brien, OTD, OTR/L, CHT

References

1. Chesterton LS, van der Windt DA, Sim J, et al. Transcutaneous electrical nerve stimulation for the management of tennis elbow: a pragmatic randomized controlled trial: the TATE trial (ISRCTN 87141084). *BMC Musculoskelet Disord.* 2009;10:156, file:///C:/Users/Computer/Documents/JHS.YrBk/Chesteron%20et%20al.2009.study%20protocol.TE.TENS.pdf. Accessed February 15, 2015.
2. Chesteron LS, Lewis AM, Sim J, et al. Transcutaneous electrical nerve stimulation as adjunct to primary care management for tennis elbow: pragmatic randomized controlled trial (TATE trial). *BMJ.* 2013;347:f5160, file:///C:/Users/Computer/Documents/JHS.YrBk/Chesterton%20et%20al.2013.TE.TENs%20TATE%20study.pdf. Accessed February 15, 2015.

Delayed-Onset Ulnar Neuritis After Release of Elbow Contractures: Clinical Presentation, Pathological Findings, and Treatment

Blonna D, Huffmann GR, O'Driscoll SW (Mayo Clinic, Rochester, MN; et al)

Am J Sports Med 42:2113-2121, 2014

Background.—Little information exists regarding delayed-onset ulnar neuritis (DOUN) after arthroscopic release of elbow contractures.

Purpose.—To describe, in a large cohort of patients, the clinical presentation of and risk factors for developing DOUN after arthroscopic release of elbow contractures.

Study Design.—Case-control study; Level of evidence, 3.

Methods.—A retrospective study of 565 consecutive arthroscopic releases of elbow contractures was conducted. Essentially, DOUN was defined as ulnar neuritis or neuropathy, or worsening of pre-existing ulnar nerve symptoms, that developed postoperatively in patients with normal neurological examination findings immediately after surgery. After inclusion and exclusion criteria were met, 235 contracture releases in patients who had not undergone any ulnar nerve surgery remained and were used for the analysis of risk factors with a multivariate logistic regression analysis.

Results.—Twenty-six patients (11%) developed DOUN. The patients fell into 1 of 3 distinct groups. Fifteen (58%) presented with rapidly progressive DOUN, characterized by rapidly progressive sensorimotor ulnar neuropathy, increasing pain at the cubital tunnel during end-range flexion and/or extension, and rapidly deteriorating range of motion within the first week after surgery. Urgent ulnar subcutaneous nerve transposition was performed within 1 or 2 days of diagnosis. Eight (31%) presented with nonprogressive DOUN, characterized by mild sensory ulnar neuropathy, neither motor weakness nor substantial pain at the cubital tunnel, or loss of motion. Three (12%) presented with slowly progressive DOUN, characterized by the insidious onset of mild ulnar neuropathy. Significant risk factors for DOUN included a diagnosis of heterotopic ossification (odds ratio, 31; 95% CI, 5-191; $P < .001$), preoperative neurological symptoms (odds ratio, 6; 95% CI, 2-19; $P = .001$), and preoperative arc of motion (odds ratio, 0.97 per degree of motion; 95% CI, 0.96-0.99; $P = .02$).

Conclusion.—Delayed-onset ulnar neuritis is an important complication of arthroscopic release of elbow contractures. We recommend a high index of suspicion and monitoring patients with progressive loss of elbow motion and end-range pain for evidence of subclinical ulnar neuritis.

▶ This large retrospective study by Blonna and colleagues is an important study for any surgeon who performs arthroscopic contracture release in the elbow. They describe and categorize ulnar neuritis after arthroscopic release of elbow contractors. Although the risk for neuromuscular injury after elbow arthroscopy is well known, the risk for delayed-onset ulnar neuritis (DOUN) is less widely discussed. In this study, the rate of presentation of DOUN was low but not insignificant at 11%. In this series, it was also emphasized that all these patients had normal findings on neurologic examination immediately after the surgery, so these were not a result of the surgical procedure itself and were truly a delayed phenomenon. Identified risk factors from this study included increased tourniquet time (more than 100 minutes) and larger deficits in motion preoperatively.

It is useful to realize that the presentation of DOUN is varied, with some cases progressing rapidly (58% of cases) and others progressing more slowly. The authors recommended urgent (within 48 hours of diagnosis) subcutaneous transposition for treatment of the rapid-onset cases because of their effect on motion and neurologic status. Based on these data, it is prudent to have close follow-up with these patients to assess neurologic status in the first few days after surgery. If a patient has a rapid increase in pain, numbness, and tingling and rapid loss of motion, the nerve should be transposed urgently.

All of the patients in this series followed a protocol that involved the use of a continuous passive motion (CPM) machine and a nerve catheter or single-shot regional block. No data analysis was performed on whether the use of CPM itself contributed to the development of this condition. I have not made CPM a regular part of my protocol for this procedure, and I have not identified any cases of such delayed-onset ulnar neuritis. Although my series of cases is nowhere near the size of this series, I cannot help but wonder if strapping a patient into a machine continuously for range of motion for up to 4 weeks might have some role in the development of this condition.

L. T. Kroonen, MD

Outcomes of an Open Autologous Osteochondral Plug Graft for Capitellar Osteochondritis Dissecans: Time to Return to Sports

Maruyama M, Takahara M, Harada M, et al (Yamagata Univ Faculty of Medicine, Japan; Izumi Orthopaedic Hosp, Sendai, Japan)
Am J Sports Med 42:2122-2127, 2014

Background.—Autologous osteochondral plug grafts have been used for capitellar osteochondritis dissecans (OCD), and good clinical results have been described. However, little is known about the optimal timing of return to sports.

Purpose.—To investigate the clinical outcomes of open autologous osteochondral plug grafts for capitellar OCD and to address the timing of return to sports.

Study Design.—Case series; Level of evidence, 4.

Methods.—Thirty-three male patients with a mean age at the time of surgery of 13.6 years (range, 11-17 years) and with advanced lesions of capitellar OCD underwent a procedure using open autologous osteochondral plug grafts. All patients played baseball, and the lesion affected their throwing side. Thirteen lesions were arthroscopically classified as International Cartilage Repair Society (ICRS) OCD III and 20 lesions as ICRS OCD IV. The mean size of the lesions (sagittal × coronal) was 16 × 14 mm. One to 3 osteochondral plug grafts, with a mean diameter of 7 mm (range, 5-9 mm), were harvested from the lateral femoral condyle and transplanted to the defects. Patients were allowed to begin throwing after 3 months and to return to sports after 6 months. The mean follow-up was 28.4 months (range, 12-76 months), during which elbow pain, Timmerman and Andrews scores, return to sports, and radiographs were evaluated.

Results.—After surgery, 30 patients (91%) had no elbow pain, and 3 patients (9%) had occasional mild throwing pain. The mean total arc of elbow motion increased significantly from 116° to 133° ($P < .05$). The mean Timmerman and Andrews score improved significantly from 143 to 190 ($P < .05$). All except 2 patients returned to a competitive level at which they had previously played after a mean of 6.9 months (range, 6-14 months). One patient chose another sport, and another retired from baseball after high school graduation. All patients achieved graft incorporation, and there was no postoperative enlargement of osteophytes on radiographs. One patient had mild anterior knee pain at the donor site during exercise. The remaining patients had no knee pain. The mean Lysholm score was 99.8.

Conclusion.—The results of this study indicate that an open autologous osteochondral plug graft allows a return to the previous competitive level of throwing by a mean of 7 months postoperatively.

▶ In this level 4 study, the authors report their outcomes with open autologous osteochondral plug grafts for capitellar osteochondritis dissecans. More importantly, they share their experience with time to return to sport. Graft incorporation was determined by radiographs and averaged 3.8 months. This influenced the return to sport time.

Given the younger age of this population, one question that must be asked is, does graft incorporation occur earlier than 3 months? Could CT scan be used to evaluate graft incorporation at 2 months? If these findings did show earlier healing, one could argue for earlier motion and perhaps earlier return to sport.

Additionally, their population of players affirms that osteochondritis dissecans is not a condition that only affects pitchers. In my practice, I treat baseball players who play other positions almost as frequently as pitchers.

The authors identified 7 mm to be the ideal graft plug size but don't define what is ideal about it. They mention early incorporation of the graft as being ideal with a 7-mm graft, but they used a range of sizes with an average of 7 mm. Regardless, a more than 90% return to sport is a respectable outcome.

J. Ortiz, Jr, MD

Endoscopic Cubital Tunnel Release

Fowler JR (Univ of Pittsburgh, PA)
J Hand Surg Am 39:2064-2066, 2014

Background.—Ulnar neuropathy at the elbow occurs with an incidence of 25 cases per 100,000 person-years, making it the second most common peripheral mononeuropathy of the upper extremity. Between 50,000 and 75,000 cubital tunnel decompressions are done in the United States annually, with anterior transposition, either submuscular or subcutaneous, the current standard approach. However, less invasive procedures have become more attractive, with endoscopic cubital tunnel release (ECUTR) offering an alternative to open in situ release. Appropriate equipment has been developed to permit the use of the less-invasive approach.

Patient Description.—Laborer, 48, has intermittent numbness of the little and ring fingers that he has managed with night splints and elbow pads for 3 months but with little relief. Ulnar nerve conduction velocity is 40 m/sec across the elbow, and denervation is absent. Physical examination reveals no nerve subluxation, two-point discrimination of 6 mm over the little finger, and no weakness or atrophy of the first dorsal interosseous muscle. The patient is interested in ECUTR because it offers the hope of returning to work sooner than if an open decompression is done.

Analysis.—Studies indicate high levels of success with ECUTR, usually achieving good to excellent results in 81% to 94% of patients. Most patients have complete resolution of weakness, pain, and numbness. Sensory losses are resolved, and motor conduction velocities and two-point discrimination return to normal in the majority of cases. Complication rates range from 7% to 18%. Included in the list of complications are hematoma, superficial infection, persistent symptoms, antecubital superficial thrombophlebitis, medial antebrachial cutaneous nerve paresthesia, and disproportionate pain and disability (complex regional pain syndrome). Return-to-work times are between 1 and 3 weeks. Patient satisfaction, pain, numbness, and weakness appear to be comparable between patients having ECUTR or open decompression.

The data on ECUTR must be interpreted cautiously because of the wide variety of equipment and techniques used as well as the fact that most studies are small, retrospective case series that involve patients whose disease severity and duration of symptoms vary considerably. In addition, many measures of success are subjective, including patient satisfaction, return-to-work times, and the need for repeat surgery. No prospective, randomized trials compare treatment options.

Recommendations.—For the patient described, open in situ cubital tunnel release would be the best option. The slightly smaller incision, earlier return to work, and greater patient satisfaction associated with ECUTR are statistically and clinically insignificant and subject to surgeon and patient bias. ECUTR requires greater use of resources and carries an unknown risk of nerve injury. High-volume centers and surgeons who have created devices and techniques will likely have higher rates of safety and efficacy using ECUTR than most centers and surgeons. Reliably good results and acceptable return-to-work times can be achieved with the standard open in situ release.

▶ The author gives an expert opinion in conjunction with a literature review of endoscopic cubital tunnel and assesses in his opinion if endoscopic cubital tunnel release is an approach he would use in his own patient compared with an open in situ decompression of the ulnar nerve. One small study comparing 20 patients with endoscopic cubital tunnel with those with open in situ decompression was cited with no difference in outcome. Dutzmann et al[1] also compared a larger study of 114 patients with endoscopic vs open cubital tunnel and found no significant difference in the outcomes of recovery and pain postoperatively.

The return-to-work data for the controls of many of the endoscopic studies are historical data based on an open anterior subcutaneous transposition, which is not a similar comparison to an open in situ decompression. Further larger studies comparing endoscopic with open in situ decompression are needed, including cost, return to work, patient satisfaction, and recovery time analyses.

C. Heinrich, MD

Reference

1. Dützmann S, Martin KD, Sobottka S, et al. Open vs retractor-endoscopic in situ decompression of the ulnar nerve in cubital tunnel syndrome: a retrospective cohort study. *Neurosurgery.* 2013;72:605-616.

Non-surgical treatment of lateral epicondylitis: a systematic review of randomized controlled trials

Sims SEG, Miller K, Elfar JC, et al (Univ of Rochester Med Ctr, NY; Univ of Rochester School of Medicine and Dentistry, NY)
Hand 9:419-446, 2014

Background.—Non-surgical approaches to treatment of lateral epicondylitis are numerous. The aim of this systematic review is to examine randomized, controlled trials of these treatments.

Methods.—Numerous databases were systematically searched from earliest records to February 2013. Search terms included "lateral epicondylitis," "lateral elbow pain," "tennis elbow," "lateral epicondylalgia," and "elbow tendinopathy" combined with "randomized controlled trial." Two reviewers examined the literature for eligibility via article abstract and full text.

Results.—Fifty-eight articles met eligibility criteria: (1) a target population of patients with symptoms of lateral epicondylitis; (2) evaluation of treatment of lateral epicondylitis with the following non-surgical techniques: corticosteroid injection, injection technique, iontophoresis, botulinum toxin A injection, prolotherapy, platelet-rich plasma or autologous blood injection, bracing, physical therapy, shockwave therapy, or laser therapy; and (3) a randomized controlled trial design. Lateral epicondylitis is a condition that is usually self-limited. There may be a short-term pain relief advantage found with the application of corticosteroids, but no demonstrable long-term pain relief. Injection of botulinum toxin A and prolotherapy are superior to placebo but not to corticosteroids, and botulinum toxin A is likely to produce concomitant extensor weakness. Platelet-rich plasma or autologous blood injections have been found to be both more and less effective than corticosteroid injections. Non-invasive treatment methods such as bracing, physical therapy, and extracorporeal shockwave therapy do not appear to provide definitive benefit regarding pain relief. Some studies of low-level laser therapy show superiority to placebo whereas others do not.

Conclusions.—There are multiple randomized controlled trials for non-surgical management of lateral epicondylitis, but the existing literature does not provide conclusive evidence that there is one preferred method of non-surgical treatment for this condition. Lateral epicondylitis is a condition that is usually self-limited, resolving over a 12- to 18-month period without treatment.

Level of Evidence.—Therapeutic Level II. See Instructions to Authors for a complete description of level of evidence.

▶ Patients with lateral epicondylitis are seen frequently in the orthopedic surgeon's clinic, and often the visit is equally frustrating for the patient and the treating physician. Symptoms are generally self-limited but may take 12 to 18 months to resolve without intervention. The authors performed a systematic review and meta-analysis of double-blind, randomized, controlled trials and single-blind studies that evaluate nonoperative treatment techniques for symptomatic lateral epicondylitis. Despite the inherent limitations of a meta-analysis, the authors have provided meaningful conclusions that continue to support the challenges in treating this irritating problem. There is no single intervention that has proven superior in resolving the symptoms associated with this condition. In my practice, I continue to use several of these treatments including anti-inflammatories, bracing, and physical therapy. Although there is no definitive evidence to support bracing or physical therapy, the risks of treatment are minimal in my opinion. My use of corticosteroid injections has continued to decrease for this diagnosis, especially in light of the newer studies that have indicated a worse prognosis at 1 year compared with placebo or the wait-and-see approach.[1,2] Despite the high level of evidence in the analyzed studies, physicians are left without a definitive nonoperative treatment solution. Perhaps education, observation, and reassurance should become the mainstay of management.

A. Moeller, MD

References

1. Bisset L, Beller E, Jull G, Brooks P, Darnell R, Vicenzino B. Mobilisation with movement and exercise, corticosteroid injection, or wait and see for tennis elbow: randomised trial. *BMJ*. 2006;333:939.
2. Coombes BK, Bisset L, Brooks P, Khan A, Vicenzino B. Effect of corticosteroid injection, physiotherapy, or both on clinical outcomes in patients with unilateral lateral epicondylalgia: a randomized controlled trial. *JAMA*. 2013;309:461-469.

Medial Collateral Ligament of the Elbow: Acute Deterioration in Throwing Athletes

Stachowicz RZ, Agnoda AM, Baratz ME (Crystal Clinic Orthopaedic Ctr, Akron, OH; Orthopaedic Specialist UPMC, Bethel Park, PA)

J Hand Surg Am 39:1603-1605, 2014

Background.—Medial collateral ligament (MCL) insufficiency generally occurs only in elite throwing athletes. It commonly manifests as acute deterioration, but actually results from long-term attenuation with acute symptoms, perhaps related to failure of the remaining ligament. Nonsurgical or surgical treatments are available, but fewer than 50% of overhead athletes with acute or chronic MCL insufficiency perform at previous levels.

Nonsurgical Management.—Nonsurgical treatment requires an average of 24 weeks. The two-stage program includes 3 months of rest plus stretching exercises to improve elbow extension, then a stage of strengthening exercises for all muscle groups in the upper extremity followed 12 weeks of graduated throwing.

Surgical Management.—Ligament repair has yielded mixed results. Good to excellent outcomes have been achieved in 69% of athletes with acute symptoms and 31% of those with chronic symptoms, or between 50% and 70% of those treated.

Among the ligament reconstruction techniques are a figure-of-8 palmaris longus tendon graft technique with detachment of the flexor-pronator mass and submuscular ulnar nerve transposition; modification to retract the humeral head of the flexor carpi ulnaris to expose the sublime tubercle and use a subcutaneous rather than submuscular ulnar nerve transposition; a muscle-splitting approach to the MCL with the graft passed through an anterior humeral tunnel; and a docking technique without ulnar nerve transposition and using a muscle-splitting technique. Systematic reviews of MCL reconstruction report return to play percentages between 68% and 92% overall, with 31% to 65% among professional athletes. Returning to throwing status required 4 months and returning to play status, 12 months. The best results are achieved with the muscle-splitting approach (70% to 87% excellent results); the docking technique, which uses a three-strand graft with double anterior bundle (90% excellent results); and a modified docking technique (95% excellent results). Graft choice has not altered return to play results. Systematic reviews reveal that patients who had previous surgery have poorer chances for excellent recovery than those having reconstruction only.

Complications.—Dysfunction is the most common complication, occurring in 2% to 5% of recent series where the nerve was transposed subcutaneously or left in situ. The largest series had a 20% complication rate, including a 16% incidence of ulnar nerve neuropathy. However, most patients with ulnar nerve dysfunction recover within 6 weeks and nearly all within 1 year. Ulnar nerve dysfunction does not alter return to play time.

Recommendations.—Athletes with chronic attenuation should be treated nonsurgically, with rest until pain and tenderness resolve, flexor-pronator mass strengthening, and a throwing program emphasizing proper mechanics and lower-body strengthening. Elite throwing athletes with acute deterioration require reconstruction. Ulnar collateral ligament (UCL) repair is recommended for pediatric patients with symptomatic avulsion fracture of the medial epicondyle. The preferred surgical technique detaches the humeral but not the ulnar head of the flexor carpi ulnaris and uses a double docking technique and two-strand palmaris longus graft, leaving the ulnar nerve in situ. Elbow splinting is advised for 2 weeks, then a hinge brace and stretching exercises are begun. Flexor pronator mass strengthening begins 6 to 8 weeks after surgery; throwing is initiated 3 to 4 months after surgery, aiming for a return to play in 9 to 12 months.

▶ The authors share a relatively uncommon yet clinically challenging condition. Among the many technical aspects that need to be addressed, patients' realistic expectations stand out as the most significant concern.

Like the authors, I favor a conservative approach to throwers with chronic insufficiency. Surgically, I prefer a muscle splitting technique. I have also achieved improved results with distal humeral docking and have found this easier to perform. I have evolved to leaving the ulnar nerve in situ, and, as reported, I have found fewer unlar nerve concerns. I prefer the palmaris longus for my graft, but when absent, I have found success with a split semitendinosis graft.

Whether treated conservatively or surgically, having an honest discussion with the patient about the risks, outcomes, and time investment is paramount. With such a discussion, it is not unusual to find an athlete that is willing to discontinue throwing in one sport, so that they can be ready to participate in a different nonthrowing sport.

J. Ortiz, Jr, MD

Postoperative Ulnar Neuropathy is not Necessarily Iatrogenic: A Prospective Study on Dynamic Ulnar Nerve Dislocation at The Elbow

Billmann FG, Bokor-Billmann TT, Burnett CA, et al (St. Vincentius Kliniken, Karlsruhe, Germany; Universitätsklinikum Freiburg, Freiburg im Breisgau, Germany)

World J Surg 38:1978-1983, 2014

Background.—Patients who undergo surgery may develop ulnar neuropathy. Although the mechanism of ulnar neuropathy is still not clear, ulnar neuropathies are common causes of successful lawsuits against surgeons. Recently, the concept developed that endogenous patient factors can lead to postoperative peripheral neuropathies. We hypothesize that dynamic ulnar nerve dislocation at the elbow (DUNDE) may be a predisposing factor for ulnar irritation (i.e. neuropathy) in normal subjects.

Methods.—In a prospective investigation, patients aged 20 years and older presenting in our emergency department were asked to participate. Three physicians examined both elbows of subjects included in our study for evidence of DUNDE (through clinical and sonographic examination) and for clinical symptoms related to ulnar neuropathy.

Results.—Dynamic ulnar nerve dislocation was observed in 29.3 % of examined subjects. No significant difference in its occurrence was observed in relation to gender or dominant side. Physical examination with provocation tests demonstrated significantly more positive Tinel tests and spontaneous signs of neuropathy in patients with dynamic dislocating ulnar nerves (14.7 vs. 1.1 %).

Conclusion.—Dynamic ulnar nerve dislocation may be linked to ulnar nerve irritability (i.e. ulnar neuropathy) in normal subjects without history of trauma, surgical procedure, or anesthesia. Considering the high incidence of this variant in the general population, our study supports previous investigations suggesting that many postoperative ulnar nerve deficits are traceable to chronic patient conditions. Our study suggests that dynamic ulnar nerve dislocation is a predisposing factor in the development of ulnar neuropathy in the postoperative period.

Notes.—(1) neuropathy should be viewed as a broad definition as signs of nerve irritation/inflammation, and independently of the pathophysiology and etiology; (2) because no specific term exists in the international anatomic nomenclature (Nomina Anatomica) to designate this variant, several synonyms have been used in the literature, leading to confusion and misleading conclusions concerning its traumatic etiologies and their consequences: (a) recurrent or habitual ulnar nerve luxation (or subluxation); (b) recurrent or habitual ulnar nerve dislocation; (c) ulnar nerve instability; (d) laxity of the ulnar nerve; and (e) ulnar nerve hypermobility.

▶ The authors present a prospective clinical anatomy study in which they evaluate the incidence of dynamic ulnar nerve dislocation in the general population of patients not presenting with ulnar nerve-related symptoms. The diagnosis of dynamic ulnar nerve dislocation was made based on clinical examination as well as ultrasound scan of the nerve. The incidence of dynamic ulnar nerve dislocation reported in a study of 1235 patients was 29.3%, and the incidence of ulnar nerve neuropathy was 17.5% in dislocating ulnar nerves compared with 1.4% in nondislocating ulnar nerves. Although the authors try to associate the high incidence of dynamic ulnar nerve dislocation with postoperative ulnar nerve neuropathy based on this study, it is a difficult to draw that conclusion. However, this study shows that there is a high incidence of undiagnosed dynamic ulnar nerve instability in the population that should be recognized and considered in the preoperative evaluation of patients.

C. Heinrich, MD

Clinical Results After Arthroscopic Treatment for Septic Arthritis of the Elbow Joint

Moon J-G, Bilaris S, Jeong W-K, et al (Korea Univ Guro Hosp, Seoul)
Arthroscopy 30:673-678, 2014

Purpose.—The purpose of this study was to examine clinical findings of septic arthritis of the elbow joint in a series of immunocompetent patients and to evaluate the outcomes after arthroscopic treatment.

Methods.—Between October 2006 and January 2012, 11 patients with septic arthritis of the elbow underwent arthroscopic surgery. History, laboratory findings, and radiologic findings were reviewed. Functional outcomes were evaluated using the Mayo Elbow Performance Score (MEPS).

Results.—The study included 5 men and 6 women with a mean age of 45 years. An underlying medical disease was present in 1 patient (diabetes). *Staphylococcus aureus* was the most common organism identified (5 patients). There was 1 reoperation and no complications related to the arthroscopic procedure. Eight of 11 patients had excellent results assessed by MEPS at the final follow-up. The mean MEPS was 94.5 at the final follow-up.

Conclusions.—Septic arthritis of the elbow joint can occur in otherwise healthy patients without pre-existing elbow disease. Arthroscopic irrigation and synovectomy are safe and effective in patients with septic arthritis and result in good functional outcomes.

Level of Evidence.—Level IV, therapeutic case series.

▶ This retrospective case series of patients with septic arthritis of the elbow treated with arthroscopic irrigation and debridement describes an experience with a difficult but uncommon clinical problem, for which there is limited guidance in the literature.

The study is notable for the presentation of 11 healthy patients who had septic arthritis without preexisting elbow pathology. This report serves as a reminder that septic arthritis of the elbow must be considered in patients with acute elbow joint pain, effusion, and limited range or motion, even in the absence of identifiable risk factors. A synovial fluid white blood cell count greater than 50 000 cells per microliter and positive cultures were not present in all patients in this series. Therefore, a high index of suspicion should be maintained, and the synovial fluid cell count and cultures should both be used to make the diagnosis of septic arthritis in the elbow.

Interestingly, all of the patients in this series had either ultrasound scan or MRI, in addition to a standard elbow X-ray series. The authors describe these studies as confirming the presence of a fluid collection in or around the elbow joint. It would be helpful to know whether the ultrasound scan and MRI studies changed or informed the management of these patients.

The technique described for arthroscopic management of septic arthritis of the elbow includes a thorough synovectomy and debridement of the joint. Reassuringly, the only complication reported was reoperation in one patient at 4 weeks, which supports the safety of arthroscopic management of this infection. The average length of admission (15 days) did seem long when compared with the average 2-week course of intravenous antibiotics. In the discussion, the authors note the potential advantages of home intravenous antibiotic therapy. Further investigation on the length of inpatient and outpatient antibiotic therapy needed to treat septic arthritis of the elbow would be beneficial.

E. Kinnucan, MD

The Fascial Elevation and Tendon Origin Resection Technique for the Treatment of Chronic Recalcitrant Medial Epicondylitis

Kwon BC, Kwon YS, Bae KJ (Hallym Univ Sacred Heart Hosp, Anyang, South Korea; Hallym Univ Chuncheon Sacred Heart Hosp, South Korea)

Am J Sports Med 42:1731-1737, 2014

Background.—Medial epicondylitis is a tendinopathy of the common flexor-pronator origin, and surgical treatment is required when this condition fails to respond to nonoperative methods. This study details the development of a new technique, termed fascial elevation and tendon origin resection (FETOR), which facilitates the complete visualization and resection of the CFPO with limited soft tissue dissection.

Purpose.—To evaluate the outcomes of FETOR for the treatment of chronic recalcitrant medial epicondylitis.

Study Design.—Case series; Level of evidence, 4.

Methods.—The electronic medical records of patients who underwent FETOR from January 2008 to July 2011 were retrospectively reviewed. Outcome assessments included the visual analog scale (VAS) for average pain, pain at rest, and pain experienced during hard work or heavy lifting; the Disabilities of the Arm, Shoulder and Hand (DASH) questionnaire; and pain-free grip strength. Preoperative and postoperative data were compared.

Results.—A total of 22 elbows in 20 patients with a mean age of 48.8 years (range, 29-58 years) were included. At a mean follow-up of 35.6 months (range, 16-77 months), the VAS score decreased by 93% for average pain, 94% for pain at rest, and 83% for pain during hard work or heavy lifting ($P < .001$). The patients' perception of arm function as assessed using the DASH recovered to the level of the healthy population (from a mean of 51.6 ± 18.0 to 8.0 ± 11.1; $P < .001$). The mean pain-free grip strength improved significantly from 53.7% ± 30.3% to 97.3% ± 19.8% of the uninvolved arm ($P < .001$). Eighteen (90%) patients were satisfied with the surgical outcomes, while 2 patients changed their jobs because of decreased elbow function. No major complications occurred.

Conclusion.—The FETOR technique is an effective and safe method for the treatment of chronic recalcitrant medial epicondylitis.

▶ The authors present a retrospective case series of patients who underwent a limited surgical approach with fascial elevation and tendon origin resection for treatment of medial epicondylitis. All patients had diagnosis based on clinical examination and ultrasound scan to identify the degenerate tendon origin and had 3 months of nonoperative treatment. This study tries to correlate with historical controls of other studies; however, the other studies looked primarily at pain and grip strength but did not use the Disabilities of the Arm, Shoulder and Hand (DASH) or other standardized evaluations, which makes it difficult to compare.

Overall, the authors were able to show significant improvement in pain, motion, and DASH score postoperatively in this small study group. However, conclusions as to whether it is better than the Jobe approach or the Nirschl technique cannot be drawn from this study.

C. Heinrich, MD

Long-term Outcomes After Ulnar Collateral Ligament Reconstruction in Competitive Baseball Players: Minimum 10-Year Follow-up

Osbahr DC, Cain EL Jr, Raines BT, et al (Orlando Health Orthopedic Inst, FL; American Sports Medicine Inst, Birmingham, AL; Univ of Alabama at Birmingham School of Medicine)

Am J Sports Med 42:1333-1342, 2014

Background.—Ulnar collateral ligament reconstruction (UCLR) has afforded baseball players with excellent results; however, previous studies have described only short-term outcomes.

Purpose.—To evaluate long-term outcomes after UCLR in baseball players.

Study Design.—Case series; Level of evidence, 4.

Methods.—All UCLRs performed on competitive baseball players with a minimum 10-year follow-up were identified. Surgical data were collected prospectively and patients were surveyed by telephone follow-up, during which scoring systems were used to assess baseball career and post—baseball career outcomes.

Results.—Of 313 patients, 256 (82%) were contacted at an average of 12.6 years; 83% of these baseball players (90% pitchers) were able to return to the same or higher level of competition in less than 1 year, but results varied according to preoperative level of play. Baseball career longevity was 3.6 years in general and 2.9 years at the same or higher level of play, but major and minor league players returned for longer than did collegiate and high school players after surgery ($P < .001$). Baseball retirement typically occurred for reasons other than elbow problems (86%). Many players had shoulder problems (34%) or surgery (25%) during their baseball career, and these occurrences most often resulted in retirement attributable to shoulder problems ($P < .001$). For post—baseball career outcomes, 92% of patients were able to throw without pain, and 98% were still able to participate in throwing at least on a recreational level. The 10-year minimum follow-up scores (mean ± standard deviation) for the Disabilities of the Arm, Shoulder and Hand (DASH), DASH work module, and DASH sports module were 0.80 ± 4.43, 1.10 ± 6.90, and 2.88 ± 11.91, respectively. Overall, 93% of patients were satisfied, with few reports of persistent elbow pain (3%) or limitation of function (5%).

Conclusion.—Long-term follow-up of UCLRs in baseball players indicates that most patients were satisfied, with few reports of persistent elbow pain or limitation of function. During their baseball career, most of these athletes were able to return to the same or higher level of competition in less than 1 year, with acceptable career longevity and retirement typically for reasons other than the elbow. According to a standardized disability and outcome scale, patients also had excellent results after UCLR during daily, work, and sporting activities.

▶ Osbahr et al provide what will prove to be a landmark study for the outcomes of ulnar collateral ligament (UCL) reconstruction in a throwing population. They provided a minimum 10-year follow-up on more than 250 baseball players, the majority being pitchers, and were able to provide hard numbers that are encouraging for the elbow surgeon with more than 80% of athletes and 90% of pitchers able to return to the same or higher level of play.

One of the weaknesses of the study is that the series presented was that of a single, very experienced surgeon, using a figure-of-8 autograft technique and a consistent rehabilitation protocol. My personal preference for this surgery has been for an anatomic reconstruction using a docking technique. In this study, although all patients underwent a figure-of-8 technique procedure, the data analysis did not suggest any difference based on graft choice, and it would be reasonable to assume that results with a docking technique would be similarly promising.

Surprisingly, the need for concomitant procedures at the time of UCL reconstruction did not seem to affect overall outcome. However, as the authors astutely point out, it is important to stratify these additional conditions. The outcomes for a player with concomitant injury of the flexor-pronator musculature is much poorer, whereas concomitant debridement of olecranon osteophytes would be expected to do well.

The other important correlation is with shoulder pathology. In this series, more than one-third of players had associated shoulder pathology, and although the reason for retirement was rarely related to elbow pathology (10%), the shoulder played a role in more than twice that (24%). Thus, thorough assessment and treatment for shoulder pathology in these athletes might be more critical to their overall longevity than their elbow, which almost universally does well.

At least in the hands of the authors, this article confirms that UCL reconstruction is a successful and durable operation that will more often than not be successful in returning a player to baseball.

L. T. Kroonen, MD

Radial Head Reconstruction in Elbow Fracture-Dislocation: Monopolar or Bipolar Prosthesis?

Hartzler RU, Morrey BF, Steinmann SP, et al (San Antonio Orthopaedic Group, TX; Mayo Clinic Rochester, MN; et al)

Clin Orthop Relat Res 472:2144-2150, 2014

Background.—Monopolar and bipolar radial head prosthetic arthroplasties have been used successfully to treat elbow fracture-dislocation with unsalvageable radial head fractures. The relative stability of these two designs in different clinical situations is a topic of ongoing investigation.

Questions/Purposes.—We tested the effects of monopolar and bipolar fixed-neck prosthetic radial head implants on improvement in elbow coronal and axial plane laxity in a terrible triad biomechanical model that accounted for lateral collateral ligament integrity and the presence of a transverse coronoid fracture.

Methods.—Kinematic data were collected on six fresh-frozen cadaveric upper extremities tested with passive motion throughout the flexion arc. Varus and valgus gravity stress were applied with the wrist in neutral position. A lateral collateral ligament reconstruction was simulated. We assessed instability after radial head resection and reconstruction with either a monopolar or bipolar implant in the presence of a transversely fractured (Regan and Morrey Type 2) or fixed coronoid process.

Results.—With collateral ligament integrity, no difference was detected, with the numbers available, in valgus laxity between implants under valgus stress ($p = 1.0$). Laxity improvement with each prosthesis was higher when the coronoid was fractured (mean ± SD: monopolar: 7.4° ± 1.6°, $p < 0.001$; bipolar: 6.4° ± 1.6°, $p = 0.003$) than when it was fixed (monopolar: 4.0° ± 1.6°, $p = 0.02$; bipolar: 4.2° ± 1.6°, $p = 0.01$). With the numbers available, there was no difference in external rotation laxity between implants under valgus stress ($p = 1.0$). The greatest stabilizing effect of the prostheses occurred when the coronoid was fractured (monopolar: 3.3° ± 1.2°, $p = 0.15$; bipolar: 3.3° ± 1.2°, $p = 0.17$). Radial head arthroplasty offered no substantial stability under varus stress for varus or internal rotation laxity.

Conclusions.—In our terrible triad cadaveric model, coronoid fixation was effective in improving varus laxity with a monopolar or bipolar prosthesis in place. Also, both types of prostheses were effective in improving valgus and external rotation laxity to the elbow, regardless of coronoid status. With collateral ligaments reconstructed, no large kinematic differences were noted between implants regardless of the varus-valgus position or whether the coronoid was fractured or fixed.

Clinical Relevance.—The data from our cadaveric model support the use of either implant type in terrible triad injuries if the collateral ligaments are intact or reconstructed.

► Elbow stability can be difficult to achieve in the setting of complex elbow trauma. However, unless stability is achieved, early range of motion cannot begin, resulting in a guarded prognosis for the patient. Radial head arthroplasty is commonly used to address the unreconstructable radial head fracture, and this study aims to test 2 of the more commonly used prosthesis types. This study used a clinically relevant biomechanical model, one in which the lateral collateral ligaments were repaired, with or without coronoid fixation. The authors' conclusions are sound; they stress the clinical insignificance of differences in joint angle of only a degree even though they may have achieved statistical significance. They also make note of concerns related to cost of the various prosthesis and report that their data do not support the use of a more expensive implant for the injuries simulated in their study. Consideration must be given to the fact that stability was only tested with the wrist in neutral rotation, and effects of pronation and supination were not evaluated. Additionally, the simulated lateral collateral repair, which was performed as a lateral epicondyle osteotomy, is likely more robust than the typical repair after a traumatic injury. Personally, I have not used a bipolar implant. I have been happy with the monoblock design but must emphasize the importance of achieving stability before leaving the operating room so that early range of motion can begin. I believe that this is the key to the successful outcomes, and unless a large-scale randomized trial is performed, we will likely be unable to identify any significant differences between the prosthesis types.

R. Grewal, MD

Deficits in Glenohumeral Passive Range of Motion Increase Risk of Elbow Injury in Professional Baseball Pitchers: A Prospective Study

Wilk KE, Macrina LC, Fleisig GS, et al (Champion Sports Medicine, Birmingham, AL; American Sports Medicine Inst, Birmingham, AL)

Am J Sports Med 42:2075-2081, 2014

Background.—Injuries to the elbow joint in baseball pitchers appear common. There appears to be a correlation between shoulder range of motion and elbow injuries.

Purpose.—To prospectively determine whether decreased ROM of the throwing shoulder is correlated with the onset of elbow injuries in professional baseball pitchers.

Study Design.—Cohort study; Level of evidence, 2.

Methods.—For 8 consecutive years (2005-2012), passive range of motion of both the throwing and nonthrowing shoulders of all major and minor league pitchers within a single professional baseball organization were measured by using a bubble goniometer during spring training. In total, 505 examinations were conducted on 296 pitchers. Glenohumeral external rotation and internal rotation were assessed in the supine position with the arm at 90° of abduction and in the plane of the scapula. The scapula was stabilized per methods previously established. Total rotation was defined as the sum of external rotation and internal rotation. Passive shoulder flexion was assessed with the subject supine and the scapula stabilized per methods previously established. Elbow injuries and days missed because of elbow injuries were assessed and recorded by the medical staff of the team. Throwing and nonthrowing shoulder measurements were compared by using Student *t* tests; 1-tailed Fisher exact tests were performed to identify significant associations between shoulder motion and elbow injury. Nominal logistic regression was performed to determine the odds of elbow injury.

Results.—Significant differences were noted during side-to-side comparisons within subjects. There were 49 elbow injuries and 8 surgeries in 38 players, accounting for a total of 2551 days missed. Neither glenohumeral internal rotation deficit nor external rotation insufficiency was correlated with elbow injuries. Pitchers with deficits of >5° in total rotation in their throwing shoulders had a 2.6 times greater risk for injury. Pitchers with deficit of ≥5° in flexion of the throwing shoulder had a 2.8 times greater risk for injury.

Conclusion.—Bilateral differences in shoulder total rotation and flexion had a significant effect on the risk for elbow injuries in pitchers. Clinicians need to be aware of these findings and plan preventive programs that address these issues in hopes of reducing elbow injuries.

► This is an interesting article. An association between decreased passive shoulder range of motion and presence of elbow injury was found to be significant. This is of great clinical significance because it suggests the possibility of developing a prevention program by increasing shoulder range of motion in those players who may be at risk. The study's main strength is the prospective characteristic and thorough follow-up. In addition, the study represents a large cohort of patients. Its main weakness is that the only measure of the severity of injury is represented as days on the disabled list. Another weakness is that passive range of motion was measured before any exercise, warm-up, or throwing activities. This might not represent the true passive shoulder range of motion that is present during the real injury phase. Nonetheless, if stretching exercises and increasing passive range of motion could potentially avoid elbow injury, it should be recommended to any throwing athlete, and this is now among the things I recommend my patients to do.

J. P. Simone, MD

Selective 360° Percutaneous Extensor Carpi Radialis Brevis Tendon Release for Tennis Elbow: An Experimental Study

Capa-Grasa A, Rojo-Manaute JM, Rodriguez-Maruri G, et al (Univ Hosp La Paz, Madrid, Spain; Hosp Gregorio Marañón, Madrid, Spain; et al)

J Ultrasound Med 31:1193-1201, 2012

Objectives.—The purpose of this study was to define in volunteers and cadavers the positions of structures at risk and the extensor carpi radialis brevis (ECRB) origin limits for sonographically guided percutaneous tendon release in tennis elbow.

Methods.—First, in volunteers, we used Doppler sonography to determine the position (danger zone) of the structures at risk (neurovascular bundle and radial collateral ligament) from the most lateral point of the epicondyle (point of entry). Second, in cadavers, we studied the footprint of the ECRB's origin for finally performing sonographically guided tendon release (1- to 2-mm incision) away from the danger zone. Efficacy was measured in terms of detachment ratios for the ECRB and safety as the absence of neurovascular bundle or radial collateral ligament injuries.

Results.—In 10 volunteers (20 elbows), the neurovascular bundle was located 18.1 mm or greater anteromedially from the point of entry. The neurovascular bundle was not in direct contact with the bone. In 13 formaldehyde-embalmed cadaver elbows, the distance between the origin of the ECRB and the radial collateral ligament was 0 mm or greater. The anterior origin of the ECRB did not contact the neurovascular bundle. The maximum attachment limits of the ECRB were at 15, 5, 15, and 16 mm from the point of entry (anterior, posterior, proximal, and distal margins, respectively). Average detachment ratios were excellent for anterior and distal margins and good for posterior and proximal margins, without neurovascular bundle or radial collateral ligament injuries.

Conclusions.—This study determined a danger zone to avoid and an area of probability in which to enclose most of the ECRB's origin for sonographically guided percutaneous tendon release. A 360° ECRB detachment can be performed safely and effectively. Clinically, sonographically guided percutaneous tendon release should selectively target pathologic regions.

▶ This interesting original study was performed in Madrid, Spain, and reported in the *Journal of Ultrasound Medicine*. The article actually represents 2 separate studies, a descriptive anatomic study and an experimental or interventional study. The purpose of these 2 separate limbs was (1) to define in healthy volunteers the anatomic boundaries where a percutaneous extensor carpi radialis brevis (ECRB) detachment may be performed safely and (2) to perform sonographically guided percutaneous tendon release of the ECRB's origin in cadavers and determine its safety and efficacy.

To define critical structures at risk including the radial recurrent vessels, radial nerve, radial collateral ligament, and posterior cutaneous nerves, Doppler sonography was used to determine the position or danger zone of the aforementioned structures at risk from the most lateral point of the epicondyle (point of entry). Second, in cadavers, the authors studied the footprint of the ECRB's origin for finally performing sonographically guided tendon release (1- to 2-mm incision) away from the danger zone. The authors report that efficacy was measured in terms of detachment ratios (DR) for the ECRB and safety as the absence of neurovascular bundle or radial collateral ligament injuries. The authors' DRs were as follows: excellent (≥0.85), good (0.75–0.84), fair (0.75–0.84), poor (<0.65), and very poor and unsafe (neurovascular or radial collateral ligament injury).

With regard to the descriptive portion of the study, I applaud the authors for recognizing the potential lack of precision and complications of blind percutaneous techniques that have been recently been reported. In this study, the authors attribute an etiologic role to the ECRB and offer a detailed analysis regarding a safe zone to perform a percutaneous release. Specifically, the authors report that the maximum attachment limits of the ECRB were at 15, 5, 15, and 16 mm from the point of entry (anterior, posterior, proximal, and distal margins, respectively).

In the intervention portion of this study, 12 patients each with >3 months' follow-up were reported. They exhibited relatively rapid return of range of motion, strength, improved pain, subjective improvement, and no documented complications. Based on these data, the authors assert the efficacy, safety, and accuracy of sonographically guided surgery as a promising alternative for hand surgery in the ambulatory setting.

In sum, this is a useful study that identifies a safe zone for percutaneous release of the ECRB tendon in the treatment of tennis elbow. Unfortunately, to perform this procedure with equal efficacy as was reported in this study, the operator must be skilled in ultrasound principles, including the identification of critical structures as well as percutaneous release based on real-time ultrasonography. According to the authors, future randomized controlled studies are underway. It will be interesting to view the results of this technique vs that of standard open and arthroscopic tennis-elbow debridements.

S. M. Jacoby, MD

Radiocapitellar Joint Contact Pressures Following Radial Head Arthroplasty

Cohn M, Glait SA, Sapienza A, et al (NYU Hosp for Joint Diseases)
J Hand Surg Am 39:1566-1571, 2014

Purpose.—To determine the radial head arthroplasty length that best replicates the native radiocapitellar contact pressure.

Methods.—Eight cadaveric elbows (4 matched pairs) with an average age of 73 years were tested. All specimens were ligamentously stable and without visible cartilage wear. Radiocapitellar contact pressures were digitally analyzed during simulated joint loading at 0°, 45°, and 90° of elbow flexion and neutral rotation in the intact specimens and after ligament-preserving radial head arthroplasty at -2 mm, 0 mm, and +2 mm of the native length. The results were analyzed using 1-way analysis of variance and post hoc Tukey pairwise comparison tests.

Results.—Paired analysis demonstrated significantly decreased mean contact pressures when comparing the native versus the minus 2 groups. Significantly decreased maximum contact pressures were also noted between the native and the minus 2 groups. Examining the mean contact pressures showed no significant difference between the native and the zero group and the native and the plus 2 groups. As for the maximum contact pressures, there was also no significant difference between the native and the zero group and the native and the plus 2 group.

Conclusions.—Up to 2 mm of overlengthening may be tolerated under simulated loading conditions without significantly increasing contact pressures of the radiocapitellar joint. Surgeons can use this knowledge along with radiographic parameters and intraoperative examination of elbow stability to gauge the appropriate size of the radial head implant to be used in order to decrease the risk of overstuffing the joint and minimizing radiocapitellar chondral wear.

Type of Study/Level of Evidence.—Prognostic IV.

▶ Radial head arthroplasty resulting in pain and stiffness is often attributed to overstuffing of the radiocapitellar joint by overlengthening the implant relative to the native radial head causing articular damage. This article reports on the contact pressures with 3 lengths of radial head prosthetic.

Although the conclusion is that 2 mm of overlengthening may be tolerated, the authors are careful to caution, appropriately, that surgeons should continue to adhere to principles of correct placement, including using the coronoid, visual gapping of the ulnohumeral joint, and elbow stability as the guide to proper implant size. The trend of increasing contact pressures was certainly shown with increasing length.

The model used was based on validated elbow joint-loading protocols at multiple flexion angles in neutral rotation. Adding stress testing or forearm rotation during the evaluation could enhance the data obtained. Testing of additional sizes and implant types or brands would also be useful.

Additionally, application to clinical scenario may be difficult. It would be helpful to see how these lengths correlated with radiographic findings, which are typically used for intraoperative sizing. Also, often radial head arthroplasty occurs in a setting with associated ligament or other bony injury that may influence contact pressures both by their injury and changes associated with repair.

Although some reassurance may be offered to surgeons who inadvertently lengthen or overstuff the radial head during arthroplasty, this cadaveric model may not allow for physiologic conditions. This is a relevant body of work that addresses a common pathology, and expanding this work may increase its applicability.

J. Geissler, MD

Discovery Elbow System: 2- to 5-Year Results in Distal Humerus Fractures and Posttraumatic Conditions: A Prospective Study on 24 Patients

Giannicola G, Scacchi M, Polimanti D, et al ("Sapienza" Univ of Rome, Italy)
J Hand Surg Am 39:1746-1756, 2014

Purpose.—To prospectively evaluate preliminary results of the Discovery Elbow System (DES) used for acute distal humerus fractures and posttraumatic conditions.

Methods.—We analyzed 24 patients (9 men and 15 women), with a mean age of 69 years (range, 45–89 y). Ten had comminuted distal humerus fractures (group I), and 14 had severe posttraumatic arthritis, chronic instability, or nonunion (group II). Clinical and radiographic evaluations were performed. The preoperative (group II) and postoperative (both groups) evaluations were assessed with the Mayo Elbow Performance Score and Mayo Elbow Performance Index, the Quick Disabilities of the Arm, Shoulder, and Hand score, and the modified American Shoulder and Elbow Surgeons score. Patient satisfaction was evaluated on a 4-point scale.

Results.—Mean follow-up was 41 months (range, 29–63 mo). At the last evaluation, average flexion, extension, pronation, and supination were 136°, 17°, 80°, and 83°, respectively. The average Mayo Elbow Performance Score, Quick Disabilities of the Arm, Shoulder, and Hand score, and the modified American Shoulder and Elbow Surgeons score were 96, 20, and 84, respectively, and without significant intergroup differences. According to the Mayo Elbow Performance Index, there were 20 excellent, 3 good, and 1 fair result. Twenty patients were very satisfied or satisfied with the outcome. A significant increase in the functional scores was observed in group II compared with preoperative results. Radiological evaluation showed 1 patient with progressive radiolucency and 1 with a nonprogressive radiolucency at the final follow-up. No mechanical failures were observed. Two transient ulnar neuropathies, 1 wound infection, and 1 epicondyle fracture were observed.

Conclusions.—The DES yielded promising 2- to 5-year results in the treatment of acute fractures and posttraumatic conditions regarding pain relief, functional improvement, and patient satisfaction, achieving excellent results in most cases. The DES may represent an effective linked-implant option for total elbow replacement in such patients. However, long-term studies are needed.

Type of Study/Level of Evidence.—Therapeutic IV.

▶ Middle-age patients with unreconstructable distal humerus fractures or posttraumatic elbow arthritis remain a challenge to treat. Several newer elbow prostheses have been designed to combat this challenge, but few have midterm-reported outcomes. The use of elbow arthroplasty in the low-demand rheumatoid patient is well documented as successful and durable. The current study, to the commentator's knowledge, is the first to report midterm outcome results for the Biomet Discovery Elbow System (DES) in traumatic and posttraumatic patients. The report is novel, as there are little data available on the nonrheumatoid patient group and little published outcome on the DES prosthesis. The study's limitations are listed within the article and include the small number of patients, lack of a control group, and the relative short clinical follow-up to evaluate implant survivorship. However, the study does use clinically relevant patient-reported outcomes that allow near direct comparison to the more widely used Coonrad-Morrey prosthesis.

For the elderly patient with posttraumatic arthritis or a distal humerus fracture, the decision for a total elbow arthroplasty remains simple. When a younger patient presents with posttraumatic arthritis, the decision to proceed with a total elbow arthroplasty remains more complicated. The subgroup of patients in this study is less than elderly, with an average age of 69 and a minimum age of 45. Other options for surgical intervention in these younger patients with posttraumatic arthritis include interposition arthroplasty, as it delays the time to a total elbow arthroplasty. The results of this procedure are inconsistent, but conversion to arthroplasty is fairly predictable. A previous study by Blaine et al[1] found excellent results for total elbow arthroplasty after interposition arthroplasty. This study, however, does allow physicians to provide better information to their patients to make informed decisions about potential surgery. This article reports excellent range of motion (136°-17°) and no cases of mechanical failure at a minimum follow-up of 2 years. However, there were 2 cases of radiolucency seen, one being progressive. As with many aspects of medicine, newer technology has advanced so quickly that evidence-based medicine has failed to keep pace. Orthopedic surgeons should regard this early/midterm follow-up with cautious optimism, but longer follow-up is needed to make broader conclusions.

M. B. Gottschalk, MD
J. T. Capo, MD

Reference

1. Blaine TA, Adams R, Morrey BF. Total elbow arthroplasty after interposition arthroplasty for elbow arthritis. *J Bone Joint Surg Am*. 2005;87:286-292.

Radial Head Replacement for Acute Complex Fractures: What Are the Rate and Risks Factors for Revision or Removal?

Duckworth AD, Wickramasinghe NR, Clement ND, et al (Royal Infirmary of Edinburgh, UK)
Clin Orthop Relat Res 472:2136-2143, 2014

Background.—When treating complex radial head fractures, important goals include prevention of elbow or forearm instability, with restoration of radiocapitellar contact essential. When open reduction and internal fixation cannot achieve this, radial head replacement is routinely employed, but the frequency of and risk factors for prosthesis revision or removal are not well defined.

Questions/Purposes.—We determined (1) the frequency of prosthesis revision or removal after radial head replacement for acute complex unstable radial head fractures, (2) risk factors for revision or removal, and (3) functional outcomes after radial head replacement.

Methods.—We identified from our prospective trauma database all patients over a 16-year period managed acutely for unstable complex radial head fractures with primary radial head replacement. Of the 119 patients identified, 105 (88%) met our inclusion criteria; mean age was 50 years (range, 16–93 years) and 57 (54%) were female. All implants were uncemented monopolar prostheses, of which 86% were metallic and 14% silastic. We recorded further procedures for prosthesis revision or removal for any cause, with a minimum followup of 1 year (n = 105). Cox regression analysis was used to determine independent factors associated with revision or removal when controlling for baseline patient (age, sex, comorbidities) and fracture (location, classification, associated injury) characteristics. Short-term functional outcomes (Broberg and Morrey score, ROM) were determined from retrospective review of clinic followup (n = 74), with a minimum followup of 3 months.

Results.—Twenty-nine patients (28%) underwent prosthesis revision (n = 3) or removal (n = 26) at a mean of 6.7 years (range, 1.8–18 years) after injury. Independent risk factors for removal or revision were silastic implant type and lower age. At a mean of 1.1 years (range, 0.3–5.5 years) after surgery, mean Broberg and Morrey score was 80 out of 100 (range, 40–99). Mean elbow flexion was 133° (range, 90°–159°; SD, 13°), extension 21° (range, 0°–80°; SD, 17°), flexion arc 112° (range, 10°–140°; SD, 25°), pronation 84° (range, 0°–90°; SD, 18°), supination 73° (range, 0°–90°; SD, 28°), and forearm rotation arc 156° (range, 0°–180°; SD, 38°).

Conclusions.—We demonstrated a high removal or revision rate after radial head replacement for acute unstable complex fractures, with lower age and silastic implants independent risk factors. Younger patients should be counseled regarding the increased risk of requiring further surgery after radial head replacement. Future work should focus on long-term patient-reported outcomes after these injuries.

Level of Evidence.—Level IV, therapeutic study. See Instructions for Authors for a complete description of levels of evidence.

► McQueen et al present a useful retrospective study examining the rate of revision of radial head prostheses as well as the risk factors for failure and functional outcomes. Although the article has many limitations, the overall message is beneficial. The strengths of this study include the inclusion of patients from a prospective trauma registry managed with a similar algorithm and its relatively large size (105 patients). The revision rate was surprisingly high to me at 28%. That said, the inclusion of patients having undergone silicone arthroplasty only served to muddy the results for me because, in my opinion, that is now of historical interest only. The complications of silicone radial head arthroplasty have been well documented (and are supported in this series having had a 60% revision rate of the silicone implants), and I am unaware of anyone currently using them in their practice. The issues of injury pattern, implant design, and functional outcomes merit further discussion.

Injury Patterns: Only 63% of patients in this series had initial radiographs, making the injury classification as a true predictor of failure of little true benefit. Of those patients in whom injuries were classified, the injuries varied with about one-third being higher injury and two-thirds lower injury. The associations of coronoid fractures, terrible triad, ligamentous injury, among others, highlight the difficulty in grouping these injuries and generalizing outcomes of radial head prosthesis when the injury patterns are so vastly different in many cases. One consistent finding of this study that is of benefit for me (and that I now counsel patients specifically about) is the higher risk of explantation in younger patients. This was consistent when analyzing the data for only metallic radial head fractures and controlling for comorbidities and injury patterns.

Implant Design: Prosthetic design may certainly influence failure rate of metallic radial head arthroplasty, although there are a paucity of data comparing varying implants. Stems may be smooth, ingrowth, or cemented. Heads may be monopolar or bipolar and can be monoblock or modular in their association with the stem. In this series, only smooth stem, monoblock prostheses were used. Generalizing these results to other implant designs is not possible, nor is comparison between different implant designs. I personally favor a smooth stem design as well, and if removal is required, the procedure is much easier compared with ingrowth or cemented stems.

Functional Outcomes: Functional outcome data to me was limited in this article because of short follow-up inclusion (3 months) and limited data collection (only 74 of 105 patients). Furthermore, the authors routinely immobilized patients for 2 to 3 weeks before beginning range of motion, which is extremely different from my practice of 2 to 3 days of immobilization; therefore, these data are less generalizable to my practice. It is interesting that 41% of early revisions in this series were due to stiffness. Perhaps early motion could limit this number?

In the end, this article highlights the need to counsel patients, particularly younger patients, of the potential need for revision surgery and implant removal. I do routinely use radial head arthroplasty in my practice for elbow fractures and fracture dislocations in a similar algorithm to that of the authors; I feel at present that any implant other than silicone is reasonable but personally favor a smooth stem unipolar, modular design. I believe earlier institution of motion (at 2–3 days) is beneficial and wonder if this may decrease the revision rate reported by the authors.

G. Gaston, MD

9 Brachial Plexus

Surgical correction of shoulder rotation deformity in brachial plexus birth palsy: long-term results in 118 patients

Hultgren T, Jönsson K, Roos F, et al (Karolinska Inst, Stockholm, Sweden)

Bone Joint J 96-B:1411-1418, 2014

We present the long-term results of open surgery for internal shoulder rotational deformity in brachial plexus birth palsy (BPBP).

From 1997 to 2005, 207 patients (107 females, 100 males, mean age 6.2 (0.6 to 34)) were operated on with subscapularis elongation and/or latissimus dorsi to infraspinatus transfer. Incongruent shoulder joints were relocated. The early results of these patients has been reported previously. We analysed 118 (64 females, 54 males, mean age 15.1 (7.6 to 34)) of the original patient cohort at a mean of 10.4 years (7.0 to 15.1) post-operatively. A third of patients with relocated joints had undergone secondary internal rotational osteotomy of the humerus.

A mixed effects models approach was used to evaluate the effects of surgery on shoulder rotation, abduction, and the Mallet score. Independent factors were time (pre-and post-surgery), gender, age, joint category (congruent, relocated, relocated plus osteotomy) and whether or not a transfer had been performed. Data from a previously published short-term evaluation were reworked in order to obtain pre-operative values.

The mean improvement in external rotation from pre-surgery to the long-term follow-up was 66.5° (95% confidence interval (CI) 61.5 to 71.6). The internal rotation had decreased by a mean of 22.6° (95% CI -18.7 to -26.5). The mean improvement in the three-grade aggregate Mallet score was 3.1 (95% CI 2.7 to 3.4), from 8.7 (95% CI 8.4 to 9.0) to 11.8 (11.5 to 12.1).

Our results show that open subscapularis elongation achieves good long-term results for patients with BPBP and an internal rotation contracture, providing lasting joint congruency and resolution of the trumpet sign, but with a moderate mean loss of internal rotation.

▶ This is a long-term follow-up of previously published short-term results in patients with brachial plexus birth palsies who underwent open surgery for internal shoulder rotational deformity.[1] The study analyzes functional outcomes of a large cohort of patients. The study is well done with reasonable follow-up. The authors use a mixed-effects model to evaluate the effect of surgery on shoulder function over time. These models are able to accommodate missing data and integrate time-varying factors.

The authors reference their initial publication to communicate their algorithm for determining surgical treatment.[1] Follow-up for 118 patients (short-term results published on 270 patients) was conducted with measurements taken for shoulder motion and function. Results show that shoulder joint relocation was achieved in 63 of 66 joints. Additionally, since the 1-year follow-up study, 23 of the 63 patients also required an internally rotating osteotomy of the proximal humerus (18 of which were indicated for active internal rotation of $< 30°$, causing difficulty in their daily activities and 5 for recurrent humeral head subluxation.)

Latissimus dorsi transfer was an isolated procedure for an initial 8 patients with full passive mobility. Five of these patients subsequently had a rotational contracture necessitating a second operation consisting of subscapularis elongation.

The authors found good long-term improvement in the mean external rotation after subscapularis elongation with effective correction in the trumpet sign (mean improvement in Mallet score, 3.1 units), no clinically relevant change in mean abduction, and an acceptable mean loss of internal rotation. They did find, however, that the long-term improvement in external rotation was similar in the group with subscapularis elongation alone and the group with a combined subscapularis elongation and latissimus dorsi transfer. They have since modified their algorithm so that latissimus dorsi transfers are not performed in combination with subscapularis elongation. If necessary, it is performed as a second procedure.

Further evaluation was performed to determine functional impairment in these patients. Three activities were used for evaluations: unbuttoning/buttoning a shirt, putting their hand in trouser pocket, and washing the opposite axilla. All patients could button a shirt, 3 of 107 were unable to put their hand in the trouser pocket, and 7 of 107 could not wash the contralateral axilla without the aid of the other hand.

Clinically, this study nicely shows long-term follow-up of a cohort of challenging patients and the durability of shoulder-stabilizing procedures. Additionally, the outcome data regarding the long-term improvement in patients who receive subscapularis lengthening latissimus dorsi transfer are similar, perhaps influencing patient care and obviating the need for the transfer as an index procedure. Additionally, the data caution against expectations in patients who require shoulder relocation, as additional surgery is often necessary in this group.

E. Lawler, MD

Reference

1. Hultgren T, Jonsson K, Pettersson H, Hammarberg H. Surgical correction of a rotational deformity of teh shoulder in patients with obstetric brachial plexus palsy: short-term results in 270 patients. *Bone Joint J*. 2013;95-B:1432-1438.

The Role of Subscapularis Muscle Denervation in the Pathogenesis of Shoulder Internal Rotation Contracture after Neonatal Brachial Plexus Palsy: A Study in a Rat Model

Mascarenhas VV, Casaccia M, Fernandez-Martin A, et al (Centro de Imagiologia, Portugal, Spain; Universitat Autònoma de Barcelona, Spain; et al)
J Orthop Res 32:1675-1679, 2014

We assessed the role of subscapularis muscle denervation in the development of shoulder internal rotation contracture in neonatal brachial plexus injury. Seventeen newborn rats underwent selective denervation of the subscapular muscle. The rats were evaluated at weekly intervals to measure passive shoulder external rotation. After 4 weeks, the animals were euthanized. The subscapularis thickness was measured using 7.2T MRI axial images. The subscapularis muscle was then studied grossly, and its mass was registered. The fiber area and the area of fibrosis were measured using collagen-I inmunostained muscle sections. Significant progressive decrease in passive shoulder external rotation was noted with a mean loss of 58° at four weeks. A significant decrease in thickness and mass of the subscapularis muscles in the involved shoulders was also found with a mean loss of 69%. Subscapularis muscle fiber size decreased significantly, while the area of fibrosis remained unchanged. Our study shows that subscapularis denervation, per se, could explain shoulder contracture after neonatal brachial plexus injury, though its relevance compared to other pathogenic factors needs further investigation.

▶ This study examines the effect of selective denervation of the subscapularis in a rat model. The subscapularis muscle has been implicated as a primary deforming force leading to the development of shoulder internal rotation contracture and glenohumeral dysplasia. The mechanism by which this occurs has been hypothesized as either imbalance or denervation. The imbalance theory explains subscapularis contracture by lack of stretching in absence of active external rotation. The denervation hypothesis points to progressive muscle fibrosis, shortening, and contracture.

This study performed a neurectomy of the inferior and superior subscapular nerves in 5-day old rats. The shoulders were then examined for passive range of motion weekly for four weeks. Subsequently, MRI was performed to determine thickness followed by anatomic dissection to determine mass. Finally, histologic evaluation was performed to examine for fibrosis.

The authors found that in these denervated rats, a significant decrease in passive shoulder external rotation occurred starting in the second week after surgery. Additionally, a significant decrease in muscle thickness was noted on MRI, and a significant decrease in muscle mass was noted on dissection. Histologic evaluation, however, did not show differences in fibrosis.

This study differs from previous ones in that the subscapularis was selectively denervated as prior studies had denervated both the subscapularis and the external rotators.[1] Additionally, the lack of fibrosis in the early stages shows that fibrosis is a later finding after muscle shortening and stiffness.

Clinically, this finding may support the idea of passive range-of-motion exercises in a denervated muscle to help prevent contracture. Because fibrosis is not occurring in the early stages, passive range of motion may continue to prevent contractures and joint subluxation. At our institution, babies with brachial plexus birth palsies are started on scapular stabilization and passive range of motion emphasizing external rotation.

One criticism of this model, however, is the complete neurectomy and its relevance in clinical settings. Many brachial plexus birth injuries are incomplete, and, thus, this model of the subscapularis may not be completely accurate. The model assumes a complete transection of the nerve when in clinical practice the injury may be a neuropraxia.

E. Lawler, MD

Reference

1. Nikolaou S, Hu L, Tuttle LJ, et al. The contribution of denervated muscle to contractures following neonatal brachial plexus injury: not just muscle fibrosis. *Muscle Nerve*. 2013;49:398-404.

Ultrasound-guided supraclavicular brachial plexus block in upper limb surgery: outcomes and patient satisfaction

Gamo K, Kuriyama K, Higuchi H, et al (Hoshigaoka Koseinenkin Hosp, Osaka, Japan)

Bone Joint J 96-B:795-799, 2014

We examined the outcomes and levels of patient satisfaction in 202 consecutive cases of ultrasound-guided supraclavicular brachial plexus block (SBPB) in upper limb surgery performed between September 2007 and March 2010.

All blocks were performed by orthopaedic surgeons using ultrasound visualisation with a high-frequency linear probe. The probe was placed in the coronal–oblique plane in the supraclavicular fossa, and the puncture was 'in-plane' from lateral to medial. Most of the blocks were performed with 0.75% ropivacaine/1% lidocaine (1:1), with or without adrenaline in 1:200 000 dilution. In 201 patients (99.5%) the brachial plexus block permitted surgery without conversion to general anaesthesia. The mean procedure time for block was 3.9 min (2 to 12), the mean waiting time for surgery was 34.1 min (10 to 64), the mean surgical time was 75.2 min (6 to 232), and the mean duration of post-anaesthetic analgesia was 437 min (171 to 992). A total of 20 patients (10%) developed a transient Horner's syndrome. No nerve injury, pneumothorax, arterial puncture or systemic anaesthetic toxicity were recorded. Most patients (96.7%) were satisfied with ultrasound-guided SBPB. This study demonstrates the efficacy and safety of ultrasound-guided SBPB for orthopaedic surgery on the upper limb.

► In my practice, most surgical procedures are performed with either monitored anesthesia care with local or with an upper extremity block. In our facility, the anesthesiologist performs the blocks. Over the last few years, they have been adopting the use of ultrasound-assisted supraclavicular blocks, which have now become the standard.

Although I have not specifically looked at patient satisfaction during this transition, I can tell you that surgeon satisfaction has increased significantly. Like the authors, I occasionally have to supplement the incision with local anesthetic prior to commencement. However, in my experience, this has been necessary in about 10% of cases, less frequent than reported here. It is insightful to see the authors report that ultrasound-guided supraclavicular blocks also improve the patient experience.

Additionally, the use of ultrasound scan with supraclavicular blocks has increased the confidence of my anesthesia colleagues. Even those who would often be resistant to performing a block and would often suggest a general anesthetic have now been inclined to perform a block.

This technique is a win for the surgeon, the anesthesiologist, and most importantly for the patient.

J. Ortiz, Jr, MD

Reconstruction of Pediatric Brachial Plexus Injuries With Nerve Grafts and Nerve Transfers

Chim H, Kircher MF, Spinner RJ, et al (Mayo Clinic, Rochester, MN)
J Hand Surg Am 39:1771-1778, 2014

Purpose.—To review the demographics and injury patterns in consecutive pediatric patients with traumatic brachial plexus injury presenting to a single center over a 16-year period and to review the outcomes of nerve grafting and nerve transfers for reconstruction of shoulder abduction and elbow flexion in these patients.

Methods.—Forty-five pediatric patients presented for treatment of traumatic Brachial plexus injury from 1996 to 2012. Subgroup analysis of patients who had nerve grafting or nerve transfers for restoration of shoulder abduction and elbow flexion was carried out to compare outcomes of Medical Research Council (MRC) motor grading.

Results.—The mean age of patients was 13.8 years (range, 3–17 y). Panplexal injuries (62%) and upper plexus injuries (16%) were particularly common. There was a very high proportion of preganglionic injuries (91%). Six of the 10 of patients who underwent intraplexal nerve grafting only for restoration of shoulder abduction achieved grade 3 or better power compared with 42% (5/12) of patients who had nerve transfers. When contralateral C7 was used as a donor for nerve transfer in restoration of shoulder abduction, 1 of the 5 patients achieved grade 3 or better shoulder abduction. All 4 patients who had nerve grafts for restoration of elbow flexion achieved grade 3 or better power, compared with 11 of 12 patients who had nerve transfers. There was no statistical difference in outcome (MRC grade 3 or 4) between patients who had nerve grafts and those who had nerve transfers.

Conclusions.—This study shows that nerve grafts can result in similar outcomes (MRC grading) to nerve transfers for restoration of shoulder abduction and elbow flexion in traumatic pediatric BPI. The findings of this study do not support the use of contralateral C7 as a donor for nerve transfer in reconstruction of shoulder abduction in this age group.

▶ The authors present a retrospective review of pediatric patients who sustained traumatic brachial plexus injuries and underwent reconstruction to achieve shoulder abduction and elbow flexion with nerve grafting, nerve transfers, or a combination of both. One goal of the study was to determine whether better outcomes were achieved with nerve grafting or nerve transfers. The cohort consisted of a large number of patients given the injury in question (n = 36 with enough data for analysis); however, no statistical differences were noted between the groups. This is different from recent studies of adult brachial plexus injuries in which nerve transfers appear to result in better outcomes than nerve grafting procedures. The small sample size may have led to no differences being identified, or the ability of pediatric patients to heal nerve injuries may have led to no significant differences being present, thus indicating that both procedures are equally effective. In my practice, younger patients, those under 5 years of age, are treated in a similar manner to brachial plexus birth palsy patients and typically undergo nerve grafting procedures if possible, with preferential treatment made to restore hand function over more proximal innervation. In patients over 5 years of age, nerve transfers are used to provide neural input closer to the target muscle, and preferential treatment is provided to restore elbow flexion and shoulder function/stability.

J. Abzug, MD

Median nerve fascicle transfer versus ulnar nerve fascicle transfer to the biceps motor branch in C5-C6 and C5-C7 brachial plexus injuries: Nonrandomized prospective study of 23 consecutive patients

Cho AB, Paulos RG, de Resende MR, et al (Univ of São Paulo, Brazil)

Microsurgery 34:511-515, 2014

The purpose of this study was to observe whether the results of the median nerve fascicle transfer to the biceps are equivalent to the classical ulnar nerve fascicle transfer, in terms of elbow flexion strength and donor nerve morbidity. Twenty-five consecutive patients were operated between March 2007 and July 2013. The patients were divided into two groups. In Group 1 ($n = 8$), the patients received an ulnar nerve fascicle transfer to the biceps motor branch. In Group 2 ($n = 15$), the patients received a median nerve fascicle transfer to the biceps motor branch. Two patients with follow-up less than six months were excluded. Both groups were similar regarding age ($P = 0.070$), interval of injury ($P = 0.185$), and follow-up period ($P = 0.477$). Elbow flexion against gravity was achieved in 7 of 8 (87.5%) patients in Group 1, versus 14 of 15 (93.3%) patients in Group 2 ($P = 1.000$). The level of injury (C5-C6 or C5-C7) did not affect antigravity elbow flexion recovery in both the groups ($P = 1.000$). It was concluded that the median nerve fascicle transfer to the biceps is as good as the ulnar nerve fascicle transfer, even in C5-C7 injuries.

► Cho and colleagues describe their experience with the ulnar nerve fascicular and median nerve fascicular transfer to the biceps motor branch for restoration of elbow flexion in upper brachial plexus injuries. In a small series of 25 consecutive patients, equivalent results as assessed by Medical Research Council grading were obtained. Given the low prevalence of brachial plexus injuries in many countries, a strength of the study is the significant number of patients who had surgery at a single center. Although there were marginally better outcomes for median nerve fascicular transfer, the significance of this finding is difficult to interpret with the small number of patients in the series. A potential confounder in the study is the performance of concomitant nerve procedures through a supraclavicular approach, such as sural cable grafting from C5 to the upper trunk in 2 patients in Group 1 and 1 patient in Group 2. However, this is probably an unavoidable consequence because of the necessity of restoring as much function as possible in brachial plexus surgery. Overall, this is an interesting contribution to the brachial plexus literature that supports the increased use of median nerve fascicular transfer when this is an option for treatment.

H. Chim, MD

Thoracodorsal Nerve Transfer for Elbow Flexion Reconstruction in Infraclavicular Brachial Plexus Injuries

Soldado F, Ghizoni MF, Bertelli J (Universitat de Barcelona, Spain; Univ of the South of Santa Catarina (Unisul), Tubarão; Governador Celso Ramos Hosp, Santa Catarina, Brazil)

J. Hand Surg Am 39:1766-1770, 2014

Purpose.—To report the clinical results of thoracodorsal nerve (TDN) transfer to the biceps nerve for elbow flexion restoration in infraclavicular brachial plexus injuries.

Methods.—Five male patients, mean age 33 years and affected with infraclavicular brachial plexus injuries, underwent a direct coaptation of the TDN to the nerve to the biceps an average of 8 months after injury. The procedure included the transfer of a branch of the TDN to the musculocutaneous nerve in 2 patients.

Results.—All patients achieved M4 elbow flexion strength according to the British Medical Research Council scale at a mean follow-up of 22 months.

Conclusions.—Direct TDN transfer seems to be a useful surgical procedure for restoring elbowflexion in patients with infraclavicular brachial plexus injuries.

Type of Study/Level of Evidence.—Therapeutic IV.

▶ Soldado and colleagues report the results of thoracodorsal nerve transfer to the biceps nerve for restoration of elbow flexion in a small series of 5 patients with infraclavicular brachial plexus injuries. Good results were achieved in all patients with M4 power at a mean follow-up of 22 months. The authors explain their selection criteria for use of the thoracodorsal nerve as a donor and also describe their surgical technique, in patients where an Oberlin transfer is not possible due to poor finger flexion or an ulnar nerve lesion. The thoracodorsal nerve is preferred by the authors as a donor compared with the intercostal nerves, for which the likelihood of elbow flexion recovery is low and the medial pectoral nerve where direct coaptation to the musculocutaneous nerve is not possible.

Although the number of patients in the series is small and the patients in the series had different associated procedures, this is a necessary limitation in all brachial plexus research. Surgeons who perform brachial plexus reconstruction should keep the thoracodorsal nerve in mind as a donor for restoration of elbow flexion.

H. Chim, MD

Neonatal Brachial Plexus Palsy with Neurotmesis of C5 and Avulsion of C6: Supraclavicular Reconstruction Strategies and Outcome

Malessy MJA, Pondaag W (Leiden Univ Med Ctr, the Netherlands)

J Bone Joint Surg Am 96:e174(1-9), 2014

Background.—Nerve reconstruction strategies for restoration of elbow flexion and shoulder function in patients with neonatal brachial plexus palsy with neurotmesis of C5 and avulsion of C6 are not well defined and the outcomes are unclear.

Methods.—From 1990 to 2008, nerve surgery was performed in 421 patients with neonatal brachial plexus palsy. This study focused on thirty-four infants who had a neurotmetic lesion of C5 and avulsion or intraforaminal neurotmesis of C6, irrespective of C7. The C8 and T1 functions were intact. Intraplexal transfer of C6 to C5 with direct coaptation was preferred for restoration of elbow flexion. The suprascapular nerve was reconnected either by extra-intraplexal transfer of the accessory nerve or by grafting from C5 to restore shoulder function. Additional grafts were attached from C5 to the C5 contribution of the posterior division of the superior trunk when technically possible.

Results.—Transfer of either the C6 anterior root filaments or the entire C6 nerve to C5 was performed in seventeen patients (group A) with direct coaptation in fifteen of them. Grafting from C5 to the anterior division of the superior trunk was performed in the remaining seventeen infants (group B). An accessory-to-suprascapular nerve transfer was applied in twenty-nine infants. The suprascapular nerve was reconnected in five patients by grafting from C5. It was possible to attach one, two, or three additional grafts from C5 to the posterior division of the superior trunk in twenty-one patients. All infants had biceps muscle recovery to a Medical Research Council (MRC) grade of ≥4, twenty-two (65%) of the thirty-four patients obtained Mallet grade-IV abduction, and eleven (32%) of the thirty-four obtained Mallet grade-IV external rotation.

Conclusions.—In patients with neonatal brachial plexus palsy who have neurotmesis of C5 and avulsion of C6, elbow flexion can be successfully restored with supraclavicular intraplexal reconstruction with use of C5 as the proximal outlet. However, shoulder function recovery following suprascapular nerve reinnervation and additional grafting from C5 to the posterior division of the superior trunk is less successful.

Level of Evidence.—Therapeutic Level III. See Instructions for Authors for a complete description of levels of evidence (Fig 2).

▶ The authors address a specific injury pattern occurring in infants with an upper-type birth brachial plexus palsy, rupture of C5 root, and avulsion of C6 root. They describe what to me is a unique reconstructive strategy, direct coaptation of the anterior (motor) rootlet component of the C6 root to the C5 root stump, and show 2 nice diagrams of the procedure (Fig 2A, B). I've been able to directly coapt an avulsed C8 root to the C7 stump, but I have not performed the procedure the authors describe. Perhaps this is because, in my experience, the avulsed C6 root with attached rootlets, or perhaps it is a very high and thus irreparable C6 rupture that has been, along with the ruptured C5 root, a block of scar with no easy morphologic definition. Certainly, it is nothing like what is shown in Fig 1 in the original article. After resecting the scar

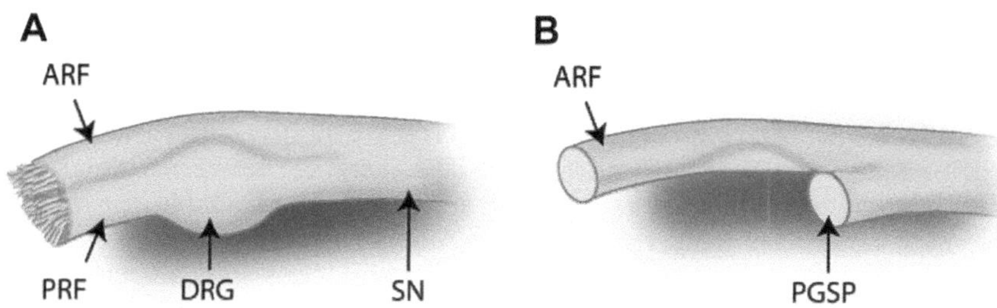

FIGURE 2.—**A** The proximal part of an avulsed spinal nerve (SN), with morphological identification of the dorsal root ganglion (DRG), the anterior root filaments (ARF), and the posterior root filaments (PRF). **B** A spinal nerve after the ganglion was dissected and removed, dividing the nerve into two parts: the anterior root filaments, which is a purely motor part, and the postganglionic pure sensory part (PGSP). (Reprinted from Malessy MJA, Pondaag W. Neonatal brachial plexus palsy with neurotmesis of C5 and Avulsion of C6: supraclavicular reconstruction strategies and outcome. *J Bone Joint Surg Am.* 2014;96:e174(1-9), with permission from The Journal of Bone and Joint Surgery, Incorporated.)

(typically a neuroma in continuity), the healthy C6 contribution to the superior trunk in no way will reach the healthy-appearing stump of the C5 root. In 34 cases, the authors were able to achieve this only 6 times. I'll look more closely at the injured roots in the future. The authors' results for restoring elbow flexion and shoulder abduction are similar to others, and they experience the same disappointing results in restoring external rotation. This is an unsolved problem because the principal pathologic sequelae of this injury, leading to more secondary operations than any other, is the development of an internal rotation contracture. The authors show a possible surgical strategy for these patients, using a branch of the medial pectoral nerve to restore elbow flexion. This procedure is of historic value for patients with a totally normal hand and wrist for whom an Oberlin transfer is not only possible but preferred.

V. R. Hentz, MD

Double Fascicular Nerve Transfer for Elbow Flexion and Extension

Yang PR, Brunworth LS, Gray RR, et al (Univ of Miami Miller School of Medicine, FL)

J Reconstr Microsurg 30:343-348, 2014

Traumatic brachial plexus injuries are life changing, often leaving affected individuals with severe functional deficits. Recent advances in nerve transfers have allowed surgeons to improve elbow flexion, shoulder abduction, and prehension of the hand in some patients. We hypothesize that in a patient who lacks both biceps and triceps function, a double fascicular transfer may be the key to restore elbow flexion and extension. In three cadaver upper limbs, we transferred the expendable motor fascicle of the ulnar nerve to the biceps branch of the musculocutaneous nerve, and the expendable motor fascicle of the median nerve to the triceps (ulnar collateral) branch of the radial nerve. We evaluated the feasibility of this double nerve transfer via a medial approach, and elucidated the anatomy. The transfers were easily performed and were tension-free throughout full range of motion at the elbow. The triceps branch of the radial nerve that we utilized has a length of approximately 4.9 cm, and is best found between 3.5 and 6 cm from the anterior axillary line. We consistently identified a relatively avascular plane in the region between 7.5 and 11 cm from the anterior axillary line, which corresponds with the recipient sites of the medial head of the triceps. The distance between the triceps branch to the median nerve was an average of 2.5 cm. Transfer of expendable motor fascicles from the ulnar and median nerves to the biceps and triceps nerve branches can be successfully and consistently performed through a medial approach in a cadaver.

▶ The authors report on a new nerve transfer alternative building on the partial ulnar nerve transfer to the biceps.. In addition to transferring ulnar nerve fascicles innervating the flexor carpi ulnaris muscle, the authors have identified an additional transfer that uses expendable median motor fascicles supplying to the flexor carpi radialis, transferring these to a triceps branch of the radial nerve. The authors showed the feasibility of the transfer in this study using 4 fresh-frozen cadavers.

In this article, the authors point out several helpful techniques, including measurements of structures from identifiable surface anatomy landmarks. They imply that an extensile, 15-cm incision is necessary for the operation. In my experience, with the partial ulnar transfer, such an extensile incision is not needed. I find it useful to estimate the location of the biceps branch of the musculocutaneous nerve by identifying a region 10 to 12 cm from the tip of the acromion. The insertion of the biceps branch of the musculocutaneous nerve into the biceps muscle is predictably found at this level.

Ultimately, at issue with this combination of transfer is the need for the restoration of triceps function in the setting of absent or severely limited shoulder function as would be expected in patients with C5, 6, or 7 brachial plexus injury. Another consideration, given the nerve root composition of the median nerve, is whether median nerve function could be at risk with this intrafascicular dissection and whether the use of these expendable median nerve fascicles could be better made by transferring these to the brachialis muscle to further augment elbow animation.

P. Murray, MD

10 Shoulder: Rotator Cuff

Rotator Cuff Tear Degeneration and Cell Apoptosis in Smokers Versus Nonsmokers

Lundgreen K, Lian ØB, Scott A, et al (Lovisenberg Diaconal Hosp, Oslo, Norway; Kristiansund Hosp HNR, Norway; Univ of British Columbia, Vancouver, Canada)

Arthroscopy 30:936-941, 2014

Purpose.—The purpose of this study was to assess the effect of smoking on supraspinatus tendon degeneration, including cellular alterations, proliferation, and apoptosis of tendon cells.

Methods.—Supraspinatus tendon samples of 10 smokers and 15 nonsmokers with full-thickness tears were compared, focusing on the severity of tendon histopathology including apoptosis (programmed cell death), cellularity, and proliferation. Immunohistochemistry was used to assess the density of apoptotic cells and proliferation. The extent of tendon degeneration was classified according to a revised version of the Bonar tendon histopathology score.

Results.—The smokers were younger ($P = .01$). The symptom duration among smokers was longer ($P < .05$). The supraspinatus tendons from the smokers presented significantly more advanced degenerative changes (Bonar score, 13.5 [interquartile range, 1.4] *v* 9 [interquartile range, 3]; $P < .001$). The smokers' tendons showed increased density of apoptotic cells (0.108 [SE, 0.038] *v* 0.0107 [SE, 0.007]; $P = .024$) accompanied by reduced tenocyte density ($P = .019$) and upregulation of proliferative activity ($P < .0001$).

Conclusions.—Smoking is associated with worsened supraspinatus tendon histopathology and increased apoptosis.

Clinical Relevance.—Pronounced degenerative changes, reduced tendon cellularity, and increased apoptosis may indicate reduced tendon healing capacity in smokers.

► This well-done study gives treating surgeons further impetus to implore patients to quit smoking. Interestingly (but not surprisingly), finding 2 comparable groups resulted in having a younger cohort of smokers. Intuitively, this makes sense, as most would agree that smokers are "physiologically older" than their nonsmoking counterparts.

The torn edge of rotator cuff tissue in smokers shows a statistically significant higher amount of apoptosis (programmed cell death) compared with torn tissue from nonsmokers. This study reminds us of the importance of smoking cessation counseling to patients to potentially improve surgical outcomes.

R. Papandrea, MD

Arthroscopic-Assisted Latissimus Dorsi Transfer for the Management of Irreparable Rotator Cuff Tears: Short-Term Results

Castricini R, Longo UG, De Benedetto M, et al (Villa Maria Cecilia Hosp, Ravenna, Italy; Campus Bio-Medico Univ, Rome, Italy; et al)

J Bone Joint Surg Am 96:e119.1-e119.6, 2014

Background.—Irreparable rotator cuff tears associated with shoulder functional impairment represent a challenge, especially in young and active patients. Latissimus dorsi muscle-tendon transfer is performed to replace the irreversibly lost contractile elements in patients with irreparable tears of the posterosuperior aspect of the rotator cuff.

Methods.—From 2008 to 2010, we enrolled twenty-seven patients (mean age, sixty years; range, forty-six to sixty-seven years) with irreparable, full-thickness rotator cuff tears involving at least two tendons who underwent arthroscopicassisted latissimus dorsi muscle-tendon transfer. Outcome measures included the Constant and Murley score, shoulder range of motion in external rotation, and muscle strength in forward elevation. The mean duration of follow-up was twentyseven months (range, twenty-four to thirty-six months).

Results.—There was a significant improvement ($p < 0.05$) in the mean Constant and Murley score, pain score, muscle strength in forward elevation, and range of motion in external rotation at the time of the last follow-up. There was no significant correlation between the mean preoperative range of motion, pain, and strength and the mean postoperative Constant and Murley score. There was no significant osteoarthritis progression and proximal migration of the humeral head after surgery in the time period studied.

Conclusions.—Arthroscopic-assisted latissimus dorsi muscle-tendon transfer at short-term follow-up is an effective alternative to open surgery for the management of painful irreparable posterosuperior rotator cuff tears refractory to conservative management.

Level of Evidence.—Therapeutic Level IV. See Instructions for Authors for a complete description of levels of evidence.

► This is an interesting technique to augment latissimus dorsi muscle transfers. The arthroscopic addition is used only for the passage of the graft and the fixation to the humeral head. The surgical description includes a technique for creating the graft passage tunnel with a Hegar uterine retractor. Images and more detail here would have been helpful, as this reviewer finds creating a wide enough tunnel labor intensive.

The described technique does not change the tendon harvest, which can be difficult, especially in large, muscular patients. For those surgeons that only take the latissimus and do not transfer the teres major, this technique is intriguing but does not change or simplify the most challenging portions of a potentially difficult and labor-intensive surgery.

R. Papandrea, MD

Three-Dimensional Analysis of Acromial Morphologic Characteristics in Patients With and Without Rotator Cuff Tears Using a Reconstructed Computed Tomography Model

Fujisawa Y, Mihata T, Murase T, et al (Osaka Med College, Takatsuki, Japan; Osaka Univ, Suita, Japan)

Am J Sports Med 42:2621-2626, 2014

Background.—The relationship between rotator cuff tears and acromial shape has yet to be clarified. As a result, the most suitable location for acromioplasty for the treatment of rotator cuff tears is not known.

Purpose.—To determine whether any particular change in acromial shape is significantly associated with the presence of rotator cuff tears.

Study Design.—Cross-sectional study; Level of evidence, 3.

Methods.—From 2007 to 2010, we examined 25 consecutive patients with unilateral full-thickness rotator cuff tears who underwent arthroscopic repair and 17 consecutive patients with adhesive capsulitis but intact rotator cuffs who underwent arthroscopic capsular release. Before surgery, a reconstructed 3-dimensional computed tomography model was used to evaluate the acromial structure. Changes in the shape of the affected scapula were qualitatively evaluated relative to the unaffected, contralateral scapula by use of proximity mapping. Differences in acromial structure between affected and unaffected shoulders were assessed at the anterior, lateral, and medial edges and the inferior surface. The association between rotator cuff tear size and change in acromial structure was also evaluated.

Results.—Rates of bony projection at the anterior (>2 mm) and lateral (>3 mm) edges of the acromion in patients with rotator cuff tears were significantly greater compared with rates in patients without rotator cuff tears ($P < .01$). Tear size was not correlated with changes in acromial structure ($P = .37\text{-}.73$).

Conclusion.—Bone spurs at the anterior and lateral edges of the acromion are associated with the presence of full-thickness rotator cuff tears in symptomatic patients.

► This is a well-conceived and executed study that attempts to shed more light on the role that acromial morphology plays in rotator cuff pathology. The authors took the added step of performing a power analysis to ensure adequate sample size and developed a useful 3-dimensional system comparing affected scapulae with the normal contralateral. In the end, their conclusion that lateral and anterior bones are related to rotator cuff tears still does not prove causation.

It is interesting to note that the location of bone that was felt to be related to rotator cuff pathology was not inferior, such that, in this reviewer's opinion, it is unlikely to be removed with standard arthroscopic acromioplasty. In this time of increasing evidence of the limited benefit of acromioplasty and decreased relative value unit assignment for the procedure, this study may create more questions than it answers. It is still a valuable addition to the debate on external impingement.

R. Papandrea, MD

Tendon Repair Compared with Physiotherapy in the Treatment of Rotator Cuff Tears: A Randomized Controlled Study in 103 Cases with a Five-Year Follow-up

Moosmayer S, Lund G, Seljom US, et al (Martina Hansens Hosp, Sandvika, Norway; et al)
J Bone Joint Surg Am 96:1504-1514, 2014

Background.—There is limited Level-I evidence that compares operative and nonoperative treatment of rotator cuff tears. We compared outcomes of patients treated with primary tendon repair with outcomes of those treated with physiotherapy and optional secondary tendon repair if needed.

Methods.—A single-center, pragmatic, randomized controlled study with follow-ups after six months and one, two, and five years was conducted in a secondary-care institution. One hundred and three patients with a rotator cuff tear not exceeding 3 cm were randomized to primary tendon repair (n = 52) or physiotherapy (n = 51). The primary outcome measure was the Constant score. Secondary outcome measures included the self-report section of the American Shoulder and Elbow Surgeons score; the physical component summary measure of the Short Form 36 Health Survey; the measurement of pain, strength, and shoulder motion; patient satisfaction; and findings from magnetic resonance imaging and sonography. Analysis was by intention to treat.

Results.—The five-year follow-up rate was 98%. Twelve of the fifty-one patients in the physiotherapy group were treated with secondary tendon repair. The results from primary tendon repair were superior to those from physiotherapy plus secondary repair, with between-group mean differences of 5.3 points on the Constant score ($p = 0.05$), 9.0 points on the American Shoulder and Elbow Surgeons score ($p < 0.001$), 1.1 cm on a 10-cm visual analog scale for pain ($p < 0.001$), and 1.0 cm on a 10-cm visual analog scale for patient satisfaction ($p = 0.03$). In 37% of tears treated with physiotherapy only, there were increasing tear sizes on ultrasound of >5 mm, over five years, associated with an inferior outcome.

Conclusions.—Although primary repair of small and medium-sized rotator cuff tears was associated with better outcome than physiotherapy treatment, the differences were small and may be below clinical importance. In the physiotherapy treatment group, there were increasing tear sizes and inferior outcomes in one-third of patients who did not undergo repair.

▶ This is a Level 1 study directly comparing mini-open rotator cuff repair with physiotherapy program for rotator cuff tears. The hypothesis was that a substantial number of patients in the physiotherapy group would have secondary tendon repair and that analysis by intention to treat would show comparable treatment benefits in the 2 study groups. Both the primary repair group and the physiotherapy plus optional secondary repair group improved from baseline to the 5-year follow-up. Interestingly, results were better for the primary tendon repair group, but the differences were small and might not represent clinical importance. Tear size in the 38 patients treated with physiotherapy increased in most patients. There was a strong trend for an inferior outcome for the group with an increasing tear size. This supports a primary trial of physiotherapy for most of these patients. Nevertheless, it must be noted that unrepaired tears are at risk of anatomic deterioration, which is associated with an inferior functional outcome. The limitations include that physiotherapy and surgery were not completely standardized. Physiotherapy was based on a protocol consisting of 52 exercises among which the therapists could select treatment measures according to the individual patient. Patients with rotator cuff injuries usually differ according to postural alterations, muscle imbalances, muscle weaknesses, and muscle activation patterns. Physiotherapy is given individually, on the basis of examination findings, such as pain tolerance, and the capacity of the patient for periscapular muscular compensation. The same applies to surgical treatment in which the approach, handling of the biceps tendon, and number and placement of sutures had to be adapted to individual findings. Since the beginning of this clinical trial, the surgical treatment of rotator cuff tears has changed from open or mini-open to all arthroscopic techniques, which may make the results less relevant. However, the results from mini-open and all-arthroscopic repairs have been reported to be comparable. Traumatic and atraumatic rotator cuff tears were included in the current study. Although they could not detect differences in treatment responses between these subgroups, existing differences may have contributed to the outcomes.

E. Cheung, MD

Effect of the Interposition of Calcium Phosphate Materials on Tendon-Bone Healing During Repair of Chronic Rotator Cuff Tear

Zhao S, Peng L, Xie G, et al (Shanghai Jiao Tong Univ, P.R. China; Shanghai Inst of Ceramics, P.R. China)

Am J Sports Med 42:1920-1929, 2014

Background.—The current nature of tendon-bone healing after rotator cuff (RC) repair is still the formation of granulation tissue at the tendon-bone interface rather than the formation of fibrocartilage, which is the crucial structure in native tendon insertion and can be observed after knee ligament reconstruction. The interposition of calcium phosphate materials has been found to be able to enhance tendon-bone healing in knee ligament reconstruction. However, whether the interposition of these kinds of materials can enhance tendon-bone healing or even change the current nature of tendon-bone healing after RC repair still needs to be explored.

Hypothesis.—The interposition of calcium phosphate materials during RC repair would enhance tendon-bone healing or change its current nature of granulation tissue formation into a more favorable process.

Study Design.—Controlled laboratory study.

Methods.—A total of 144 male Sprague-Dawley rats underwent unilateral detachment of the supraspinatus tendon, followed by delayed repair after 3 weeks. The animals were allocated into 1 of 3 groups: (1) repair alone, (2) repair with $Ca_5(PO_4)_2SiO_4$ (CPS) bioceramic interposition, or (3) repair with hydroxyapatite (HA) bioceramic interposition at the tendon-bone interface. Animals were sacrificed at 2, 4, or 8 weeks postoperatively, and microcomputed tomography (micro-CT) was used to quantify the new bone formation at the repair site. New fibrocartilage formation and collagen organization at the tendon-bone interface was evaluated by histomorphometric analysis. Biomechanical testing of the supraspinatus tendon-bone complex was performed. Statistical analysis was performed using 1-way analysis of variance. Significance was set at $P < .05$.

Results.—The micro-CT analysis demonstrated remarkable osteogenic activity and osteoconductivity to promote new bone formation and ingrowth of CPS and HA bioceramic, with CPS bioceramic showing better results than HA. Histological observations indicated that CPS bioceramic had excellent biocompatibility and biodegradability. At early time points after the RC repair, CPS bioceramic significantly increased the area of fibrocartilage at the tendon-bone interface compared with the control and HA groups. Moreover, CPS and HA bioceramics had significantly improved collagen organization. Biomechanical tests indicated that the CPS and HA groups have greater ultimate load to failure and stiffness than the control group at 4 and 8 weeks, and the CPS specimens exhibited the maximum ultimate load to failure, stiffness, and stress of the healing enthesis.

Conclusion.—Both CPS and HA bioceramics aid in cell attachment and proliferation and accelerate new bone formation, and CPS bioceramic has a more prominent effect on tendon-to-bone healing.

Clinical Relevance.—Local application of CPS and HA bioceramic at the tendon-bone interface shows promise in improving healing after rotator cuff tear repair

▶ Tendon-to-bone healing depends on bone ingrowth into the granulation tissue formed at the healing rotator cuff tendon–bone interface. Traditional rotator cuff repairs result in a fibrovascular scar formation rather than 4-layered organized tendon insertion into bone. This study aimed at changing the formation of granulation tissue into fibrocartilage so that a native tendon—bone insertion site can be recreated by using calcium phosphate-based biomaterial powders. Based on the findings reported, the biomaterials (especially $Ca_5(PO_4)_2SiO_4$ compared with hydroxyapatite) elicited a biocompatible host tissue response, with improvements in the area of fibrocartilage and collagen organization, leading to improved mechanical strength. It seems like the osteoconductive and osteogenic nature of these biomaterials, in addition to their biodegradability during the healing process, possibly creates an ideal augmentative matrix for cuff repairs. Further research is needed to understand whether these findings can be extrapolated to humans, which might lead to a significant improvement of the retear rates after rotator cuff repairs.

A. Cil, MD

Tendon Repair Compared with Physiotherapy in the Treatment of Rotator Cuff Tears: A Randomized Controlled Study in 103 Cases with a Five-Year Follow-up

Moosmayer S, Lund G, Seljom US, et al (Martina Hansens Hosp, Sandvika, Norway; et al)

J Bone Joint Surg Am 96:1504-1514, 2014

Background.—There is limited Level-I evidence that compares operative and nonoperative treatment of rotator cuff tears. We compared outcomes of patients treated with primary tendon repair with outcomes of those treated with physiotherapy and optional secondary tendon repair if needed.

Methods.—A single-center, pragmatic, randomized controlled study with follow-ups after six months and one, two, and five years was conducted in a secondary-care institution. One hundred and three patients with a rotator cuff tear not exceeding 3 cm were randomized to primary tendon repair (n = 52) or physiotherapy (n = 51). The primary outcome measure was the Constant score. Secondary outcome measures included the self-report section of the American Shoulder and Elbow Surgeons score; the physical component summary measure of the Short Form 36 Health Survey; the measurement of pain, strength, and shoulder motion; patient satisfaction; and findings from magnetic resonance imaging and sonography. Analysis was by intention to treat.

Results.—The five-year follow-up rate was 98%. Twelve of the fifty-one patients in the physiotherapy group were treated with secondary tendon repair. The results from primary tendon repair were superior to those from physiotherapy plus secondary repair, with between-group mean differences of 5.3 points on the Constant score ($p = 0.05$), 9.0 points on the American Shoulder and Elbow Surgeons score ($p < 0.001$), 1.1 cm on a 10-cm visual analog scale for pain ($p < 0.001$), and 1.0 cm on a 10-cm visual analog scale for patient satisfaction ($p = 0.03$). In 37% of tears treated with physiotherapy only, there were increasing tear sizes on ultrasound of >5 mm, over five years, associated with an inferior outcome.

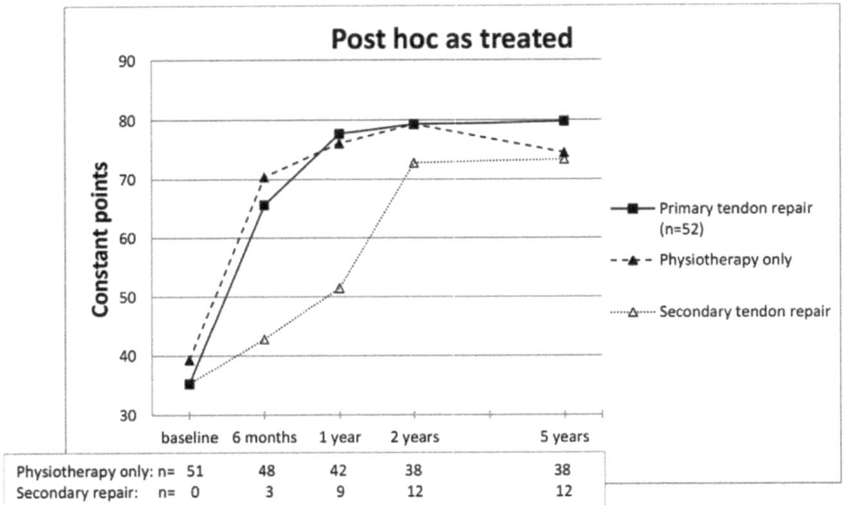

FIGURE 4.—Post hoc as-treated analysis showing mean constant scores at baseline and at the six-month, one-year, two-year, and five-year follow-ups for the primary tendon repair group, the physiotherapy-only group, and the group with secondary tendon repair because of persistent symptoms. The number of patients in the physiotherapy-only group and in the secondary tendon repair group at each follow-up is given below the x axis. (Reprinted from Moosmayer S, Lund G, Seljom US, et al. Tendon repair compared with physiotherapy in the treatment of rotator cuff tears: a randomized controlled study in 103 cases with a five-year follow-up. *J Bone Joint Surg Am.* 2014;96:1504-1514, with permission from The Journal of Bone and Joint Surgery, Incorporated.)

Conclusions.—Although primary repair of small and medium-sized rotator cuff tears was associated with better outcome than physiotherapy treatment, the differences were small and may be below clinical importance. In the physiotherapy treatment group, there were increasing tear sizes and inferior outcomes in one-third of patients who did not undergo repair (Fig 4).

▶ Several studies support the effectiveness of primary repair of or rehabilitation therapy interventions for rotator cuff tears. However, Moosmayer and colleagues are the first to compare the results of these 2 intervention approaches. In this study, 103 persons with MRI and sonography-confirmed full-thickness tears of less than 3 cm, positive clinical signs, tears no greater than 25% of the subscapularis tendon, without local/systemic disease affecting shoulder function, and without a history of previous shoulder surgery were randomly assigned to therapy ($n = 51$) or surgery ($n = 52$) intervention groups. Of those allocated, only 1 participant in the surgery group elected to not receive the intervention. The Constant Shoulder Score;[1] the self-reported section of the American Shoulder and Elbow Surgeons (ASES) Scale; the physical subscale of the 36-Item Short Form Health Survey; pain; shoulder mobility; shoulder strength; and satisfaction with treatment were the primary and secondary measures of the study and were all administered by a blinded assessor.

Those participants assigned to the surgery group underwent primary repair of the rotator cuff tendons and acromioplasty through open or mini techniques, 18 of which also required tenodesis of the long head of the biceps tendon. Postoperative therapy began on an inpatient basis on postoperative day 1 and was sustained until 12 or more weeks postoperatively.

The therapy group received outpatient rehabilitation services, which were grounded in procedures supported by the literature. The therapy regimen included 52 different exercises, which focused on postural correction and restoration of scapulothoracic and scapulohumeral control and stability. The protocol was delivered in a patient-centered fashion in which the needs of the participant were considered, as necessary, on a case-by-case basis. For the first 12 weeks, intervention sessions occurred twice weekly for 45 minutes and were, depending on the needs of the participant, tapered down across the subsequent 6 to 12 weeks. When mastery of given exercises in the clinic was demonstrated, participants were assigned these as a part of a home program. The frequency and intensity of the home program, however, was not described.

If after 15 sessions of therapy the therapy group participant was unsatisfied in his or her outcomes and clinical findings were unimproved, tendon repair was offered. The clinical criteria, however, were not explicitly operationalized.

Within the 5-year evaluation period, 12 of the 51 therapy group participants elected to undergo tendon repair after undergoing at least 15 therapy sessions. The baseline visual analog scale for pain (VAS) and ASES scores of these 12 were significantly higher ($P = .04$) and lower ($P = .03$), respectively, indicating that these participants were experiencing more pain and dysfunction at baseline than those who did not elect for surgery. At 5 years after surgery, when controlling for the effects of time, the main effects of intervention type on Constant ($P = .05$), ASES ($P < .001$), and VAS ($P < .001$) scores was significant and in favor of the primary surgery group. The main effects of the intervention type on pain-free movement, strength, and the physical subscale of the 36-Item Short Form Health Survey was nonsignificant.

The authors report that, when separating out the Constant scores of those who received therapy but elected to have surgery, those in the primary surgery group had higher ($P = .006$) Constant scores than those who completed the therapy intervention; however, the Constant scores of those in the primary surgery group and those who received therapy but later sought surgery were not different ($P = .23$). This assertion, however, is not supported by the results presented in Fig 4 of the article.

In the therapy-only group, an advancement of rotator cuff tears of less than 5 mm was noted in 24 participants and greater than 5 in 14 at 5 years of follow-up. Those with an increased tear size of 5 mm or greater were found to have a reduction in (1) Constant scores that were approaching significance ($P = .06$) and (2) shoulder strength ($P = .02$) when compared with those with a smaller change in tear size. Sixty participants who received primary or secondary repairs underwent sonography of their repair at 5 years, and full-thickness tears were apparent in 8, while partial-thickness tears were evident in 7. Based on the totality of these findings, the authors concluded that the outcomes of the therapy group were, in many cases, statistically inferior but not necessarily to the extent that the differences are clinically meaningful.

These conclusions aside, a major limitation of the study's design is that the primary surgery group actually received a combined intervention. Given that primary repair of the rotator cuff involved immediate and sustained postoperative therapy for 12 or more weeks, the authors are truly comparing the results of a primary surgery plus therapy intervention with therapy alone. For the case to be made that surgery alone is more effective than rehabilitation, the surgery group should not have received any postoperative rehabilitation. However, the ethics of such a design are quite questionable. Regardless, because of this design flaw, the results should be interpreted cautiously.

Another missing piece in the design of this study is a measure of therapy adherence and motivation. If those randomly assigned to the therapy group would have preferred a primary surgery group assignment and were aware that after 15 therapy sessions, surgery was an option, it's quite likely that therapy adherence and motivation were poor.

Ultimately, given the absence of between-group differences that are greater than what is known to be clinically meaningful, the authors ascribed that a primary trial of rehabilitation is recommended prior to considering surgery for persons with small to medium-sized full-thickness rotator cuff tears. The findings of this study also suggest that baseline ASES and VAS pain scores may be indicators of therapy responsiveness. Further exploration on (1) alternative designs to address this study's methodologic limitations and (2) use of these tools as screens for therapy responsiveness is required.

C. McGee, PhD, OTR/L, CHT

Reference

1. Constant C, Murley A. A clinical method of functional assessment of the shoulder. *Clin Orthop Relat Res.* 1987;214:160-164.

A Survey of Expert Opinion Regarding Rotator Cuff Repair

Acevedo DC, Paxton ES, Williams GR, et al (Thomas Jefferson Univ, Philadelphia, PA)

J Bone Joint Surg Am 96:e123.1-e123.7, 2014

Many patients with rotator cuff tears have questions for their surgeons regarding the surgical procedure, perioperative management, restrictions, therapy, and ability to work after a rotator cuff repair. The purpose of our study was to determine common clinical practices among experts regarding rotator cuff repair and to assist them in counseling patients. We surveyed 372 members of the American Shoulder and Elbow Surgeons (ASES) and the Association of Clinical Elbow and Shoulder Surgeons (ACESS); 111 members (29.8%) completed all or part of the survey, and 92.8% of the respondents answered every question. A consensus response (>50% agreement) was achieved on 49% (24 of 49) of the questions. Variability in responses likely reflects the fact that clinical practices have evolved over time based on clinical experience.

▶ This article provides detailed insight into the common practices of shoulder surgeons with regard to rotator cuff repair. Of interest is the high rate of respondents who would recommend surgery in smokers. Although it is well known that poorer outcomes can be expected in this patient cohort, it suggests that surgeons consider a surgical intervention to at least partially improve the natural history of the disease.

Surprisingly, only half of questions reached a consensus. This may be in part due to the unavailability of conclusive research supporting 1 specific practice pattern. Large variability among respondents was seen with regard to the timing of postoperative therapy. This could be a reflection of recent literature raising doubts on the benefits of early therapy.

The lack of consensus in other topics such as duration of postoperative analgesics underlines how other factors such as patient variability, regulations, and personal positions toward narcotic use may potentially play a role in shaping clinical practices. The lack of consensus on this and other topics calls for ongoing research as well as further efforts in establishing clinical guidelines.

P. Streubel, MD

Arthroscopic Repair of Full-Thickness Rotator Cuff Tears With and Without Acromioplasty: Randomized Prospective Trial With 2-Year Follow-Up

Abrams GD, Gupta AK, Hussey KE, et al (Stanford Univ, CA; Florida Orthopedic Inst, Tampa; Rush Univ Med Ctr, Chicago, IL; et al)

Am J Sports Med 42:1296-1303, 2014

Background.—Acromioplasty is commonly performed during arthroscopic rotator cuff repair, but its effect on short-term outcomes is debated.

Purpose.—To report the short-term clinical outcomes of patients undergoing arthroscopic repair of full-thickness rotator cuff tears with and without acromioplasty.

Study Design.—Randomized controlled trial; Level of evidence, 2.

Methods.—Patients undergoing arthroscopic repair of full-thickness rotator cuff tears were randomized into acromioplasty or nonacromioplasty groups. The Simple Shoulder Test (SST), American Shoulder and Elbow Surgeons (ASES) score, Constant score, University of California—Los Angeles (UCLA) score, and Short Form—12 (SF-12) health assessment were collected along with physical examination including range of motion and dynamometer strength testing. Intraoperative data including tear size, repair configuration, and concomitant procedures were recorded. Follow-up examination was performed at regular intervals up to 2 years. Preoperative imaging was reviewed to classify the acromial morphologic type, acromial angle, and lateral acromial angulation.

Results.—A total of 114 patients were initially enrolled in the study, and 95 (83%; 43 nonacromioplasty, 52 acromioplasty) were available for a minimum 2-year follow-up. There were no significant differences in baseline characteristics, including number of tendons torn, repair configuration, concomitant procedures, and acromion type and angles. Within groups, there was a significant ($P < .001$) improvement in all functional outcome scores from preoperatively to all follow-up time points, including

2 years, for the nonacromioplasty and acromioplasty groups (ASES score: 55.1-91.5, 48.8-89.0; Constant score: 48.3-75.0, 51.9-78.7, respectively). There were no significant differences in functional outcomes between nonacromioplasty and acromioplasty groups or between subjects with different acromial features at any time point.

Conclusion.—The results of this study demonstrate no difference in clinical outcomes after rotator cuff repair with or without acromioplasty at 2 years postoperatively.

▶ This randomized controlled trial adds to the mounting evidence not supporting routine acromioplasty during rotator cuff repair. The authors observed no differences at 1 and 2 years after surgery with regard to Simple Shoulder Test, American Shoulder and Elbow Surgeons, Constant, University of California–Los Angeles, and Short Form-12 scores in patients with or without acromioplasty. However, a higher rate of revision repairs was performed in patients not undergoing acromioplasty (9%), compared with those undergoing acromioplasty (2%). Although this difference was not found to be statistically significant, it does replicate results observed by other investigators.[1-4] Future studies on this topic should be powered to confirm or rule out differences on this specific complication.

P. Streubel, MD

References

1. Ketola S, Lehtinen J, Arnala I, et al. Does arthroscopic acromioplasty provide any additional value in the treatment of shoulder impingement syndrome?: a two-year randomised controlled trial. *J Bone Joint Surg Br.* 2009;91:1326-1334.
2. Ketola S, Lehtinen J, Rousi T, et al. No evidence of long-term benefits of arthroscopicacromioplasty in the treatment of shoulder impingement syndrome: five-year results of a randomised controlled trial. *Bone Joint Res.* 2013;2:132-139.
3. MacDonald P, McRae S, Leiter J, Mascarenhas R, Lapner P. Arthroscopic rotator cuff repair with and without acromioplasty in the treatment of full-thickness rotator cuff tears: a multicenter, randomized controlled trial. *J Bone Joint Surg Am.* 2011;93:1953-1960.
4. Shin SJ, Oh JH, Chung SW, Song MH. The efficacy of acromioplasty in the arthroscopic repair of small- to medium-sized rotator cuff tears without acromial spur: prospective comparative study. *Arthroscopy.* 2012;28:628-635.

The Detrimental Effects of Systemic Ibuprofen Delivery on Tendon Healing Are Time-Dependent

Connizzo BK, Yannascoli SM, Tucker JJ, et al (Univ of Pennsylvania, Philadelphia)

Clin Orthop Relat Res 472:2433-2439, 2014

Background.—Current clinical treatment after tendon repairs often includes prescribing NSAIDs to limit pain and inflammation. The negative influence of NSAIDs on bone repair is well documented, but their effects on tendon healing are less clear. While NSAIDs may be detrimental to early tendon healing, some evidence suggests that they may improve healing if administered later in the repair process.

Questions/Purposes.—We asked whether the biomechanical and histologic effects of systemic ibuprofen administration on tendon healing are influenced by either immediate or delayed drug administration.

Methods.—After bilateral supraspinatus detachment and repair surgeries, rats were divided into groups and given ibuprofen orally for either Days 0 to 7 (early) or Days 8 to 14 (delayed) after surgery; a control group did not receive ibuprofen. Healing was evaluated at 1, 2, and 4 weeks postsurgery through biomechanical testing and histologic assessment.

Results.—Biomechanical evaluation resulted in decreased stiffness and modulus at 4 weeks postsurgery for early ibuprofen delivery (mean ± SD [95% CI]: 10.8 ± 6.4 N/mm [6.7–14.8] and 8.9 ± 5.9 MPa [5.4–12.3]) when compared to control repair (20.4 ± 8.6 N/mm [16.3–24.5] and 15.7 ± 7.5 MPa [12.3–19.2]) ($p = 0.003$ and 0.013); however, there were no differences between the delayed ibuprofen group (18.1 ± 7.4 N/mm [14.2–22.1] and 11.5 ± 5.6 MPa [8.2–14.9]) and the control group. Histology confirmed mechanical results with reduced fiber reorganization over time in the early ibuprofen group.

Conclusions.—Early administration of ibuprofen in the postoperative period was detrimental to tendon healing, while delayed administration did not affect tendon healing.

Clinical Relevance.—Historically, clinicians have often prescribed ibuprofen after tendon repair, but this study suggests that the timing of ibuprofen administration is critical to adequate tendon healing. This research necessitates future clinical studies investigating the use of ibuprofen for pain control after rotator cuff repair and other tendon injuries.

► This study shows that, in a rat model, ibuprofen is detrimental to tendon healing when administered within 8 days after surgery, but this effect was not seen when ibuprofen was delivered later. The experimental conditions used are certainly different from those in humans. Healing in the rat may be faster, and the biological responses to systemic drug use could differ. Therefore, it is hard to assume that oral intake of ibuprofen is harmful to healing of the rotator cuff in human patients, much less before or after a particular day following surgery.

I am not aware of any clinical studies indicating a definite relationship between the use of ibuprofen and ruptures of a repaired rotator cuff or other tendons. However, the results of this study may indicate in general that ibuprofen is not beneficial to tendon healing. Such detrimental effects may occur if ibuprofen is administered immediately after surgery, when pain and inflammation are prominent. Use of ibuprofen is usually not necessary 2 weeks after surgery because pain is substantially relieved.

For many years, I have rarely prescribed ibuprofen because it causes stomach discomfort and pain relief is mild or inefficient. I prescribe more potent pain medications for 1 or 2 weeks after tendon repair. I do not trust ibuprofen based on feedback from my patients (and I know many of my colleagues in China do not prescribe it postoperatively either). I do not usually use it unless the patient requests it or informs me about his or her positive experience with this medication.

I do not believe ibuprofen should commonly be used after surgery. After rotator cuff repair or other tendon/ligament repairs, it may be a misconception to consider nonsteroidal anti-inflammatory drugs beneficial, because they may have insignificant or marginal effects in reducing inflammation and relieving pain.

J. B. Tang, MD

Is Double-Row Rotator Cuff Repair Clinically Superior to Single-Row Rotator Cuff Repair: A Systematic Review of Overlapping Meta-analyses

Mascarenhas R, Chalmers PN, Sayegh ET, et al (Rush Univ Med Ctr, Chicago, IL; Columbia Univ, NY; et al)

Arthroscopy 30:1156-1165, 2014

Purpose.—Multiple meta-analyses of randomized clinical trials, the highest available level of evidence, have been conducted to determine whether double-row (DR) or single-row (SR) rotator cuff repair (RCR) provides superior clinical outcomes and structural healing; however, results are discordant. The purpose of this study was to conduct a systematic review of meta-analyses comparing SR and DR RCR to elucidate the cause of discordance and to determine which meta-analysis provides the current best available evidence.

Methods.—In this study we evaluated available scientific support for SR versus DR RCR by systematically reviewing the literature for published meta-analyses. Data were extracted from these meta-analyses for patient outcomes and structural healing. Meta-analysis quality was assessed with the Oxman-Guyatt and Quality of Reporting of Meta-analyses (QUOROM) systems. The Jadad algorithm was then applied to determine which meta-analyses provided the highest level of evidence.

Results.—Eight meta-analyses met the eligibility criteria: 4 including Level I evidence and 4 including both Level I and Level II evidence. Six meta-analyses found no differences between SR and DR RCR for patient outcomes, whereas 2 favored DR RCR for tears greater than 3 cm. Two meta-analyses found no structural healing differences between SR and DR RCR, whereas 3 found DR repair to be superior for tears greater than 3 cm and 2 found DR repair to be superior for all tears. Four meta-analyses had low Oxman-Guyatt scores (<3) indicative of major flaws. After application of the Jadad algorithm, 3 concordant high-quality meta-analyses were selected, all of which found significantly better structural healing with DR compared with SR RCR.

Conclusions.—According to this systematic review of overlapping meta-analyses comparing SR and DR RCR, the current highest level of evidence suggests that DR RCR provides superior structural healing to SR RCR.

Level of Evidence.—Level II, systematic review of Level I and II studies.

▶ Several meta-analyses in the literature discuss which fixation method for rotator cuff tears is best. This article's main strength is that it selects the highest quality reviews on single vs double row rotator cuff repair. Its main weakness comes from the heterogeneity seen in different surgical techniques that might influence outcomes. Results from the highest quality reviews show that there is greater healing of rotator cuff repairs when using double row fixation methods. Certainly, however, choice of this (more costly) technique as opposed to single row repair will depend in large part on future cost-effectiveness studies. However, clinical benefits of one technique over the other has not been proved. Further research is needed to justify the use of double row repair systematically. From a personal standpoint, I tend to repair small cuff tears with single row and large and massive ones with double row. Medium tears will depend on tissue quality and tear configuration. Future cost analyses will be important to determine the most appropriate treatment, given that cost is currently an issue I have to consider for my patients and is likely to assume a greater role in decision making in the future.

J. P. Simone, MD

Effect of Postoperative Passive Motion on Rotator Cuff Reconstruction With Acellular Dermal Matrix Grafts in a Rat Model

Uezono K, Ide J, Tokunaga T, et al (Kumamoto Univ, Japan)

Am J Sports Med 42:1930-1938, 2014

Background.—Although postoperative rehabilitation is critical for rotator cuff tendon-to-bone healing and shoulder function recovery, no standardized protocol has been established.

Hypothesis.—Postoperative immediate passive motion is detrimental to tendon-to-bone remodeling and tendon maturation after rotator cuff acellular dermal matrix (ADM) grafting, although postoperative delayed passive motion does no harm.

Study Design.—Controlled laboratory study.

Methods.—Male Sprague-Dawley rats underwent rotator cuff reconstruction with ADM grafts. Their shoulders were immobilized for 2 weeks thereafter. The rats were assigned to 3 different rehabilitation protocols: (1) immobilization without passive motion (nonpassive motion [N-PM], controls), (2) immobilization with immediate passive motion (I-PM), and (3) immobilization with delayed passive motion (D-PM). Specimens obtained 2, 6, and 12 weeks postoperatively were analyzed histologically, and semiquantitative histomorphological measurements of collagen organization, vascularity, and cellularity were obtained; the area of interest was divided into 2 zones, the midsubstance of the graft and the graft-bone interface. Another set of samples taken at 12 weeks was subjected to biomechanical analysis.

Results.—At 2 weeks, there was no significant difference among the groups in terms of semiquantitative histomorphological measurements of collagen organization, vascularity, and cellularity. At 6 weeks, collagen organization at the insertion site was significantly poorer in I-PM than in N-PM and D-PM rats ($P = .0095$). At 12 weeks, collagen organization at the insertion site and midsubstance of ADM grafts was also significantly poorer in I-PM rats ($P = .0125$ and $P = .0018$, respectively), and ultimate load-to-failure was lower in this group ($P = .0043$).

Conclusion.—While postoperative immediate passive motion was detrimental to remodeled tendon-to-bone healing and to the tendon maturation of ADM grafts placed in the rotator cuff tendon defects, delayed passive motion did no harm.

Clinical Relevance.—For patients with 6-week immobilization after rotator cuff reconstruction, we recommend that early passive motion be started no sooner than 3 weeks after surgery. Immediate early passive motion should be avoided.

▶ This article is significant because it is the first to analyze the effect of passive motion on rotator cuff reconstruction with acellular dermal matrix grafts. Biological factors in rotator cuff repair are certainly the future in managing cuff disease as fixation and surgical methods seem to be reaching a closer limit. This article's main strength is that it used 3 groups to compare outcomes according to postoperative motion. Its weakness is that it employed animal specimens with healthy cuffs and probably higher healing rates than those of diseased cuffs in humans. Nonetheless, part of the aim of this study was to evaluate biomechanical response as well as biological response, which can have some significance in human subjects. From a personal standpoint, I do not allow early passive range of motion for my patients because delayed motion has shown the same clinical results in the long term with less risk of cuff retearing.

J. P. Simone, MD

11 Shoulder: Miscellaneous

Hill-Sachs Lesions in Shoulders With Traumatic Anterior Instability: Evaluation Using Computed Tomography with 3-Dimensional Reconstruction

Ozaki R, Nakagawa S, Mizuno N, et al (Toyonaka Municipal Hosp, Osaka, Japan; Yukioka Hosp, Osaka, Japan; et al)

Am J Sports Med 42:2597-2605, 2014

Background.—In patients with traumatic anterior shoulder instability, a large Hill-Sachs lesion is a risk factor for postoperative recurrence. However, there is no consensus regarding the occurrence and enlargement of Hill-Sachs lesions.

Purpose.—To investigate the influence of the number of dislocations and subluxations on the prevalence and size of Hill-Sachs lesions evaluated by computed tomography (CT) with 3-dimensional reconstruction.

Study Design.—Cohort study (diagnosis); Level of evidence, 2.

Methods.—The prevalence and size of Hill-Sachs lesions were evaluated preoperatively by CT in 142 shoulders (30 with primary instability and 112 with recurrent instability) before arthroscopic Bankart repair. First, the prevalence of Hill-Sachs lesions was compared with the arthroscopic findings. Then, the size of Hill-Sachs lesions confirmed by arthroscopy was remeasured using the previous CT data. In addition, the relationship of Hill-Sachs lesions with the number of dislocations and subluxations was investigated.

Results.—Hill-Sachs lesions were detected in 90 shoulders by initial CT evaluation and were found in 118 shoulders at arthroscopy. The Hill-Sachs lesions missed by initial CT were 15 chondral lesions and 13 osseous lesions. However, all 103 osseous Hill-Sachs lesions were detected by reviewing the CT data. In patients with primary subluxation, the prevalence of Hill-Sachs lesions was 26.7%, and the mean length, width, and depth of the lesions (calculated as a percentage of the diameter of the humeral head) were 9.0%, 5.3%, and 2.1%, respectively, while the corresponding numbers for primary dislocation were 73.3%, 27.7%, 14.8%, and 7.0%, all showing statistically significant differences. Among all 142 shoulders, the corresponding numbers were, respectively, 56.3%, 20.7%, 11.2%, and 4.8% in patients who had subluxations but never a dislocation; 83.3%, 33.4%, 19.1%, and 7.6% in patients with 1 episode of dislocation; and 87.5%, 46.8%, 22.2%, and 10.2% in patients with ≥2 episodes, all showing statistically significant differences. There were no differences in lesion measurements in relation to the number of subluxations.

Conclusion.—Computed tomography is a useful imaging modality for evaluating Hill-Sachs lesions except for purely cartilaginous lesions. Hill-Sachs lesions were more frequent and larger when the primary episode was dislocation than when it was subluxation. Among patients with recurrent episodes of complete dislocation, the prevalence of Hill-Sachs lesions is increased, and the lesions are larger.

▶ This prospective study looked to quantify the frequency and size of Hill-Sachs lesions after primary and recurrent glenohumeral dislocations. The number of previous subluxations and dislocations was also correlated with the size of the Hill-Sachs lesion. The authors prospectively evaluated CT scans in 142 shoulder before arthroscopic labral repair. They found the presence of a Hill-Sachs lesion in 27% of patients who had a primary subluxation and 73% for primary dislocation. An increasing incidence of Hill-Sachs lesions was noted with an increasing number of dislocations: subluxation without dislocation was 56%, 1 dislocation was 83%, and 2 dislocations were 88%. This prospective study helps to establish baseline data as to the frequency as well as the depth of Hill-Sachs lesions after glenohumeral subluxation and dislocation. These data will help to provide a foundation for further clinical study of this frequent problem.

J. Macalena, MD

Online Resources for Shoulder Instability: What Are Patients Reading?

Garcia GH, Taylor SA, Dy CJ, et al (Hosp for Special Surgery, NY; et al)

J Bone Joint Surg Am 96:e177(1-7), 2014

Background.—Evaluations of the medical literature suggest that many online sites provide poor-quality information. The purpose of our study was to investigate the value of online resources for patient education about shoulder instability.

Methods.—Three search terms (“shoulder instability,” “loose shoulder,” and “shoulder dislocation”) were entered into three Internet search engines. Three orthopaedic residents independently gauged the quality and accuracy of the information with use of a set of predetermined scoring criteria, in addition to noting whether or not four potential surgery options were mentioned. The readability of the web sites was evaluated with use of the Flesch-Kincaid score.

Results.—Eighty-two unique web sites were evaluated. Quality and accuracy were significantly higher with use of the term “shoulder instability” compared with the term “loose shoulder” (quality, $p < 0.001$; accuracy, $p = 0.001$). However, the reading level was significantly more advanced for the “shoulder instability” web sites ($p < 0.001$). Quality was significantly higher on web sites with reading levels above the eighth grade level ($p = 0.001$) (88% of web sites). Only twenty-three sites (28%) mentioned surgical options for shoulder instability, and of these, only eight mentioned thermal capsulorrhaphy as a primary treatment.

Conclusions.—Online information regarding shoulder instability is often inaccurate and/or at an inappropriately high reading level. The quality of information is highly dependent on the specific search term used. Clinicians need to be aware of the information that is available online and should help direct patients to proper sites and guide Internet search terms.

► Quality and accuracy of available online information is clearly variable. However, around 60% of internet users search for medical information online. This study hypothesized that the use of more medically accurate search terms would improve the overall quality and accuracy of the websites found. Findings showed that a more medically accurate diagnosis that can be communicated effectively to a patient might be a more useful and accurate way of reaching better quality websites that have higher accuracy, with a caveat of higher reading level necessary for the patient to comprehend the knowledge provided. They also found that only a handful websites present the patient with surgical treatment options, which might lead to a delay in diagnosis and treatment because of late presentation of the younger patients. More interestingly, thermal capsulorrhaphy was still being presented as a primary surgical option, although nobody probably has been using this modality for almost a decade. The most important conclusion of this study is to increase the physician authorship focusing on the layman's terms to increase reach among patients.

A. Cil, MD

The Open Latarjet Procedure Is More Reliable in Terms of Shoulder Stability Than Arthroscopic Bankart Repair

Bessière C, Trojani C, Carles M, et al (Univ of Nice-Sophia Antipolis, France)
Clin Orthop Relat Res 472:2345-2351, 2014

Background.—Arthroscopic Bankart repair and open Latarjet bone block procedure are widely considered mainstays for surgical treatment of recurrent anterior shoulder instability. The choice between these procedures depends mainly on surgeon preference or training rather than published evidence.

Questions/Purposes.—We compared patients with recurrent posttraumatic anterior shoulder instability treated with arthroscopic Bankart or open Latarjet procedure in terms of (1) frequency and timing of recurrent instability, (2) risk factors for recurrent instability, and (3) patient-reported outcomes.

Methods.—In this retrospective comparative study, we paired 93 patients undergoing open Latarjet procedures with 93 patients undergoing arthroscopic Bankart repairs over the same period for posttraumatic anterior shoulder instability by one of four surgeons at the same center. Both groups were comparable except that patients in the Latarjet group had more glenoid lesions and more instability episodes preoperatively. Minimum followup was 4 years (mean, 6 years; range, 4-10 years). Patients were assessed with a questionnaire, including stability, Rowe score, and return to sports. Recurrent instability was defined as at least one episode of recurrent dislocation or subluxation. Return to sports was evaluated using a 0% to 100% scale that patients completed after recovery from surgery. Various risk factors for recurrent instability were also analyzed.

Results.—At latest followup, 10% (nine of 93) in the Latarjet group and 22% (20 of 93) in the Bankart group demonstrated recurrent instability ($p = 0.026$; odds ratio, 0.39; 95% CI, 0.17-0.91). Ten recurrences in the Bankart group (50%) occurred after 2 years, compared to only one (11%) in the Latarjet group. Reoperation rate was 6% and 7% in the Bankart and Latarjet groups, respectively. In both groups, patients younger than 20 years had higher recurrence risk ($p = 0.019$). In the Bankart group, independent factors predictive for recurrence were practice of competitive sports and shoulder hyperlaxity (ie, passive external rotation > 85° in the contralateral uninjured shoulder). Although return to sports was not different between groups, the mean Rowe score was higher in the Latarjet group (78 versus 68, $p = 0.018$).

Conclusions.—Patients who had the open Latarjet procedure had less recurrent instability and better Rowe scores over a mean 6-year followup. We now perform isolated arthroscopic Bankart repair for carefully selected patients, including patients with an Instability Severity Index Score of 3 or less.

Level of Evidence.—Level III, therapeutic study. See Instructions for Authors for a complete description of levels of evidence.

▶ This article looks at the results of arthroscopic Bankart repairs versus Latarjet bone block procedure in a retrospective manner and uses paired matching technique to identify subjects. After a minimum of 4 years of follow-up, the authors showed that recurrence rates of instability with Bankart repairs were twice as high compared with those of the Latarjet procedure; however, the reapportion rates were very similar. One interesting finding that they outlined was that if there was recurrence, it was within the first 2 years in the Latarjet cases; however, Bankart repairs continued to become unstable and fail even after 2 years in 50% of the cases. Satisfaction among 2 groups of patients and Simple Shoulder Test values were not significantly different. The authors concluded that the open Latarjet procedure is a more reliable method to fix shoulder instability. I agree that Latarjet procedure is a very successful procedure in select indications like significant glenoid bone loss or off-track Hill-Sachs lesions. However, if we exclude these cases, the arthroscopic Bankart repairs are as successful as Latarjet procedures based on the current literature. Moreover, there is an increased incidence of degenerative changes with longer term follow-ups of Latarjet procedures, which this article has not reported, as they did not do any radiographic follow-up. Consequently, in my clinical practice, these 2 surgeries are complementary to treat the spectrum of shoulder instability rather than used interchangeably.

A. Cil, MD

Measurement of the Glenoid Track In Vivo as Investigated by 3-Dimensional Motion Analysis Using Open MRI

Omori Y, Yamamoto N, Koishi H, et al (Osaka Univ Graduate School of Medicine, Suita, Japan; Tohoku Univ School of Medicine, Sendai, Japan)

Am J Sports Med 42:1290-1295, 2014

Background.—A Hill-Sachs lesion is a common injury associated with anterior glenohumeral instability, and a Hill-Sachs lesion that engages with the anterior glenoid rim is 1 factor related to recurrent instability. In a cadaveric study in 2007, a new concept, the "glenoid track," was proposed to evaluate the risk of engagement of Hill-Sachs lesions with the glenoid.

Purpose.—To investigate the glenoid track in vivo using a custom-developed noninvasive motion analysis system.

Study Design.—Descriptive laboratory study.

Methods.—Using a wide-gantry magnetic resonance imaging (MRI) scanner, the right shoulders of 30 healthy volunteers were examined. The MRI scans were taken of the right arm in 7 static supine positions from 0° to maximum abduction, keeping maximum external rotation and horizontal extension. Using the custom motion analysis system, 3-dimensional models of the scapula and humerus were created from the MRI data. Then, the movement of the humerus and scapula was calculated using voxel-based registration of each model, and the motion of the glenoid on the humeral head was analyzed.

Results.—The models demonstrated that glenoid contact shifted from the inferomedial to the superolateral portion of the humeral head. The mean widths of the glenoid track with the arm at 60°, 90°, 120°, and 150° of abduction were 20.7 ± 4.5 mm, 19.4 ± 3.9 mm, 18.9 ± 2.7 mm, and 18.7 ± 2.5 mm (89%, 83%, 82%, and 81% of the glenoid width), respectively. The width of the glenoid track at 60° of abduction was significantly greater than those at 90°, 120°, and 150° of abduction ($P = .0472$, .0148, and .0083, respectively). There were no significant differences among widths measured at 90°, 120°, and 150° of abduction.

Conclusion.—The existence and widths of the glenoid track were confirmed in vivo.

► The glenoid track was hypothesized, based on cadaveric studies in 2007, as the path that the humeral head follows as it progresses across the glenoid. This hypothesis has not yet been shown in a clinical model. The authors created a noninvasive, custom motion analysis system in which static MR images of the glenohumeral compartment were obtained in progressive amounts of abduction. The track of the humeral head across the glenoid was then charted. The glenoid track was seen to progress from inferomedial to superolateral with progressive abduction. This study provides an in vivo correlation of a previously completed cadaveric study. It provides a mechanism for engagement of a Hill-Sachs defect with the glenoid, one of the known risk factors for repeat dislocation.

J. Macalena, MD

Arthroscopy After Locked Plating of Proximal Humeral Fractures: Implant Removal, Capsular Release, and Intra-articular Findings

Katthagen JC, Hennecke D, Jensen G, et al (Diakoniekrankenhaus Friederikenstift gGmbH, Hannover, Germany)

Arthroscopy 30:1061-1067, 2014

Purpose.—The purpose of this study was to determine the outcomes of arthroscopy after proximal humeral plating and the occurrence of concomitant pathology and avascular necrosis.

Methods.—Forty-five patients (28 women; median age, 58.5 years [range, 30 to 82 years]) underwent arthroscopies of 46 shoulders because of unsatisfactory results after locked plating of proximal humeral fractures. They were prospectively followed up for 3, 12, and 24 months postoperatively. Relevant intra-articular lesions were documented. The patients were assigned to 1 of the following groups: (1) articular screw perforation, (2) subacromial plate impingement, or (3) post-traumatic/postoperative shoulder stiffness. Shoulder range of motion and function as measured with the age- and gender-adjusted Constant-Murley score, as well as the Simple Shoulder Test, were compared among the groups.

Results.—Concomitant lesions of the articular cartilage, long head of the biceps tendon, tuberosities, and rotator cuff were found in 34 patients (75%). Two-thirds of patients (n = 31) had a partial or complete 270° capsular release. Of the patients, 84% (n = 38) underwent 3 and 12 months' follow-up and 82% (n = 37) underwent 24 months' follow-up. The active range of abduction ($P = .029$), flexion ($P = .048$), and internal rotation ($P = .0005$) had improved significantly at 24 months' follow-up compared with the preoperative status. The mean adjusted Constant-Murley score of patients with post-traumatic shoulder stiffness (n = 15, 64.2% ± 7.9%) and articular screw perforation (n = 19, 73.3% ± 8.4%) was significantly lower ($P = .0089$ and $P = .042$, respectively) than that of patients with subacromial plate impingement (n = 12, 93.4% ± 4.3%).

Conclusions.—High rates of relevant articular pathologies and the necessity of capsular release in a majority of patients with unsatisfactory results after locked plating of proximal humeral fractures make arthroscopy a valuable revision tool with promising results in cases of high plate positioning, screw perforation, and postoperative/post- traumatic shoulder stiffness.

Level of Evidence.—Level IV, therapeutic case series.

▶ Intraarticular concomitant pathologies of the articular cartilage, long head of the biceps tendon, rotator cuff, and tuberosities are thought to be common in patients with unsatisfactory results after locked plating of proximal humeral fractures. Arthroscopy in this patient population has been shown to be a valuable tool. For example, capsular release, which cannot be carried out to the same extent during common open revision surgery, may be best achieved during arthroscopy. The authors emphasize that capsular release is important during arthroscopy. Evaluation of intraoperative findings of all 46 shoulders showed 1 or more relevant concomitant intraarticular pathologies in 75% of patients. Chondral lesions (grade II–IV chondromalacia) of the articular cartilage were found in 50% of shoulders. The glenoid showed chondral damage in 18 cases and the humeral head in 13 cases. Most of the cartilage damage was intraoperatively found to be associated with articular screw perforation. In 48% of patients, a lesion of the long head of the biceps tendon was identified and treated with either debridement or tenotomy. If reasonable, the long head of the biceps tendon was debrided and preserved, especially in younger patients. Eighty-two percent were satisfied with the outcome at 24 months postoperatively and rated the arthroscopic procedure as being beneficial. The only issues that the authors did not address were the technical difficulties associated with arthroscopic release of subdeltoid adhesions, which can be substantial and also may be a factor in achieving range of motion.

In my experience, subdeltoid and subacromial adhesions can be not only extensive in surface area but also thick in consistency and difficult to excise short of using a physical incision via an open approach. Nonetheless, the authors present consistently good results with their arthroscopic technique, especially in light of the ability to achieve intraarticular capsular release, and the ability of the patient to undergo a less painful procedure and achieve an expedited recovery with the arthroscopic technique.

E. Cheung, MD

How often do surgeons intervene on shoulder labral lesions detected at MR examination? A retrospective review of MR examinations correlated with arthroscopy

Magee T (Univ of Central Florida School of Medicine, Orlando)
Br J Radiol 87:20130736, 2014

Objective.—We report the prevalence of surgical intervention on shoulder labral lesions detected at MR examinations and how surgeons describe labral tears seen at MR examinations in their arthroscopy reports.

Methods.—A retrospective review of 100 consecutive patients aged 50 years or younger who had shoulder labral tears on MR and went on to have surgery performed. It was determined whether surgical intervention was performed on the MR lesions.

Results.—Of these 100 patients, 72 had superior labral anterior to posterior (SLAP) tears, 38 had posterior labral tears and 28 had anterior labral tears on MR examination. All 100 patients went on to arthroscopy. All lesions described on MRI were described on arthroscopy. Of the 72 SLAP tears, 64 were described as fraying on arthroscopy with 51 debrided. The remaining eight SLAP tears were tacked surgically. Of the 38 posterior labral tears, 36 were described as fraying on arthroscopy with 29 debrided and 2 had surgical tacking performed. Of the 28 anterior labral tears described on MR examination, 26 had surgical tacking performed and 2 were debrided. There were four SLAP tears, two anterior labral tears and three posterior labral tears seen on arthroscopy but not seen on MR examination.

Conclusion.—In this series, a high percentage of SLAP tears and posterior labral tears described on MR examination did not have surgical tacking. Most anterior labral tears had surgical tacking. Based on the above, our surgeons request we describe superior and posterior labral lesions as fraying and/or tearing, unless we can see a displaced tear. Most anterior labral lesions are treated with surgical tacking.

Advances in Knowledge.—MRI allows for sensitive detection of labral tears. The tears often are not clinically significant.

▶ MRI is found to be sensitive and specific in the diagnosis of labral tears. This study confirms the findings in previous literature on the excellent detection power of the MRIs of labral tears. This study possibly originated from a disagreement between the radiologists and orthopedic surgeons on what is called a (clinically significant) tear. Radiologists have identified tears on the MRI, and each of those has been seen during the arthroscopy. However, some of the radiologically described tears were described as fraying rather than tearing at the time of surgery, and also some of the radiologically described tears were either ignored or simply derided and did not require repair, especially when they were involving superior or posterior labrum. There are a couple of reasons for this discrepancy. The main problem is the patient perception of how adequately a tear should be addressed by their treating physicians. If it is called a tear but the physician simply ignored it at the time of surgery, as it was clinically not important, will the patient be unsatisfied or feel something was forgotten? That is probably the most important reason the surgeons are somewhat reluctant to call some labral lesions tears, especially when they are not clinically significant. The anterior labral tears in this study were repaired, but most of the superior labral anterior to posterior (SLAP) tears and posterior labrum tears were either debrided or left alone and were not described as tears but as fraying. Anterior labral lesions are most frequently treated as expected because anterior instability at the described age group is more frequent or better understood than a posterior instability or a SLAP tear that might be symptomatic. However, based on SLAP tear classification, type 1 SLAP tears are described as fraying of the labrum, so theoretically, fraying means a type 1 SLAP tear regardless of how we would like to interpret it at the time of surgery.

A. Cil, MD

Arthroscopic Stabilization for Recurrent Shoulder Instability With Moderate Glenoid Bone Defect in Patients With Moderate to Low Functional Demand

Kim S-J, Kim S-H, Park B-K, et al (Yonsei Univ College of Medicine, Seoul, South Korea)

Arthroscopy 30:921-927, 2014

Purpose.—The purpose of this study was to investigate the functional outcomes of arthroscopic Bankart repair for recurrent shoulder instability in the setting of moderate glenoid bone defect ranging from 20% to 30% in patients with moderate to low functional demand.

Methods.—This study included 36 patients with unilateral recurrent instability and glenoid bone defects of 20% to 30% treated with arthroscopic stabilization. Glenoid bone loss was estimated on the en-face view of preoperative 3-dimensional computed tomography. Joint laxity was assessed clinically by use of the Beighton and Horan criteria, and patients were divided into 2 groups based on the presence of excessive joint laxity, group L (n = 13), or absence of excessive joint laxity, group N (n = 23). Functional assessments were performed with the patient-reported activity level; subjective shoulder value; Rowe score; and University of California, Los Angeles shoulder score.

Results.—The mean glenoid defect size was 25.1% (range, 20% to 29%), and the overall functional outcomes improved significantly after surgery. A return to greater than 90% of the premorbid activity level was reported by 72% of patients (26 of 36 patients), and patient satisfaction was 83% (30 of 36 patients). There was no significant difference in functional outcomes between groups L and N (subjective shoulder value, 85.0% for group L *v* 88.9% for group N, $P = .397$; Rowe score, 83.5 for group L *v* 92.8 for group N, $P = .537$; and University of California, Los Angeles shoulder score, 32.2 for group L *v* 31.9 for group N, $P = .697$). Recurrent instability occurred in 4 patients (11%), 3 patients in group L (3 of 13, 23%) and 1 patient in group N (1 of 23, 4%), but this difference was not statistically significant ($P = .125$).

Conclusions.—Arthroscopic stabilization for recurrent shoulder instability in patients with moderate to low functional demand produced satisfactory outcomes despite the presence of moderate glenoid bone defects of 20% to 30%. For patients with excessive joint laxity, however, arthroscopic stabilization may not be reliable, with a recurrence rate of 23%.

Level of Evidence.—Level IV, therapeutic case series.

▶ Shoulder instability in the setting of glenoid bone loss has received increased attention over the last decade, as capsulolabral repair has shown unacceptable high rates of recurrent instability, especially in contact athletes. In this setting coracoid transfer has become the mainstay of treatment, either open or arthroscopic. Autograft and allograft techniques are also described with acceptable outcomes. The authors present their results of Bankart repair in the presence of 20% to 30% glenoid bone loss in a cohort of patients with moderate and low functional demands. Their outcomes are encouraging, especially for patients without generalized ligamentous laxity. In this subgroup, stability can be reliably restored using standard capsulolabral repair. Likely one of the most difficult to treat patients, namely those with combined glenoid bone loss and generalized laxity, do not fare well with Bankart repair only. Although based on clinical functional scores alone, favorable results were recorded; recurrent instability occurred in one-fourth of these patients. Glenoid bone grafting as previously described should likely be considered in this specific patient population.

As one would expect, sample size is small from a statistical perspective. Comparisons between lax and nonlax groups are, therefore, likely underpowered. However, from a clinical perspective, this is a large cohort of a specific group of patients with a rare and complex variety of shoulder instability. Studies to further clarify this topic will likely require multicenter efforts.

P. N. Streubel, MD

Dexamethasone for pain after outpatient shoulder surgery: a randomised, double-blind, placebo-controlled trial

Bjørnholdt KT, Mønsted PN, Søballe K, et al (Horsens Regional Hosp, Denmark; Aarhus Univ Hosp, Denmark)

Acta Anaesthesiol Scand 58:751-758, 2014

Background.—Dexamethasone has analgesic properties when given intravenously before surgery, but the optimal dose has not been determined. We hypothesised that a dose of 40 mg dexamethasone would improve analgesia after outpatient shoulder surgery compared with 8 mg.

Methods.—A randomised, double-blind, placebo-controlled clinical trial was conducted at Horsens Regional Hospital, Denmark. Patients scheduled for arthroscopic subacromial decompression and/or acromioclavicular joint resection as an outpatient procedure ($n = 101$) were randomised to receive intravenous dexamethasone 40 mg (D40), 8 mg (D8) or placebo (D0) before surgery. The primary outcome was pain intensity 8 h after surgery rated on a numeric rating scale of 0 to 10. Secondary outcomes were pain intensity, analgesic consumption and side effects during the first 3 days after surgery.

Results.—Data from 73 patients were available for analysis: (D40: 25, D8: 26, D0: 22 patients). Eight hours after surgery, pain intensity were: [median (interquartile range)] group D40: 2 (1–4), group D8: 2.5 (1–5), group D0: 4 (2–7). There was no significant difference in pain intensity between group D40 and D8 after 8 h ($P = 0.46$) or at any other time. When comparing all three groups, a statistically significant dose–response relationship was seen for present, average and worst pain intensity after 8 h and on the following morning. No differences were found in analgesic consumption. No serious side effects were observed.

Conclusion.—Although our data supported a dose–response relationship, increasing the dexamethasone dose from 8 to 40 mg did not improve analgesia significantly after outpatient shoulder surgery.

▶ This is a well-designed study seeking to delineate a dose–response for dexamethasone as a pain reliever after arthroscopic shoulder surgery. Although widely used for postoperative nausea and vomiting, there is evidence to support the use of glucocorticoids in a postoperative pain regimen. However, previous literature provides limited guidance on the ideal dosage of dexamethasone as a pain reliever in outpatient orthopedic surgery.

The authors of this study identified clear primary and secondary outcomes and included a power analysis, thereby improving the likelihood that the trial will measure clinically relevant differences in postoperative pain. The results suggest an inverse relationship between the dexamethasone dose and pain intensity within the first 24 hours after surgery. However, the higher dexamethasone dose did not lead to a significant reduction in postoperative pain or analgesic use in the first 3 days after arthroscopic subacromial decompression or acromioclavicular joint resection. Therefore, the readers of this article may not choose to adopt the higher dose of dexamethasone when treating the postoperative pain of arthroscopic shoulder surgery patients.

The study also investigated the potential complications associated with dexamethasone in the perioperative setting. There were no significant differences in patient-reported side effects with or without dexamethasone, and dexamethasone was not associated with infection or delayed wound healing. These findings regarding the side effects will be reassuring for those providers who choose to use dexamethasone for postoperative nausea and vomiting and/or pain control.

E. Kinnucan, MD

Glenohumeral Contact Pressure With Simulated Anterior Labral and Osseous Defects in Cadaveric Shoulders Before and After Soft Tissue Repair

Yamamoto A, Massimini DF, DiStefano J, et al (Gunma Univ Graduate School of Medicine, Japan; Massachusetts Inst of Technology, Boston; Brigham and Women's Hosp, Boston, MA)

Am J Sports Med 42:1947-1954, 2014

Background.—Glenoid rim fractures and erosion can result from traumatic and repeated shoulder dislocations, leading to glenoid bone loss. Traditional instability surgery includes Bankart repair to restore soft tissue anatomy, although a recent trend is to address glenoid bone deficiency when appropriate with a bone block procedure.

Hypothesis/Purpose.—The purpose of this study was to quantify glenohumeral joint contact pressures as a function of anterior labral detachment, progressive anterior glenoid bone loss, and labral repair. The hypothesis was that a critical glenoid defect size exists whereby labral repair alone cannot restore joint contact pressures, therefore favoring bone block augmentation over soft tissue repair.

Study Design.—Controlled laboratory study.

Methods.—Eight fresh-frozen cadaveric shoulders were tested under a 440-N compressive load simulating glenohumeral abduction positions of 30° and 60° in neutral rotation and 60° with 90° of external rotation. Glenohumeral joint contact pressures were recorded with a Tekscan pressure sensor system in these configurations: (1) intact specimen, (2) Bankart lesion, (3) 10% anterior rim bone defect, (4) 10% bone defect with labral repair, (5) 20% bone defect, (6) 20% bone defect with labral repair, (7) 30% bone defect, and (8) 30% bone defect with labral repair. The joint contact pressures were compared at all configurations.

Results.—The Bankart lesion and 10%, 20%, and 30% glenoid defects showed significant ($P < .05$) increases in mean contact pressures over baseline values. Labral repair at 10% bone loss reduced mean contact pressures to below the intact state, and labral repair of 20% defects demonstrated normalized mean contact pressures. However, mean contact pressures remained statistically elevated compared with baseline values after labral repair of 30% glenoid defects.

Conclusion.—Glenohumeral joint contact pressures were restored to baseline values after labral repair of 10% and 20% anterior glenoid bone defects. Conversely, labral repair at 30% glenoid bone loss did not restore glenohumeral contact mechanics, yielding elevated contact pressures despite repair. Further study is warranted to investigate the stability (resistance to dislocations) of the glenohumeral joint after labral repair and bone block augmentation.

Clinical Relevance.—A critical glenoid defect size exists in which labral repair alone does not restore normal glenohumeral contact pressures. Surgeons should carefully evaluate glenoid bone loss before selecting a surgical treatment for shoulder instability.

▶ This controlled laboratory study evaluated the effects of glenoid bone loss with regard to contact pressure of the glenohumeral joint. It is a study of 8 cadaveric specimens with anterior labral tears and progressive bone defects of the anterior glenoid rim. The tested states include the intact state, Bankart tear, and 10%, 20%, and 30% bony fractures of the anterior glenoid. The authors found that labral tears and all 3 bony defects increased the glenohumeral contact pressures. The cohort with an isolated labral repair and the repaired 10% and 20% bone defects showed normalization of the contact stresses. Repair of a 30% defect did not restore the baseline contact pressures. This report suggests that there is a critical value of bone defect (between 20% and 30%) that, when present, causes an increase in contact pressure, despite repair. Further work is necessary to correlate this laboratory study with clinical experience.

J. Macalena, MD

Improper Trunk Rotation Sequence Is Associated With Increased Maximal Shoulder External Rotation Angle and Shoulder Joint Force in High School Baseball Pitchers

Oyama S, Yu B, Blackburn JT, et al (Univ of Texas San Antonio; Univ of North Carolina at Chapel Hill; et al)

Am J Sports Med 42:2089-2094, 2014

Background.—In a properly coordinated throwing motion, peak pelvic rotation velocity is reached before peak upper torso rotation velocity, so that angular momentum can be transferred effectively from the proximal (pelvis) to distal (upper torso) segment. However, the effects of trunk rotation sequence on pitching biomechanics and performance have not been investigated.

Purpose.—The aim of this study was to investigate the effects of trunk rotation sequence on ball speed and on upper extremity biomechanics that are linked to injuries in high school baseball pitchers. The hypothesis was that pitchers with improper trunk rotation sequence would demonstrate lower ball velocity and greater stress to the joint.

Study Design.—Descriptive laboratory study.

Methods.—Three-dimensional pitching kinematics data were captured from 72 high school pitchers. Subjects were considered to have proper or improper trunk rotation sequences when the peak pelvic rotation velocity was reached either before or after the peak upper torso rotation velocity beyond the margin of error (±3.7% of the time from stride-foot contact to ball release). Maximal shoulder external rotation angle, elbow extension angle at ball release, peak shoulder proximal force, shoulder internal rotation moment, and elbow varus moment were compared between groups using independent t tests ($\alpha < 0.05$).

Results.—Pitchers with improper trunk rotation sequences ($n = 33$) demonstrated greater maximal shoulder external rotation angle (mean difference, 7.2° ± 2.9°, $P = .016$) and greater shoulder proximal force (mean difference, 9.2% ± 3.9% body weight, $P = .021$) compared with those with proper trunk rotation sequences ($n = 22$). No other variables differed significantly different between groups.

Conclusion.—High school baseball pitchers who demonstrated improper trunk rotation sequences demonstrated greater maximal shoulder external rotation angle and shoulder proximal force compared with pitchers with proper trunk rotation sequences.

Clinical Relevance.—Improper sequencing of the trunk and torso alter upper extremity joint loading in ways that may influence injury risk. As such, exercises that reinforce the use of a proper trunk rotation sequence during the pitching motion may reduce the stress placed on the structures around the shoulder joint and lead to the prevention of injuries.

▶ In this study, the authors attempted to evaluate the relationship between peak pelvic rotational velocity on upper extremity throwing biomechanics and its effect on both ball speed and joint stress. They used 3-dimensional pitching kinematic data to evaluate the timing of peak pelvic rotation velocity. The authors found that pitchers with improper rotation had increased external rotation angle at the shoulder and increased peak shoulder force, potentially predisposing these athletes to injury. This study did not find a difference in pitch velocity. These findings suggest the importance of proper throwing mechanics, which should be stressed to all young pitchers during routine pitching as a preventative measure and during the rehabilitation process.

J. Macalena, MD

Comparison of 3–Dimensional Shoulder Complex Kinematics in Individuals With and Without Shoulder Pain, Part 1: Sternoclavicular, Acromioclavicular, and Scapulothoracic Joints

Lawrence RL, Braman JP, Laprade RF, et al (Univ of Minnesota, Minneapolis; Steadman Philippon Research Inst, Vail, CO)

J Orthop Sports Phys Ther 44:636-645, 2014

Study Design.—Cross-sectional.

Objectives.—To compare sternoclavicular, acromioclavicular, and scapulothoracic joint motion between symptomatic and asymptomatic individuals during shoulder motion performed in 3 planes of humerothoracic elevation.

Background.—Differences in scapulothoracic kinematics are associated with shoulder pain. Several studies have measured these differences using surface sensors, but the results of this technique may be affected by skin-motion artifact. Furthermore, previous studies have not included the simultaneous measurement of sternoclavicular and acromioclavicular joint motion.

Methods.—Transcortical bone pins were inserted into the clavicle, scapula, and humerus of 12 asymptomatic and 10 symptomatic individuals for direct, bone-fixed tracking using electromagnetic sensors. Angular positions for the sternoclavicular, acromioclavicular, and scapulothoracic joints were measured during shoulder flexion, abduction, and scapular plane abduction.

Results.—Differences between groups were found for sternoclavicular and scapulothoracic joint positions. Symptomatic individuals consistently demonstrated less sternoclavicular posterior rotation, regardless of angle, phase, or plane of shoulder motion. Symptomatic individuals also demonstrated less scapulothoracic upward rotation at 30° and 60° of humerothoracic elevation during shoulder abduction and scapular plane abduction.

Conclusion.—The results of this study show that differences in shoulder complex kinematics exist between symptomatic and asymptomatic individuals. However, the magnitude of these differences was small, and the resulting clinical implications are not yet fully understood. The biomechanical coupling of the sternoclavicular and acromioclavicular joints requires further research to better understand scapulothoracic movement

deviations and to improve manual therapy and exercise-based physical therapy interventions.

▶ Shoulder impingement syndrome has long been ascribed to theory-based anatomic and mechanical pathology of the shoulder girdle. In recent years, 3-dimensional analyses have illustrated differences in the motion of the scapula relative to the thorax in persons with and without shoulder symptoms. Methodologically speaking, these studies have been limited by technology that was prone to movement artifact and the incomplete modeling of the shoulder complex. In this article, Lawrence et al sought to investigate whether differences in sternoclavicular (SC) and acromioclavicular (AC) joint motions accompany scapulothoracic (ST) differences between those with and without shoulder pain. Moreover, they sought to improve on earlier methodology through using transcortical bone pins to better stabilize markers used for 3-dimensional modeling of the shoulder.

Twelve adults without a history of prior or current shoulder symptoms/injury, positive shoulder provocative results, abnormal asymmetrical loss of shoulder motion, and any observable scapular dyskinesis and 10 adults with shoulder pain symptoms, 2 or more positive provocative test results for impingement, observable scapular dyskinesis, no history of traumatic injury to shoulder, negative tests for superior labrum anterior and posterior lesions or rotator cuff tear, and the absence of rheumatoid arthritis/shoulder osteoarthritis participated in this study. Transcortical pins/markers were placed, as per International Society of Biomechanics recommendations, in the humerus, scapula, and clavicle on the affected shoulder in the symptomatic group and on the participants' preferred side in the asymptomatic group. After which, kinematics (in degrees) of the ST, AC, and SC joints were analyzed during 2 trials of elevation and lowering of the humerus in the plane of the scapula (ie, scaption) in flexion and in abduction.

The between-trials repeatability of the measures were good to excellent, and within-subject trial-to-trial error was generally less than 2 degrees. As expected, the symptomatic group possessed reduced scapula-humeral rhythm in that they displayed significantly reduced scapular upward rotation during early elevation and lowering of the humerus in abduction and in early phases of humeral elevation during scaption. Additionally, the authors noted that, through all planes, angles, and phases (ie, elevation vs lowering) of humeral movement, a significant reduction of SC posterior rotation was present in those with symptomatic shoulders when compared to those without. These differences were all outside of the standard error of the mean and, therefore, represent a real difference.

The findings help to partially substantiate theory that describes a coupling effect between sternoclavicular and scapulothoracic motion in that deficits in scapular upward rotation were mirrored by deficits in sternoclavicular posterior rotation in the symptomatic group. These findings also help to substantiate theory that mechanical impingement is often a result of reduced synergy between humeral elevation and scapular upward rotation in early phases of humeral elevation. During the phases of humeral elevation in which the rotator cuff (RTC) tendons are known to be between the humeral head and acromion,[1] the symptomatic group displayed significantly less scapular upward rotation than did their asymptomatic counterparts. Although not directly measured in this study, the implication of this dysfunctional synergy pattern would be reduced subacromial space and increased risk of RTC tendon entrapment.

Moreover, the findings illustrated a normalization of scapular upward rotation in the symptomatic group beyond 90° of humeral elevation. This was likely explained by a compensatory 3° increase in SC joint upward rotation between 60° and 90° of humeral elevation in the symptomatic group relative to the asymptomatic group. The authors speculated that this is likely related to diminished upper trapezius activation during early-phase elevation and greater activation in later phases; however, no electromyographic measures were used in the study to validate such.

The pervasive reduction in SC posterior rotation during humeral elevation of the symptomatic group might have been explained by (1) AC or coracoclavicular ligamentous laxity or (2) tightness in the clavicular fibers of pectoralis major or in the upper trapezius. Further research is needed.

Lastly, the authors suggest that the within-group variability in the kinematics of those with symptomatic shoulders support that there are likely several mechanisms contributing to impingement and that, should further research support that subgroups of shoulder impingement exist, exercise protocols should be specific to the pathomechanics associated with each group.

Surgeons and therapists can apply these findings to clinical practice by including the assessment of scapular upward rotation for clients with shoulder impingement and comparing findings to the uninvolved side. One reliable procedure for measuring such is inclinometry.[2] Axial rotation of the SC joint also deserves attention but is challenging to quantify in clinical settings. Further research is required to learn more on the coupling of AC, SC, and ST movement as well as the muscle activity associated with such to better support the development of targeted manual and exercise-based therapy interventions.

C. McGee, PhD, OTR/L, CHT

References

1. Giphart JE, Jvan der Meijden OA, Millett PJ. The effects of arm elevation on the 3-dimensional acromiohumeral distance: a biplane fluoroscopy study with normative data. *J Shoulder Elbow Surg*. 2012;21:1593-1600.
2. Watson L, Balster SM, Finch C, Dalziel R. Measurement of scapula upward rotation: a reliable clinical procedure. *Br J Sports Med.* 2005;39:599-603.

Is there a relationship between subacromial impingement syndrome and scapular orientation? A systematic review

Ratcliffe E, Pickering S, McLean S, et al (Chelsea & Westminster Hosp, London, UK; Deakin Univ, Geelong, Victoria, Australia; Sheffield Hallam Univ, UK; et al)

Br J Sports Med 48:1251-1256, 2014

Background.—Alterations in scapular orientation and dynamic control, specifically involving increased anterior tilt and downward rotation, are considered to play a substantial role in contributing to a subacromial impingement syndrome (SIS). Non-surgical intervention aims at restoring normal scapular posture. The research evidence supporting this practice is equivocal.

Objective.—The aim of this study was to systematically review the relevant literature to examine whether a difference exists in scapular orientation between people without shoulder symptoms and those with SIS.

Data sources.—MEDLINE, AMED, EMBASE, CINAHL, PEDro and SPORTDiscus databases were searched using relevant search terms up to August 2013. Additional studies were identified by hand-searching the reference lists of pertinent articles.

Review methods.—Of the 7445 abstracts identified, 18 were selected for further analysis. Two reviewers independently assessed the studies for inclusion, data extraction and quality, using a modified Downs and Black quality assessment tool.

Results.—10 trials were included in the review. Scapular position was determined through two-dimensional radiological measurements, 360° inclinometers and three-dimensional motion and tracking devices. The findings were inconsistent. Some studies reported patterns of reduced upward rotation, increased anterior tilting and medial rotation of the scapula. In contrast, others reported the opposite, and some identified no difference in motion when compared to asymptomatic controls.

Conclusions.—The underlying aetiology of SIS is still debated. The results of this review demonstrated a lack of consistency of study methodologies and results. Currently, there is insufficient evidence to support a clinical belief that the scapula adopts a common and consistent posture in SIS. This may reflect the complex, multifactorial nature of the syndrome. Additionally, it may be due to the methodological variations and shortfalls in the available research. It also raises the possibility that deviation from a 'normal' scapular position may not be contributory to SIS but part of normal variations. Further research is required to establish whether a common pattern exists in scapular kinematics in SIS patients or whether subgroups of patients with common patterns can be identified to guide management options. Non-surgical treatment involving rehabilitation of the scapula to an idealised normal posture is currently not supported by the available literature.

▶ This article is of significance for upper extremity surgeons because it investigates the etiology of subacromial impingement syndrome. One of the possible underlying pathophysiologies associated with impingement is scapular dyskinesis. Several studies support this theory. If this is indeed a true association, scapular orientation should be analyzed in detail and systematically corrected in every patient with shoulder pain. This article's main strength is that it is a good methodological study assessing only comparative series of patients on this matter. Inclusion and exclusion criteria are strict and allow for good clinical judgment on the topic. Its main weakness is that the papers that confine this systematic review lack methodological consistency. There is insufficient evidence to support the idea that the scapula adopts a common and consistent posture in subacromial impingement syndrome. I think that with future investigation, scapular orientation will prove to have a consistent effect on subacromial pathology. A static scapular posture may not be the reason for pathology, but if motion analyses were investigated, a pathological pattern might be found, although this type of study would surely be more challenging to perform. Altered scapular dynamics might not be the primary and only reason for pain, but it might prove to be part of a spectrum of different causes for subacromial impingement syndrome. In my personal experience, there are a lot of patients with symmetrical imaging findings such as a bilateral torn rotator cuff and only 1 symptomatic shoulder. If the symptomatic shoulder happens to have scapular dyskinesis, the patient usually improves after a rehabilitation program.

J. P. Simone, MD

12 Diagnostic Imaging

Effect of Wrist Position on Distal Radioulnar Joint Stability: A Biomechanical Study

Iida A, Omokawa S, Moritomo H, et al (Nara Med Univ, Kashihara, Japan; Osaka Yukioka College of Health Science, Japan; et al)

J Orthop Res 32:1247-1251, 2014

We investigated distal radioulnar joint (DRUJ) stability in different wrist positions and examined the relative contribution of each ligamentous component of the triangular fibrocartilage complex (TFCC) to DRUJ stability. We used nine fresh-frozen cadavers. The humerus and ulna were fixed at 90 elbow flexion. The radiocarpal unit was translated relative to the ulna in dorsopalmar directions with the wrist in five positions. Displacement of the unit was measured by an electromagnetic tracking device. Magnitudes of displacement were compared between different wrist positions in various sectioning stages: ulnocarpal ligament (UCL) sectioning, radioulnar ligaments (RUL) sectioning, and extensor carpi ulnaris (ECU) floor sectioning. Wrist position and sectioning stage significantly influenced the displacement. In intact wrists, the displacement in wrist extension was significantly lower than that in neutral. However, after UCL sectioning, there were no longer any significant differences. After RUL sectioning, the displacement in radial deviation was significantly lower than that in neutral. Following ECU floor sectioning, there were no longer any significant differences. Thus, in intact wrists, DRUJ stability in wrist extension is likely due to tightening of the UCL. After complete RUL sectioning, DRUJ is stabilized in radial deviation due to tightening of the ECU floor.

▶ The authors present a cadaveric study on how wrist position affected the stability of the distal radioulnar joint (DRUJ) and the impact of sequential sectioning of different components of the triangular fibrocartilage complex (TFCC) on DRUJ stability. This research question is clearly based on a smart clinical observation that DRUJ stability can be affected by the wrist position. The authors have designed a genius device to measure the translation of the radiocarpal unit in reference to a fixed ulna using an electromagnetic tracking device. This mechanism simulates our clinical ballottement technique on DRUJ stability, although in practice we usually translate the ulna relative to a fixed radiocarpal unit. The result was inspiring. DRUJ stability was significantly increased with the wrist in extended and radial deviated position, which was negated by sectioning of the ulnocarpal ligament (UCL). Further sectioning of the radioulnar ligament increased the instability, which could be partially compensated by radial deviation of the wrist, presumably due to tightening of the extensor carpi ulnaris (ECU) floor. Following final ECU floor sectioning, wrist positioning no longer had an impact on DRUJ stability.

I consider this study highly relevant clinically. First, DRUJ ballottement is among the most commonly used clinical tests on the wrist, but documentation is seldom possible. This measurement device gives us insight on the possible quantification of the clinical stability of DRUJ. Second, in doing the DRUJ ballottement test, we seldom pay attention to the effect of wrist position on the DRUJ stability. With this scientific data in foresight, positioning of the wrist should become an integral part of the standard DRUJ ballottement test to examine the integrity of various components of the TFCC. Third, new diagnostic criteria on partial injury of the TFCC may be developed. For example, if ulnar wrist pain is exaggerated by balloting the DRUJ with the wrist in extension, the possibility of UCL injury must be born in mind, even if no overt DRUJ instability is noted.

P. C. Ho

Osteoarthritis of the carpometacarpal joint of the thumb: a new MR imaging technique for the standardized detection of relevant ligamental lesions

Dumont C, Lerzer S, Vafa MA, et al (Univ Med Ctr Göttingen, Goettingen, Germany)

Skeletal Radiol 43:1411-1420, 2014

Objective.—To assess ligament lesions and subluxations of the carpometacarpal joints of the thumbs (CMC I) of asymptomatic volunteers and of patients with CMC I osteoarthritis using advanced magnetic resonance imaging (MRI).

Materials and Methods.—A total of 20 CMC I joints of 14 asymptomatic volunteers (6× both sides) and 28 CMC I joints of 22 patients (6× both sides) with symptomatic and X-ray-diagnosed osteoarthritis of CMC I joints were studied. During extension, flexion, abduction and adduction of the thumb, the anterior oblique (AOL), intermetacarpal (IML), posterior oblique (POL) and dorsal radial (DRL) ligaments were evaluated using 3-T MRI on two standard planes, and translation of metacarpal I (MC I) was assessed.

Results.—The MRI demonstrated that ligament lesions of the AOL and IML are frequent. Isolated rupture of the AOL was found in 6 of 28 (21%), combined rupture of the AOL + IML in 5 of 28 (18%) and isolated IML rupture in 4 of 28 (14%) joints.

The patients had a significantly increased dorsal translation of MC I during extension with a median of 6.4 mm vs. 5.4 mm in asymptomatic volunteers ($p < 0.05$).

Conclusion.—MRIs of CMC I in two standardized planes frequently show combined ligament ruptures. The dorsal subluxation of MC I, which is increased in patients, correlates with OA severity based on X-ray and can be quantified by MRI. For joint-preserving surgical procedures and for prosthesis implantation of the CMC I, we recommend performing an MRI in two planes of the thumb—extension and abduction—to evaluate the ligaments and dorsal subluxation of MC I.

▶ This study discusses the use of MRI to evaluate the carpometacarpal (CMC) joint. The authors describe not only ligament tears but also assess stability, an important component in the evaluation of early stages of CMC pathology. The authors have nicely described the ligaments of interest, have reported a standardized positioning and imaging technique, and describe a method of quantification of the dorsal translation of the metacarpal that I believe has not been done before. There was no discussion of interrater reliability or reproducibility of their technique and no discussion of sensitivity or specificity. This will be needed before the clinical applicability of this technique can be fully established. A control group that is age and sex matched to the subjects would also add strength to this study. As we move toward the increasing use of advanced imaging of the CMC joint, we need to understand which findings are normal and which are abnormal. The literature has shown us that triangular fibrocartilage complex pathology is common among asymptomatic volunteers, and over the years we have improved our understanding of clinically relevant pathology in this area. As we move toward more commonly performing MRIs for the CMC joint, it will be important to understand what findings are normal for this age group and develop an understanding of their clinical relevance.

R. Grewal, MD

Radiation Exposure to Hand Surgeons' Hands: A Practical Comparison of Large and Mini C-Arm Fluoroscopy

Vosbikian MM, Ilyas AM, Watson DD, et al (Thomas Jefferson Univ Hosp, Philadelphia, PA; Nazareth Hosp, Philadelphia, PA)

J Hand Surg Am 39:1805-1809, 2014

Purpose.—To determine and compare the radiation exposure to surgeons' hands with large and mini C-arm fluoroscopy in a practical, clinically based model.

Methods.—Two hand surgeons monitored radiation exposure to their hands with a ring dosimeter over a 14-month period using large and mini C-arm fluoroscopic units. One surgeon performed all cases with a large C-arm unit in a hospital setting, and the other performed all cases with mini C-arms in surgical centers. For each case, fluoroscopic time, the output displayed by the unit, radiation by time, and ring dosimeter absorption were recorded and analyzed.

Results.—A total of 160 consecutive cases were reviewed with 71 cases and 89 cases in the large and mini C-arm groups, respectively. The median output displayed by the large C-arm was 0.7 mGy/case, and the median output displayed by the mini C-arm was 10.0 mGy/case. With output as a product of time, the median calculated values were 0.02 mGy/s for the large C-arm group and 0.28 mGy/s for the mini C-arm group. Cumulative ring dosimeter absorption to the surgeons' hands was found to be 380 mrem for 71 cases in the large C-arm group versus 1,000 mrem for 89 cases in the mini C-arm group.

Conclusions.—In our model, the use of the mini C-arm resulted in more than a 10-fold increase in the rate of output and approximately double the dosimeter absorption to the surgeon's hand compared with the large C-arm. Although it has been shown that the mini C-arm produces less radiation scatter, in a practical model, it may not be a safer alternative with respect to the surgeon's hands. Based on these findings, we recommend that surgeons be more aware of radiation exposure risk, know their C-arm unit's specifications, and try to minimize radiation exposure.

Type of Study/Level of Evidence.—Prognostic II.

▶ The authors sought to determine and compare the amount of radiation exposure to surgeons' hands from large and mini C-arm fluoroscopy. One surgeon was assigned to use the large C-arm unit in a hospital setting, and the other surgeon performed all cases with mini C-arms in surgery centers. There is an increased use of mini C-arms in surgery centers and outpatient clinics, with the advantages of easier maneuverability, surgeon independence and lack of need for radiology technologist, reduced space requirements, and decreased cost. Previous studies have demonstrated higher radiation exposure to the surgeon's hands with the mini C-arm, likely because of a reduced source-to-extremity distance. Similarly, the current study demonstrated a more than 10-fold rate of output and double the dosimeter absorption to the surgeon's hand with the use of mini C-arm compared with the large C-arm, with 88 seconds of fluoroscopic time compared with 38 seconds. The mean exposure per case was 11 mrem/case for the mini C-arm and 5 mrem/case for the large C-arm. The authors recognized that a significant portion of the added fluoroscopic time was from lack of a laser pointer and more adjustments to center the images. Moreover, surgeons often assume that the mini C-arm leads to less radiation exposure and that more images may be taken. However, in the current study, there may be differences in the types of cases performed in the 2 groups with hospital compared with surgery center settings and the 2 surgeons' different practices.

We currently mostly use the large C-arm at our institution, both in the hospital and at the surgery center. There has been no demonstrated advantage to mini C-arms. The laser pointer that centers the image and better image resolution are both advantages of the large C-arm.

J. I. Huang, MD

13 Compressive Neuropathies

Effectiveness of Ultrasound-Guided Carpal Tunnel Injection Using In-Plane Ulnar Approach: A Prospective, Randomized, Single-Blinded Study

Lee JY, Park Y, Park KD, et al (Gachon Univ, Incheon, Korea; Inje Univ College of Medicine, Seoul, Korea)

Medicine 93:e350, 2014

The objective of this study is to evaluate the degree of symptom improvement and the change of electrophysiological and ultrasonographic findings after sonographically guided local steroid injection using an in-plane ulnar approach in carpal tunnel syndrome (CTS).

Seventy-five cases of 44 patients diagnosed with CTS were included and evaluated at baseline and at 4 and 12 weeks after injection. All patients received injection with 40 mg of triamcinolone mixed with 1 mL of 1% lidocaine into the carpal tunnel using an in-plane Ultrasound (US)- guided ulnar approach, out-plane US-guided approach, and blind injection. For clinical evaluation, we used the Boston Carpal Tunnel Questionnaire (BCTQ) and electrophysiological tests. The ultrasonographic findings were also evaluated with regard to cross-sectional area and the flattening ratio of the median nerve.

Subjective symptoms measured by BCTQ and median nerve conduction parameters showed significant improvement at 4 weeks in the in-plane ulnar approach group compared with the out-plane ulnar approach and blind injection. This improvement was still observed at 12 weeks. The flattening ratio and cross-sectional area of the median nerve showed a more significant decrease with the in-plane ulnar approach than with the out-plane ulnar approach and blind injection ($P < 0.05$).

US-guided local steroid injection using an in-plane ulnar approach in the CTS may be more effective than out-plane or blind injection (Table 5).

▶ Although this study is randomized and single blind, its strength is limited. First, the total number of patients enrolled (44) is small. Second, of the enrolled patients, only 3 were men, limiting the applicability of the findings. Third, the follow-up period is only 12 weeks. If the primary goal is to assess degree of symptom improvement, then longer follow-up is necessary in my opinion. Otherwise, the injection is providing diagnostic information rather than therapeutic information. Last, the authors assert that the in-plane approach for ultrasound

TABLE 5.—Posttreatment Complication of the Patients

Treatment Group	Nerve Insult	Vessel Insult	Skin Lesion
Blind	5	2	8
Ulnar-O	6	0	1
Ulnar-I	1	0	3

Blind = blind injection group, Ulnar-I = in-plane ulnar approach injection group, Ulnar-O = out-plane injection group. Reprinted from Lee JY, Park Y, Park KD, et al. Effectiveness of Ultrasound-Guided Carpal Tunnel Injection Using In-Plane Ulnar Approach: A Prospective, Randomized, Single-Blinded Study. Medicine. 2014;93:e350.

(US)-guided injection is safe, but there is no description or explanation as to how nerve or vessel injuries were identified. Based on the data in Table 5 nerve injuries occurred with US-guidance, which was greater than in the blind injection group. Although the US-guided injections may have improved electrodiagnostic and sonographic findings, the conclusions of this study need to be reviewed and applied with caution, as I feel there are significant flaws in the design.

In my practice, the use of corticosteroid injections for carpal tunnel syndrome is limited to diagnostic purposes and treatment in patients who are pregnant or not surgical candidates. If a corticosteroid injection is used, I am not inclined to use ultrasonography for many reasons (eg, efficiency, cost), and this study does not provide evidence necessitating a change in my current clinical practice. As a surgeon, I have an effective and reliable surgical intervention to offer patients with carpal tunnel syndrome.

A. Moeller, MD

Symptom Severity and Conservative Treatment for Carpal Tunnel Syndrome in Association With Eventual Carpal Tunnel Release

Baker NA, Livengood HM (Univ of Pittsburgh, PA)
J Hand Surg Am 39:1792-1798, 2014

Purpose.—To study the relationship between the severity of carpal tunnel syndrome (CTS) symptoms and surgery for CTS and the relationship between conservative treatments and surgery for CTS.

Methods.—A secondary analysis of baseline to 6-month data from a randomized controlled trial, which examined the effectiveness of orthosis/stretch combinations on the symptoms of CTS, was conducted for a total of 96 participants with CTS. Participants completed the Carpal Tunnel Questionnaire and posttreatment surveys. Statistical analyses included exploration of correlates of progression to surgery for CTS and logistical regression to examine the association between conservative treatments and CTS symptoms and progression to surgery for CTS.

Results.—Twenty-one participants received surgery for their CTS, and 31 participants received 1 or more conservative treatments. Severity of baseline CTS symptoms and additional treatments were indicators of progression to surgery. The randomized controlled trial intervention was inversely associated with progression to surgery.

Conclusions.—CTS that does not respond to an initial course of conservative treatment may not improve with additional treatments. More than half of the participants who received additional conservative treatment still progressed to surgery. Current intervention guidelines for CTS provide limited guidance as to the best methods to efficiently treat CTS.

Clinical Relevance.—CTS is a costly and high-burden disorder, resulting in reduced quality of life. Research should examine when and for whom conservative care is an effective choice and the association between conservative care and the eventual need for CTS surgery.

▶ The authors investigate factors predicting the probability for surgical treatment in patients with carpal tunnel syndrome. They find that patients with more severe initial symptoms are more likely to progress to surgery and that additional conservative treatment modalities do not improve outcomes after failed conservative primary treatment.

Although this study seems well designed for the primary research question, I am not sure whether the data set obtained is really adequate to answer the secondary study questions. Apart from that, I have to admit that I am often amazed with these types of studies. The decision to proceed with surgery is made on a very individual basis and is to a great extent related to personality type, communication skills, and specialty of the treating physician. I am not sure whether the decision not to proceed with surgery—in an impressing 75 out of 96 patients—was really made by a hand surgeon, although we are told in the last paragraph that the primary referral source was hand surgeons. A fundamental weakness of this study is that the authors do not include electromyographic studies in their decision making. Why shouldn't we as hand surgeons preferably suggest primary carpal tunnel release for all patients with abnormal nerve conduction studies? There is a great body of evidence that it is easy, effective, and probably even as cost effective as nonsurgical treatment.

K. Megerle, MD

Simultaneous Bilateral or Unilateral Carpal Tunnel Release? A Prospective Cohort Study of Early Outcomes and Limitations

Osei DA, Calfee RP, Stepan JG, et al (Washington Univ School of Medicine, St Louis, MO)

J Bone Joint Surg Am 96:889-896, 2014

Background.—Over 60% of patients with carpal tunnel syndrome present with symptoms and findings of nerve compression in both hands. Our goal was to compare patient-rated difficulties in performing activities of daily living in the early postoperative period between those undergoing bilateral carpal tunnel release and those undergoing unilateral carpal tunnel release.

Methods.—This prospective cohort study enrolled consecutive patients with bilateral carpal tunnel syndrome undergoing bilateral carpal tunnel release ($n = 47$) or unilateral carpal tunnel release ($n = 41$). Patient function and disease severity were measured by an abbreviated form of the Disabilities of the Arm, Shoulder and Hand questionnaire, QuickDASH, and the Boston Carpal Tunnel Questionnaire at baseline, at postoperative visit 1 at a mean time (and standard deviation) of 10 ± 3 days, and at postoperative visit 2 at a mean time (and standard deviation) of 30 ± 6 days. Patients rated their difficulty in completing fifteen activities of daily living each day for the first postoperative week. Patients reported the factors that influenced their choice of surgery.

Results.—There was no difference in baseline function or disease severity between the two groups with regard to QuickDASH and the Boston Carpal Tunnel Questionnaire. Patients in both groups improved after carpal tunnel release with no difference between groups either at postoperative visit 1 for QuickDASH ($p = 0.97$) and the Boston Carpal Tunnel Questionnaire ($p = 0.86$) or at postoperative visit 2 for QuickDASH ($p = 0.43$) and the Boston Carpal Tunnel Questionnaire ($p = 0.34$). Patients undergoing bilateral carpal tunnel release had more difficulty only during postoperative days 1 to 2 in opening jars ($p = 0.03$), cooking ($p = 0.008$), and doing household chores ($p = 0.02$). Patients in the two groups did not differ ($p > 0.05$) in their abilities to perform activities of daily living necessary for personal hygiene or independence on any day during the first seven days following surgery with regard to using the bathroom, bathing, dressing, or eating. Although the most common reason why patients chose bilateral carpal tunnel release was to avoid two surgical procedures (42%), the most common reason why patients chose unilateral carpal tunnel release was concern for self-care (36%).

Conclusions.—Patients with bilateral carpal tunnel syndrome can anticipate more severe functional impairment during the first few postoperative days with bilateral carpal tunnel release compared with unilateral carpal tunnel release, but limitations beyond postoperative day 2 or 3 are similar for bilateral and unilateral carpal tunnel release.

Level of Evidence.—Therapeutic Level II. See Instructions for Authors for a complete description of levels of evidence.

▶ Osei et al report on a study of 2 parallel, self-selected groups of patients undergoing carpal tunnel release, focusing on difficulties in activities between simultaneous bilateral surgery and unilateral release. The principal findings are that patients undergoing simultaneous release reported difficulty in activities of daily living for a surprisingly short period, 2 days. After that, difficulty with activities, including hygiene, cooking, opening jars, bathing, dressing, and eating, was not statistically different between the 2 groups.

Simultaneous bilateral carpal tunnel release is not a new idea and has been an occasional part of many hand surgeons' practices for a long time. However, the conventional wisdom has been that in the early postoperative period, patients would require help for a substantially longer period than this trial reports. It is important to remember that this was a trial, and the authors do not report the total number of patients with bilateral carpal tunnel syndrome they saw during this period. Given that 5 busy hand surgeons recruited patients for 10 months, the number of patients not offered enrollment was likely larger than those in the trial. Further, patients were not offered enrollment if they did not have help at home during the early postoperative period, and the definition of help is not clear in the report. Patients were given impervious extra-large gloves and disposable wipes to aid in hygiene and presumably toileting after surgery. Most patients felt that help at home (63%) and the gloves they were given (70%) were helpful in being able to perform their activities of daily life.

Lastly, I suspect there are cultural and regional variations in patients' willingness to accept the type of help required after bilateral hand surgery, and it is unclear if the patient population in my geographic area (urban New England) is as open to the idea of help with toileting after elective surgery.

In terms of changing the conventional wisdom regarding simultaneous bilateral surgery, I suspect a large percentage of hand surgeons already offer simultaneous carpal tunnel release to selected patients. It is clear from this study that many of us have overestimated how much longer the disability of bilateral surgery is compared with unilateral surgery, and we can feel comfortable reassuring patients who are considering selecting this option that the time period is short.

P. Blazar, MD

An Outcomes Protocol for Carpal Tunnel Release: A Comparison of Outcomes in Patients With and Without Medical Comorbidities

Cagle PJ Jr, Reams M, Agel J, et al (Univ of Minnesota, Minneapolis; TRIA Orthopaedic Ctr, Bloomington, MN)

J Hand Surg Am 39:2175-2180, 2014

Purpose.—To prospectively report the outcomes of open carpal tunnel release with respect to patient age and medical comorbidities.

Methods.—Nine hundred fifty open carpal tunnel procedures in 826 patients (age range, 21—100 y) at a high-volume orthopedic surgery center were evaluated. Self-reported symptom severity and functional scores were collected using the validated Boston Carpal Tunnel Outcomes questionnaire preoperatively, and at 2 weeks, 6 weeks, and 12 weeks postoperatively.

Results.—Patients demonstrated a significant improvement in symptom severity scores at 2 weeks and functional severity scores at 6 weeks. Documented patient medical comorbidities did not affect improvement after surgery. Patients with diabetes improved more slowly but were not significantly different at 6 weeks. Patients with workers' compensation insurance were significantly worse at baseline, 2 weeks, and 6 weeks but were not significantly different at 3 months. The risk of negative postoperative endpoints was slightly higher in patients with a medical comorbidity, though not statistically different.

Conclusions.—Significant improvements in symptom severity and hand function may be expected after open carpal tunnel release in the general population regardless of age, medical comorbidities, or workers' compensation status.

Type of Study/Level of Evidence.—Therapeutic III.

▶ Carpal tunnel syndrome is an extremely common clinical condition. In the United States, open carpal tunnel release is also a commonly performed surgery. Open release is the gold standard treatment for patients who have failed conservative treatment of carpal tunnel syndrome, and there is wide evidence of its usefulness to treat the condition.

However, the success of this surgery in the face of medical comorbidities such as diabetes is less certain because many studies of the condition and surgery exclude patients with comorbidities.

This work helps shed light on this large and important group of patients who have carpal tunnel syndrome. In this work, patients with diabetes mellitus did improve, albeit more slowly. This improvement was also seen in worker's compensation cases. These findings are consistent with other work showing that concomitant diabetes does not necessarily mean a poorer outcome following surgery.[1,2]

As the authors point out, the study period was short, with a lower number of evaluations at 3 months. Overall, only about one-third of the patients completed the 3-month evaluation. It is not known whether adding the nonresponders to the evaluation would have changed the results.

This information will help surgeons discuss outcomes following open surgery for carpal tunnel syndrome. Specific advice can be given to patients with diabetes mellitus. However, the other comorbidities such as thyroid disease, radiculopathy, inflammatory disease, and pregnancy were grouped together and occured in 32% of patients as a whole group. It was not stated how individual comorbidities affected outcome, although this may have been difficult to do in such an analysis given the small levels of symptoms and the presence of some comorbidities such as gout and polyneuropathy. This information is most helpful for North American populations, which resemble the study population. It is not clear whether the findings are generalizable to other populations.

A. Chong, MD

References

1. Mondelli M, Padua L, Reale F, Signorini AM, Romano C. Outcome of surgical release among diabetics with carpal tunnel syndrome. *Arch Phys Med Rehabil.* 2004;85:7-13.
2. Thomsen NO, Cederlund R, Rosén I, Björk J, Dahlin LB. Clinical outcomes of surgical release among diabetic patients with carpal tunnel syndrome: prospective follow-up with matched controls. *J Hand Surg Am.* 2009;34:1177-1187.

Electrophysiological Assessment of Carpal Tunnel Syndrome in Elderly Patients: One-Year Follow-Up Study

Kanatani T, Nagura I, Kurosaka M, et al (Kobe Rosai Hosp, Japan; Kobe Univ School of Medicine, Japan)

J Hand Surg Am 39:2188-2191, 2014

Purpose.—To objectively assess elderly patients with carpal tunnel syndrome to characterize their preoperative severity and prognosis after carpal tunnel release using a electrophysiological severity scale.

Methods.—Electrophysiologic assessment was performed preoperatively and 1 year postoperatively following carpal tunnel release in 112 hands in patients over 70 years of age prospectively by the use of the following electrophysiological severity scale: stage 1, normal distal motor latency (DML) and normal sensory conduction velocity (SCV); stage 2, DML ≥ 4.5 milliseconds and normal SCV; stage 3, DML ≥ 4.5 milliseconds and SCV < 40.0 m/s; stage 4, DML ≥ 4.5 milliseconds and non-measurable SCV; stage 5; non-measurable DML and non-measurable SCV. Additionally, the outcomes of clinical symptoms of pain, nocturnal symptoms, numbness, loss of 2-point discrimination in the median nerve territory, and thenar atrophy were assessed.

Results.—The mean age of patients was 77 years at the time of the operation. Preoperatively, the most common severity was stage 5 (70 of 112 hands, 63%), and clustering stage 4 and 5 together as *severe* resulted in 103 hands (92%). One year postoperatively, 97 hands (87%) demonstrated at least one stage improvement, and the numbers of *mild* (stage 1 or 2) increased from 3 (3%) to 45 hands (40%). Parallel with the electrophysiological improvement, pain and nocturnal symptoms resolved in 17 of 17 hands and 11 of 11 hands, respectively, in whom they were present preoperatively. Numbness, loss of 2-point discrimination, and thenar atrophy demonstrated the improvement in 96 of 112 (86%) hands, in 58 of 112 (52%) hands, and in 80 of 96 (83%) hands.

Conclusions.—We observed electrophysiologic improvement in 86% of elderly patients following carpal tunnel release. Electrophysiologic outcomes correlated with improvement in clinical variables.

Type of Study/Level of Evidence.—Therapeutic IV.

▶ It is well known that the elderly show improvement after carpal tunnel release from a clinical point of view, even though they do not improve as well as young patients do. The authors of this paper provide evidence that elderly patients also show improvement in electrophysiological follow-up 1 year after surgery. This finding may be of academic interest. Considering that the main diagnostic tool for carpal tunnel syndrome is clinical evaluation along with history taking and that many physicians and surgeons involved in carpal tunnel syndrome diagnosis and/or treatment do not rely on preoperative electrophysiologic diagnosis, the value of a postoperative electrophysiological testing is questionable.

It is remarkable that no patient was lost to follow-up in a patient population with such a high age (the mean age was reported to be 77).

I agree with the authors that the treatment of choice for carpal tunnel syndrome in the elderly is operative carpal tunnel release—the same as in young patients.

M. Choi, MD

Comparison of Ultrasound and Electrodiagnostic Testing for Diagnosis of Carpal Tunnel Syndrome: Study Using a Validated Clinical Tool as the Reference Standard

Fowler JR, Munsch M, Tosti R, et al (Univ of Pittsburgh, PA; Hand & UpperEx Ctr, Wexford, PA; Temple Univ Hosp, Philadelphia, PA)

J Bone Joint Surg Am 96:e148(1-4), 2014

Background.—Ultrasound examination is both accurate and cost-effective for the confirmation of a clinical diagnosis of carpal tunnel syndrome. Previous studies have shown electrodiagnostic testing and ultrasound to be similar with regard to sensitivity and specificity. The purpose of this study was to compare the sensitivity and specificity of ultrasound and electrodiagnostic testing by using a validated clinical diagnostic tool as the reference standard.

Methods.—All consecutive patients referred to an upper-extremity practice for electrodiagnostic testing for any reason over a three-month period were recruited to participate in this study. All patients were evaluated with the use of the Carpal Tunnel Syndrome 6 (CTS-6) clinical diagnostic tool, and a score of ≥12 was considered positive for carpal tunnel syndrome. A positive finding on ultrasound was considered to be a cross-sectional area of the median nerve, measured just proximal to the level of the pisiform, of ≥10 mm^2. A positive finding on electrodiagnostic testing was a distal motor latency of ≥4.2 ms and/or a distal sensory latency of ≥3.2 ms. Sensitivity, specificity, and accuracy were calculated for ultrasound and electrodiagnostic testing with use of the CTS-6 as the reference standard.

Results.—With use of the CTS-6 as the reference standard, ultrasound had a sensitivity of 89% and a specificity of 90% in our series of eighty-five patients. Electrodiagnostic testing had a sensitivity of 89% and a specificity of 80%. The positive predictive value of ultrasound was 94% compared with 89% for electrodiagnostic testing. The negative predictive value of ultrasound was 82% compared with 80% for electrodiagnostic testing. Ultrasound was accurate in seventy-six (89%) of the eighty-five cases whereas electrodiagnostic testing was accurate in seventy-three (86%) of the eighty-five cases ($p = 0.5$).

Conclusions.—While ultrasound will not replace electrodiagnostic testing in complicated or unclear cases, in a select group of patients with a positive CTS-6, ultrasound can be used to confirm the diagnosis of carpal tunnel syndrome with better specificity and equal sensitivity as compared with those of electrodiagnostic testing.

Level of Evidence.—Diagnostic Level I. See Instructions for Authors for a complete description of levels of evidence.

► This is an excellently performed study to evaluate the use of ultrasound (US) in the diagnosis of carpal tunnel syndrome (CTS). It provides level I evidence to support the use of ultrasound as a confirmatory test for CTS.

The limits of the study are the lack of comprehensive clinical data such as the treating physician's diagnosis and the outcomes of surgical treatment. Because there is no gold standard for the diagnosis of CTS, it would be nice to see which patients carried the diagnosis to the point of surgical intervention. It would also be helpful to see what the response to surgical release was and how that improvement (which you could take as confirmation of the diagnosis) correlated with the diagnostic modality.

Otherwise, the limits of the technique are included in the article. It is not a replacement for electromyogram/nerve conduction velocity for patients with uncertain diagnoses. However, in patients with good clinical evidence for CTS, this can be confirmatory.

I have not had experience yet with the use of US for CTS. Although I do have a unit available, I have not used it in this application. One issue is that I am not certified to do diagnostic ultrasonography. Although the article mentions this as one of the advantages of their study (that it does not require an ultrasonographer or radiologist to interpret the study but rather can be performed by the hand surgeon), it is an issue that clinicians need to consider. If a clinician questions the diagnosis, the paper recommends an electrodiagnostic study. If the clinical situation requires a "stamp of approval," does a diagnostic test, such as a US, performed by an unaccredited technician (the surgeon) and interpreted by an unaccredited physician (the surgeon), provide the support the physician is looking for?

T. Hughes, MD

Carpal tunnel decompression in the super-elderly: functional outcome and patient satisfaction are equal to those of their younger counterparts

Stone OD, Clement ND, Duckworth AD, et al (Queen Margaret Hosp, Dunfermline, Fife, UK; et al)

Bone Joint J 96-B:1234-1238, 2014

There is conflicting evidence about the functional outcome and rate of satisfaction of superelderly patients (≥ 80 years of age) after carpal tunnel decompression.

We compiled outcome data for 756 patients who underwent a carpal tunnel decompression over an eight-year study period, 97 of whom were super-elderly, and 659 patients who formed a younger control group (< 80 years old). There was no significant difference between the super-elderly patients and the younger control group in terms of functional outcome according to the mean (0 to 100) QuickDASH score (adjusted mean difference at one year 1.8; 95% confidence interval (CI) -3.4 to 7.0) and satisfaction rate (odds ratio (OR) 0.78; 95% CI 0.34 to 1.58). Super-elderly patients were, however, more likely to have thenar muscle atrophy at presentation (OR 9.2, 95% CI 5.8 to 14.6). When nerve conduction studies were obtained, super-elderly patients were more likely to have a severe conduction deficit (OR 12.4, 95% CI 3.0 to 51.3).

Super-elderly patients report functional outcome and satisfaction rates equal to those of their younger counterparts. They are more likely to have thenar muscle atrophy and a severe nerve conduction deficit at presentation, and may therefore warrant earlier decompression.

▶ The authors showed that those persons over 80 years old (known as the "super-elderly") who undergo carpal tunnel decompression have functional outcomes and satisfaction rates similar to those under 80 years old. This retrospective study involved a large cohort of patients (756) who underwent carpal tunnel decompression over 8 years. If the hand surgeon was apprehensive of performing carpal tunnel release decompression in a super-elderly person just because of his or her age, then this study should convince the surgeon that this reason is unfounded. As this study shows, even if thenar atrophy and severe nerve conduction deficit are present in the super-elderly patient (which should not be surprising to anyone), this patient will still benefit from carpal tunnel decompression.

There are a few reasons (eg, a bleeding diathesis) why I might not perform a carpal tunnel release on a patient who needs it, and age over 80 years old is not one of them. The procedure is simple, quick, and can be performed under local anesthesia without a tourniquet.

S. S. Shin, MD, MMSc

Clinical efficacy of simple decompression versus anterior transposition of the ulnar nerve for the treatment of cubital tunnel syndrome: A meta-analysis

Chen H-W, Ou S, Liu G-D, et al (Central Hosp of Yiwu City, China; General Hosp of Chengdu Military Command, China; Third Military Med Univ, Chongqing, China; et al)

Clin Neurol Neurosurg 126:150-155, 2014

Objectives.—The aim of this study was to evaluate the clinical efficacy of simple decompression (SD) versus anterior transposition (AT) of the ulnar nerve for the treatment of cubital tunnel syndrome.

Methods.—Seven public databases (PubMed, MEDLINE and EMBASE, Springer, Elsevier Science Direct, Cochrane Library and Google scholar) were searched from 1971 to December 2013. The overall odds ratios (OR) and their 95% confidence intervals (CI) were pooled to compare the clinical outcomes. Subgroup analysis was performed based on the region, study type, Jadad score, type of AT, and follow-up duration. Meta-analysis was conducted by using Rev. Man 5.1 and Stata 11.0 software.

Results.—Finally, we included 13 studies involved 1009 (500 patients receiving SD and 509 patients receiving AT) patients with cubital tunnel syndrome. The overall estimate (OR = 0.91, 95% CI = 0.67–1.23, $P = 0.536$) indicated that there was no significantly statistical difference between the clinical outcomes of patients treated with SD and AT. Meanwhile, subgroup analyses by region, study type, Jadad score, type of AT and follow-up duration showed the consistent results with the overall estimate. In addition, we found that the incidence of complications in patients treated by SD was significantly lower than that in patients treated by AT (OR = 0.32, 95% CI = 0.17–0.60, $P = 0.05$).

Conclusions.—In conclusion, although SD had equivalent clinical outcomes with AT for the treatment of cubital tunnel syndrome, SD should be preferred due to having lower incidence of complications.

▶ This is a meta-analysis study that aims to examine the clinical efficacy of simple decompression vs anterior transposition of the ulnar nerve for the treatment of cubital tunnel syndrome. The authors included 13 studies that included a total of 1009 patients following a search of 7 public databases. The overall odds ratios (OR) and their 95% confidence intervals were pooled to compare the clinical outcomes.

As has been shown in previous meta-analyses, simple decompression and anterior transposition yielded no significant differences with regard to clinical outcomes. Additional information gleaned from this study is the finding that the incidence of complications in patients treated with simple decompression was significantly lower than those patients treated with anterior transposition. Despite the advantages in simple decompression, one must consider that decompression is contraindicated in the setting of recurrent cases and ulnar nerve subluxation.

One of the advantages of this study relative to previous meta-analyses is the inclusion of updated studies. In addition, both the number of studies and sample size in this study were greater than those in previous iterations. The authors correctly point at the additional soft tissue trauma and vascular effacement that occurs during transposition surgery. Previous studies have additionally found a decrease in regional blood flow to the ulnar nerve for at least 3 days after transposition surgery. Based on this rationale and multiple previous meta-analyses, my preferred technique for cubital tunnel surgery is simple decompression. However, history of elbow trauma resulting in osseous deformity, ulnar nerve subluxation, and revision cubital tunnel surgery merit anterior transposition.

S. M. Jacoby, MD

An Anatomical Basis for Endoscopic Cubital Tunnel Release and Associated Clinical Outcomes

Mirza A, Mirza JB, Lee BK, et al (North Shore Surgi-Ctr, Smithtown, NY; Plainview Hosp, NY; New York Inst of Technology, Old Westbury; et al)

J Hand Surg Am 39:1363-1369, 2014

Purpose.—To study the ulnar nerve in fresh-frozen cadavers as related to endoscopic release of the cubital tunnel and to present a retrospective review of patients treated with decompression via endoscopic visualization.

Methods.—To further our understanding of relevant anatomy, we dissected 26 cadaver limbs. We paid special attention to fascial membranes as potential sites of constriction as well as the position of nerves, vessels, and aberrant anatomy. These findings facilitated our understanding of the extent of release in 80 patients (92 cases) with endoscopic cubital tunnel simple decompression. Outcome measures included Disabilities of the Arm, Shoulder, and Hand score, Gabel and Amadio score, and grip and pinch strengths.

Results.—We noted fascial bands proximal to the medial epicondyle in 12 of 26 cadaver specimens, 2 of which could be the so-called arcade of Struthers. We observed a high degree of variability in the anatomy of the flexor pronator aponeurosis distal to the medial epicondyle. Where present (n = 10), medial antebrachial cutaneous nerve branches crossed the ulnar nerve at an average distance of 2.9 cm from the medial epicondyle (range, 1.0–4.5 cm). Aberrant structures were noted in 8 of the 26 specimens, including an anconeus epitrochlearis muscle in 2 specimens, a basilic vein crossing the ulnar nerve in 4 specimens, and an accessory origin of the medial head of the triceps from the medial intermuscular septum in 2 specimens. In the clinical portion of this study, the average Disabilities of the Arm, Shoulder, and Hand score before surgery was 49 (n = 34) and after surgery was 25 (n = 56). The Gabel and Amadio outcome scores were 24 excellent, 40 good, 25 fair, and 3 poor (n = 92). Average follow-up was 8.2 months (range, 0.1–35 mo).

Conclusions.—Cadaveric dissections shed light on vulnerable anatomical structures during release, including branches of the medial antebrachial cutaneous nerve, ulnar nerve, brachial artery, fascial bands, and basilic vein. The high degree of anatomical variability in this study highlights the advantage of endoscopic visualization in allowing surgeons to minimize surgical trauma.

Type of Study/Level of Evidence.—Therapeutic IV.

▶ This is a level 4 study that serves a dual purpose by reviewing the topography of ulnar nerve sites of compression in 26 fresh frozen cadavers in addition to detailing the authors' experiences with a specific endoscopic cubital tunnel release system. The authors hypothesize that improvements in endoscopic instrumentation and technique, along with the awareness of vulnerable anatomy, will result in specific advantages including minimal dissection, reduced nerve revascularization, decreased potential for iatrogenic trauma, minimal manipulation of the nerve, and a cosmetically pleasant-appearing scar.

One of the strengths of this report is the finding that most of the variable sites of ulnar nerve compression exist distal to the medial epicondyle. Specifically, the authors report that 24 of 26 specimens presented variability in the number and location of compressive facial bands. In addition, the medial antebrachial cutaneous nerve was found to cross the ulnar nerve in 10 specimens at an average distance of 2.9 cm from the medical epicondyle. I find this to be a critical point, as injury to this structure is a common cause of postoperative pain and complaint. Aberrant structures (including anconeus epitrochlearis, basilica vein, and accessory origin of medical head of triceps) were noted in 8 of 26 specimens.

With regard to clinical outcomes, the authors report that 80 patients (92 cases) of ulnar nerve decompression were treated with no injuries noted. However, 11 patients experienced ulnar nerve subluxation after decompression, 10 of whom ultimately required medical epicondylectomy and the other required anterior transposition. The procedure overall resulted in the usual spread of expected outcomes based on Disabilities of the Arm, Shoulder, and Hand scores and Gabel/Amadio scoring system (24, excellent; 40, good; 25, fair; 3, poor).

This report is in order with other endoscopic methods that have produced similar outcomes data. One should consider that the senior author of this report is involved in the proprietary aspect of the device used in this study. Nonetheless, much like an in situ technique, endoscopic cubital tunnel release is minimally invasive and results in less surgical trauma relative to nerve transposition and even medical epicondylectomy in the treatment of cubital tunnel. There is a steep learning curve with this technique, no matter the system of choice, so I would caution potential users of this technology to hone their skills in the laboratory environment prior to clinical adaptation. Finally, long-term comparative studies will be helpful to investigate the relative risks and benefits of endoscopic cubital tunnel release compared with the other surgical options.

S. M. Jacoby, MD

Retractor-Endoscopic Nerve Decompression in Carpal and Cubital Tunnel Syndromes: Outcomes in a Small Series

Martin KD, Dützmann S, Sobottka SB, et al (Carl Gustav Carus Univ Hosp, Dresden, Germany; Johann Wolfgang Goethe Univ, Frankfurt, Germany; et al)

World Neurosurg 82:e361-e370, 2014

Objective.—To present midterm to long-term results obtained in carpal tunnel release, in situ decompression, and anterior transposition of the ulnar nerve using the retractor integrated endoscope.

Methods.—During the period 2000–2010, 145 patients underwent endoscopic carpal tunnel releases ($n = 47$), endoscopic in situ decompression of the ulnar nerve ($n = 55$), and endoscopic anterior transposition of the ulnar nerve ($n = 52$). Bilateral surgery was performed in 9 patients.

Independent examinations at 24 months after surgery were used for objective results (Bishop score). Subjective results were procured using a questionnaire.

Results.—After endoscopic carpal tunnel release, 59.6% of patients showed excellent results, 21.2% showed good results, 12.8% showed fair results, and 6.4% showed poor results according to objective scoring. In 85% of patients, subjective improvement was noted after surgery; symptoms were the same as before surgery in 12.8% of patients and were worse in 2.1% of patients after surgery. After endoscopic in situ decompression, 56.4% of patients showed excellent results on objective scoring, 32.7% showed good results, 9.1% showed fair results, and 1.8% showed poor results. On subjective questioning, 72.7% of patients reported improvement, 20% reported no change in symptoms, and 7.3% reported worse symptoms. After endoscopic anterior transposition of the ulnar nerve, 48.1% of patients showed excellent results on objective scoring, 26.9% showed good results, 23.1% showed fair results, and 1.9% showed poor results. Subjectively, 65.4% of patients reported improvement, 26.9% reported no change in symptoms, and 7.7% reported worse symptoms. Patients with symptom duration of <9 months before surgery showed better results than patients with symptom duration of >9 months.

Conclusions.—The retractor-endoscopic technique provides good long-term results after carpal tunnel release, in situ decompression, and anterior subcutaneous transposition of the ulnar nerve. Outcomes showed some correlation to the duration of preoperative symptoms.

▶ Carpal tunnel syndrome and cubital tunnel syndrome are the most common peripheral nerve entrapments. Hand surgeons, plastic surgeons, orthopedic surgeons, and neurosurgeons commonly treat both conditions. Although there are 2 generally accepted approaches (open or endoscopic), numerous variations and modifications exist. Most modifications attempt to decrease the size of incisions and make the procedure as minimally invasive as is safe.

The authors describe their results with the use of retractor-assisted endoscopic approach for carpal tunnel release, in situ ulnar nerve decompression, and anterior transposition of the ulnar nerve. Krishnan et al previously reported their technique and outcomes in 3 papers.[1-3] In this series, they have accomplished this with 2-year follow-up and an excellent subjective data and objective outcome via the Bishop scoring system. With regard to the carpal tunnel release, a more precise survey, such as the Boston Carpal Tunnel Questionnaire, may have been used to access symptoms more specific to this condition. Further, the methodology regarding the decision to perform an anterior transposition of the ulnar nerve considered only tenderness at the medial elbow and need for revision. Despite recent literature that has concluded that simple decompression is as effective as transposition,[4] a commonly discussed indication such as ulnar nerve subluxation was not addressed.

In practice, I could envision hesitation in performing this procedure in revision situations at the cubital tunnel given the loss of natural tissue planes.

Second, despite a smaller incision, the subcutaneous dissection seems to be just as extensive. Regardless of my comments, the authors of this study should be applauded for performing 147 procedures using their endoscopic-assisted technique with comparable long-term results to other open and endoscopic techniques. In addition, they were able to realize this with a complication rate comparable to that of an open technique. Future studies for this group to strengthen their data would include prospective studies comparing to a traditional open technique with standard outcome measures.

J. C. Saillant, MD

References

1. Dützmann S, Martin KD, Sobottka S, et al. Open vs retractor-endoscopic in situ decompression of the ulnar nerve in cubital tunnel syndrome: a retrospective cohort study. *Neurosurgery.* 2013;72:605-616.
2. Krishnan KG, Pinzer T, Schackert G. A novel endoscopic technique in treating single nerve entrapment syndromes with special attention to ulnar nerve transposition and tarsal tunnel release: clinical application. *Neurosurgery.* 2006;59: ONS89-ONS100.
3. Krishnan KG, Pinzer T, Reber F, Schackert G. Endoscopic exploration of the brachial plexus: technique and topographic anatomy—a study in fresh human cadavers. *Neurosurgery.* 2004;54:401-408.
4. Caliandro P, La Torre G, Padua R, Giannini F, Padua L. Treatment for ulnar neuropathy at the elbow. *Cochrane Database Syst Rev.* 2012;(11):CD006839.

Carpal Tunnel Syndrome Diagnosis and Treatment: A Survey of Members of the American Society for Surgery of the Hand

Lane LB, Starecki M, Olson A, et al (North Shore Univ Hosp, Manhasset, NY; Long Island Jewish Med Ctr, New Hyde Park, NY; North Shore-LIJ Health System, Manhasset, NY)

J Hand Surg Am 39:2181-2187, 2014

Purpose.—In 2007 and 2009, the American Academy of Orthopaedic Surgeons released Clinical Practice Guidelines (CPG) for diagnosis and treatment of carpal tunnel syndrome (CTS) based upon review of the literature. The lack of consistently high-level evidence resulted in several recommendations, some strongly supported, some weakly supported, and others controversial. We postulated that a survey of American Society for Surgery of the Hand (ASSH) members would provide insight into practice patterns among hand surgeons treating CTS and demonstrate the extent to which the CPG influenced practice behavior.

Methods.—A multiple-choice questionnaire including detailed commonly observed clinical scenarios was developed, pre-tested, and approved by our institutional review board and the ASSH Web site committee chair. An anonymous electronic survey was emailed to ASSH members.

Results.—Surveys were sent to 2,650 eligible ASSH members, and 27% responded. Seventy-two percent would advise a patient to have carpal tunnel release (CTR) if the patient had both classic history/examination of

CTS and complete relief following cortisone injection. Forty-seven percent responded that in this scenario electrodiagnostic testing (EDX) is rarely or never necessary to recommend CTR. Seventy-nine percent of respondents were at least slightly more likely to order EDX based on CPG recommendations. Of these respondents, 57% replied that this was because of potential medicolegal ramifications.

Conclusions.—Although the CPG recommended EDX before surgery, and although most responding ASSH members use EDX to advise CTR, a majority answered that a supporting history and physical examination alone can be sufficient to recommend surgery, that a positive response to a cortisone injection can be sufficient indication for CTR, that EDX is not necessary in all cases of CTS, and that they would perform CTR in face of normal EDX if cortisone temporarily resolved symptoms. Among respondents more likely to order EDX based on the CPG, 57% answered that it was in some circumstances due to potential medicolegal ramifications.

Type of Study/Level of Evidence.—Economic and decision analysis III.

▶ The authors present a survey of members of the American Society for Surgery of the Hand attempting to determine practice patterns regarding diagnosis and treatment of carpal tunnel syndrome. This survey was intended to compare current methods of diagnosis and treatment with the American Academy of Orthopedic Surgery's (AAOS) Clinical Practice Guidelines (CPG) from 2007 and 2009. There was a 27% response rate, of which 83% had a primary specialty of Orthopedics, 60% practiced in a private setting, and 79% were currently or formerly certified in hand surgery. The AAOS CPG of 2007 recommended that electrodiagnostic testing should be obtained before surgical intervention. The authors of this study found that a majority of respondents felt that a supportive history and physical examination, combined with symptomatic relief from a corticosteroid injection, were at least occasionally sufficient indications for carpal tunnel release. The respondents felt that in these scenarios, electrodiagnostic testing was unnecessary to confirm diagnosis. Respondents relied more heavily on response to corticosteroid injection and physical exam than electrodiagnostic testing when indicating patients for surgical intervention. The authors found that respondents felt they could provide an appropriate prognosis of relief of symptoms after carpal tunnel release based on response to corticosteroid injection and results of electrodiagnostic testing. The responses regarding prognosis were subjective, with no outcomes measures. More than half of the respondents who have begun obtaining electrodiagnostic testing since the AAOS CPG were released state that it is due to "potential medical-legal ramifications created by the guidelines."

In my practice, I regularly obtain electrodiagnostic testing before surgery. I have found that patients appreciate having an objective measure of their nerve function before proceeding with an invasive procedure. In addition, I find it useful, should patients state that their symptoms have not changed after a period of time, to compare preoperative and postoperative tests to show improvement.

M. Kessler, MD

Diagnostic criteria of carpal tunnel syndrome using high-resolution ultrasonography: correlation with nerve conduction studies

Ooi CC, Wong SK, Tan ABH, et al (Singapore General Hosp)

Skeletal Radiol 43:1387-1394, 2014

The aim of this work was to evaluate the diagnostic performance of grey-scale, color Doppler, and dynamic ultrasound (US) for diagnosing carpal tunnel syndrome (CTS) using the medical diagnostic test called nerve conduction study (NCS) as the reference standard, and to correlate the increase in median nerve (MN) cross-sectional area (CSA) with severity of CTS. Fifty-one patients (95 wrists) with clinical symptoms of idiopathic CTS were recruited. The CSA and flattening ratio of the MN were measured at the distal radio-ulnar joint, pisiform, and hamate levels; bowing of the flexor retinaculum was determined at the hamate level. The hypervascularity of the MN was evaluated. The transverse sliding of the MN was observed dynamically and recorded as being either normal or restricted/absent. Another 15 healthy volunteers (30 wrists) were recruited as controls. Interoperator reliability was established for all criteria. CTS was confirmed in 75 wrists (75/95: 79%; 14 minimal, 21 mild, 23 moderate, 17 severe). CSA at the pisiform level was found to be the most reliable and accurate grey-scale criterion to diagnose CTS (optimum threshold: 9.8 mm^2). There was a good correlation between the severity of NCS and CSA ($r = 0.78$, $p < 0.001$). The sensitivity and specificity of color-Doppler and dynamic US in detecting CTS was 69, 95, 58, and 86%, respectively. Combination of these subjective criteria with CSA increases the sensitivity to 98.3%. US measurement of CSA provides additional information about the severity of MN involvement. Color-Doppler and dynamic US are useful supporting criteria that may expand the utility of US as a screening tool for CTS.

▶ The authors provide a thorough and interesting perspective on comparing high-resolution ultrasonography with nerve conduction studies with respect to diagnostic criteria for carpal tunnel syndrome. The authors acknowledge that there is no gold standard method of diagnosis for carpal tunnel syndrome, with physical exam findings, such as a positive Tinel or Phalen signs, being limited and that nerve conduction studies have a high false-negative rate. Their hypothesis was that the ultrasound evaluation could provide additional information for false-negative electrodiagnostic studies and may clarify the diagnosis. Ultrasound-guided median nerve evaluation consisted of measuring the cross-sectional area and flattening ratio of the median nerve at the level of the distal radio-ulnar joint, pisiform, and hamate levels. Also, bowing of the flexor retinaculum was measured at the hamate level. Dynamic transverse sliding of the median nerve at the carpal tunnel was evaluated as either normal or restricted/absent. Results showed that the cross-sectional area was significantly larger in carpal tunnel patients at all 3 levels compared with controls. In addition, there was significantly increased flattening ratio and bowing of the flexor retinaculum at the pisiform and hamate levels. Additionally, there was good correlation between the severity of nerve conduction studies with median nerve swelling and hypervascularity. Patients with carpal tunnel syndrome had significantly decreased median nerve mobility compared with controls. In my practice, I regularly obtain nerve conduction studies to supplement a thorough history and physical examination. I, like many others, find false-negative electrodiagnostic test results to be frustrating. The use of ultrasound appears promising as an additional test to consider in these patients who do not exhibit a clear diagnosis based on our current standard methods of evaluation.

M. Kessler, MD

Ulnar nerve deep branch compression by a ganglion: a review of nine cases

Wang B, Zhao Y, Lu A, et al (The Second Hosp of Tangshan, PR China; Chinese PLA General Hosp, Beijing, PR China; Kailuan General Hosp, Tangshan, PR China)

Injury 45:1126-1130, 2014

Background and Aim.—Ulnar nerve compression is common at the elbow, but less common at the wrist. The purposes of this study were to report a series of nine patients with pure ulnar nerve deep branch compression by a ganglion and to evaluate the outcome following a surgical treatment.

Methods.—A retrospective study was conducted with nine patients from 2000 to 2011. The patients included four male and five female patients. The mean duration of symptoms before surgery was 16 months (range, 5–32 months). Different degrees of muscular atrophy and weakness of the interossei and adductor pollicis muscles were present without sensory loss in the hand. Ganglion excision and decompression of Guyon's canal were performed in all patients. We evaluated postoperative results of this uncommon nerve lesion based on the modified Bishop's scoring system.

Results.—The ganglion compressing the deep branch originated from the pisohamate joint in eight cases and from the midpalmar space in one case. At the mean follow-up of 23 months (range, 17–31 months), strength improvement of the grip and tip pinch was achieved in all patients. In comparison, grip strength improved from a mean of 63% of the unaffected side preoperatively to 88% of the unaffected side postoperatively. Tip pinch strength improved from a mean of 61% to 87%. According to the modified Bishop's scoring system, six patients (67%) obtained excellent results, two (22%) had good results, and only one (11%) had a fair result.

Conclusions.—A ganglion causing ulnar nerve deep branch compression is rare. Early surgical treatment can result in satisfactory functional recovery.

▶ Compression of the deep branch of the ulnar nerve at the wrist is fairly uncommon. Furthermore, studies have been limited to isolated case reports.

This article is unique given the number of patients reported for this very specific and unusual entity. The authors did a nice job illustrating and noting the anatomic considerations of both the origin of the ganglions in their series and their surgical approach.

There are certain aspects of this work that left me questioning their methodology. For instance, although the authors comment on the potential use of magnetic resonance imaging or ultrasound for diagnosis, they fail to mention which, if either, they used in their evaluations. Furthermore, it would seem useful to perform electrodiagnostics on each patient; however, 3 patients did not receive such testing. Finally, if the purpose of the series is to report outcomes, readers would be better served by aligning preoperative findings such as grip strength, motor grade, and evidence of atrophy with the respective postoperative outcome of the same patient.

Although this represents a small series of patients, I do find their experience with the origin of ganglions in Guyon canal helpful. Furthermore, it is useful from a counseling standpoint to be armed with some ability to prognosticate patient outcomes.

J. C. Saillant, MD

Does the Ulnar Nerve Enlarge After Surgical Transposition?

Vosbikian MM, Tarity TD, Nazarian LN, et al (Thomas Jefferson Univ Hosp, Philadelphia, PA)

J Ultrasound Med 33:1647-1652, 2014

Objectives.—The purpose of this study was to test the hypothesis that symptomatic transposed ulnar nerves have a larger average cross-sectional area (CSA) than symptomatic in situ ulnar nerves.

Methods.—We conducted a retrospective review of the charts and sonograms of 68 patients who had failed ulnar nerve transposition compared to 48 patients with cubital tunnel syndrome who had not undergone surgical management. In addition, postoperative sonograms were compared with preoperative studies when available. Failure was defined as persistence or recurrence of symptoms of ulnar neuropathy postoperatively. The cross-sectional area of the nerve, subjective echogenicity, and residual sites of compression were recorded. Groups were subsequently compared by t tests.

Results.—The failed ulnar nerve transposition group showed a mean cross-sectional area ± SD of 17.26 ± 9.93 mm^2, whereas the control group showed a mean cross-sectional area of 13.45 ± 7.33 mm^2. This difference was statistically significant ($P = .018$). Nontransposed nerves were more likely to have identifiable sites of compression ($P < .05$). There was a trend toward postoperative enlargement in the 6 patients with available preoperative imaging ($P = .17$). No difference in subjective echogenicity was found in this analysis.

Conclusions.—Patients with failed ulnar nerve transposition show a significantly enlarged cross-sectional area when compared to symptomatic nerves in situ. Although a specific etiology for this difference cannot be determined, the data suggest that the reference ranges for the cross-sectional area of the ulnar nerve may need to be revised for those who have undergone surgery.

▶ Ultrasonography can be a tremendously versatile diagnostic tool. Although it has been used extensively in other fields, its use in orthopedics has gained popularity first in sports medicine and now in the field of hand and upper extremity surgery. Specifically, the cross-sectional area of peripheral nerves on ultrasound has been useful for diagnosis of compression neuropathies. The authors of this article have taken this idea a step further to evaluate postsurgical changes and ulnar nerve size after transposition in patients who remain symptomatic.

The authors of this study have done an excellent job of proving that the dimensions of the ulnar nerve after transposition in their patient population were in fact enlarged compared with a control group of symptomatic patients. However, we are unable to obtain any information regarding the actual change in size of the symptomatic nerve because we are not comparing the same patients' nerve pre- and posttransposition. In fact, I would surmise that the normal and pathologic size of the ulnar nerve in situ is quite variable among a given population. Furthermore, as the authors point out, patients who required transposition surgery are likely to have had more advanced disease and long-standing compression compared with a control group with patients who haven't yet had a surgical intervention. Electromyogram and nerve conduction data would have been helpful in comparing groups because the diagnosis and inclusion criteria were subjective in nature. Finally, as the authors also mention, the significance or etiology of an enlarged ulnar nerve after transposition is not clear and may represent alterations in the extrinsic blood supply to the nerve.

Although this study certainly has some merit regarding the use of ultrasound to accessing the ulnar at the elbow, readers may find themselves reaching for its applicability to clinical situations and decision making. There is no doubt that further evidence and use of ultrasound in the evaluation of peripheral nerve compressions will become a valuable tool.

J. C. Saillant, MD

Ulnar Neuropathy as a Result of Anconeus Epitrochlearis

Nellans K, Galdi B, Kim HM, et al (Columbia Univ, NY)
Orthopedics 37:e743-e745, 2014

After carpal tunnel syndrome, cubital tunnel syndrome is the second most common compression neuropathy in the upper extremity. Various sites of ulnar nerve compression at the elbow exist, with the most common being between the 2 heads of the flexor carpi ulnaris. Other potential sites include the arcade of Struthers, the space between Osborne's ligament and the medial ulnar collateral ligament, the medial epicondyle, the medial head of the triceps, and the medial intermuscular septum. The anconeus epitrochlearis, an anomalous muscle that runs between the medial aspect of the olecranon and the medial epicondyle, is found in up to 28% of cadavers. Although it is far less common, it must be considered when evaluating a patient with cubital tunnel syndrome. The authors report a 19-year-old man with a 2-month history of atraumatic left elbow pain accompanied by distal motor and sensory symptoms that significantly affected his activities of daily living and quality of life. After a short course of conservative management, surgical excision of the anomalous muscle, along with decompression of the ulnar nerve, was performed because of progression of symptoms. The patient had immediate improvement in subjective symptoms and strength on removal of the anconeus epitrochlearis. As shown in this case report, recovery of both motor and sensory nerve function can be achieved if the source of compression is an anomalous muscle and is treated with early surgical removal.

► The authors present a case report of cubital tunnel syndrome caused by an anomalous anconeus epitrochlearis muscle, in a 19-year-old male student with an acute onset of symptoms over a 2-month period. In situ decompression with resection of the anconeus epitrochlearis was performed, with subsequent complete resolution of symptoms. The authors review the literature, which suggests that excision of the anomalous muscle is sufficient to treat the ulnar nerve compression. Overall, this is an interesting case report with a rare cause of cubital tunnel syndrome that should be addressed by surgical excision if encountered intraoperatively.

H. Chim, MD

Outcomes of Revision Surgery for Cubital Tunnel Syndrome

Aleem AW, Krogue JD, Calfee RP (Washington Univ School of Medicine, St Louis, MO)

J Hand Surg Am 39:2141-2149, 2014

Purpose.—To compare both validated patient-rated and objective outcomes of patients following revision cubital tunnel surgery to a similar group of patients who underwent primary surgery.

Methods.—This case-control investigation enrolled 56 patients treated surgically for cubital tunnel syndrome (28 revision cases, 28 primary controls) at a tertiary center. Patients with a minimum of 2 years of follow-up were eligible. All patients completed an in-office study evaluation. Revision participants represented 55% of potential patients in our practice and controls (treated only with primary surgery) were chosen at random from our practice to reach a 1:1 case to control ratio. Preoperative McGowan grading was confirmed similar between the groups. Outcome measures included validated patient outcome questionnaires (Patient-Rated Elbow Evaluation, Levine-Katz questionnaire), symptoms, and physical examination findings. Statistical analyses were conducted to compare the patient groups.

Results.—Despite 79% of revision patients reporting symptomatic improvement, revision patients reported worse outcomes on all measured standardized questionnaires compared with primary patients. The Levine-Katz questionnaire indicated mild residual symptoms in the primary group (1.6) versus moderate remaining symptoms following revision surgery (2.3). The Patient-Rated Elbow Evaluation also indicated superior results for the control group (9 ± 10) compared with the revision group (32 ± 22). Revision patients had a higher frequency of constant symptoms, elevated 2-point discrimination, and diminished pinch strength. McGowan grading improved after 25% of revision surgeries versus 64% of primary surgeries, and 21% of revision patients had deterioration of their McGowan grade.

Conclusions.—Subjective and objective outcomes of revision patients in this cohort were inferior to outcomes of similar patients following primary surgery. Revision surgery can be offered in the setting of persistent or recurrent symptoms that are unexplained by an alternative diagnosis, but patients should be counseled that complete resolution of symptoms is unlikely.

Type of Study/Level of Evidence.—Therapeutic III.

▶ Cubital tunnel syndrome represents the second most common compression neuropathy in the upper extremity. Despite its prevalence, a standardized approach to surgical treatment has not been adopted. Even in the presence of meta-analyses of the existing literature, a consensus on treatment of primary and revision cases has not been reached.[1]

The authors have done an impressive job of collecting data from a large number of patients in a methodical fashion, addressing patient demographics, electrodiagnostic data, physical examination findings, McGowan grading, and subjective concerns of the patient. In addition, the strength of this study and level of evidence is increased by having a control group that underwent surgery by the same surgeons. Limitations of the report include possible selection bias in which 23 of the patients who underwent revision were not included in the data. Furthermore, retrospective collection of data from patients and medical records is often subject to recall bias and collection error.

It is commonly believed that failure of primary surgery for cubital tunnel syndrome is often related to subluxation of the ulnar nerve over the medial epicondyle or residual sites of compression. Interestingly, the authors found in their revision cases that only 5 of 26 patients had an identifiable cause of failure. It seems to be that the reason for initial failure is often unclear and could represent intrinsic nerve dysfunction, perineural scaring, or associated persistent compression. With 75% of revision patients having an equal or worse McGowan grade, 53% noting constant symptoms, and 21% reporting no symptomatic relief, we as surgeons need to realize that revision surgery for failed cubital tunnel syndrome is not simply a backup plan. These data will guide us in counseling the unhappy patient after a primary cubital tunnel release.

This study represents the first well-designed attempt to affirm that revision cubital tunnel surgery does not provide similar results to primary surgery and is not without shortcomings if the initial decompression is not effective.

J. C. Saillant, MD

Reference

1. Zlowodzki M, Chan S, Bhandari M, Kalliainen L, Schubert W. Anterior transposition compared with simple decompression for treatment of cubital tunnel syndrome. A meta-analysis of randomized, controlled trials. *J Bone Joint Surg Am.* 2007;89:2591-2598.

14 Nerve

Comparison of Nerve, Vessel, and Cartilage Grafts in Promoting Peripheral Nerve Regeneration

Firat C, Geyik Y, Aytekin AH, et al (Inonu Univ School of Medicine, Malatya, Turkey)

Ann Plast Surg 73:54-61, 2014

Peripheral nerve injury primarily occurs due to trauma as well as factors such as tumors, inflammatory diseases, congenital deformities, infections, and surgical interventions. The surgical procedure to be performed as treatment depends on the etiology, type of injury, and the anatomic region. The goal of treatment is to minimize loss of function due to motor and sensory nerve loss at the distal part of the injury. Regardless of the cause of the injury, the abnormal nerve regeneration due to incomplete nerve regeneration, optimal treatment of peripheral nerve injuries should provide adequate coaptation of proximal and distal sides without tension, preserving the neurotrophic factors within the repair line. The gold standard for the treatment of nerve defects is the autograft; however, due to denervation of the donor site, scarring, and neuroma formation, many studies have aimed to develop simpler methods, better functional results, and less morbidity. In this study, a defect 1 cm in length was created on the sciatic nerve of rats. The rats were treated with the following procedures: group 1, autograft; group 2, allogeneic aorta graft; group 3, diced cartilage graft in allogeneic aorta graft; and group 4, tubularized cartilage graft in allogeneic aorta graft. Group 5 was the control group. The effects of cartilage tissue in nerve regeneration were evaluated by functional and histomorphological methods.

Group 1, for which the repair was performed with an autograft, was evaluated to be the most similar to the control group. There was not a statistically significant difference in myelination and Schwann cell rates between group 2, in which an allogeneic aorta graft was used, and group 3, in which diced cartilage in an allogeneic aorta graft was used. In group 4, myelination and Schwann cell formation were observed; however, they were scattered and irregular, likely due to increased fibrosis.

In all of the groups, nerve regeneration at various rates was observed both functionally and histomorphologically. This study demonstrates that cartilage tissue has promoting effects in nerve regeneration (Figs 2 and 4).

▶ The authors report on a laboratory study comparing nerve regeneration with autograft, allograft aorta as a conduit and with autograft cartilage, and a

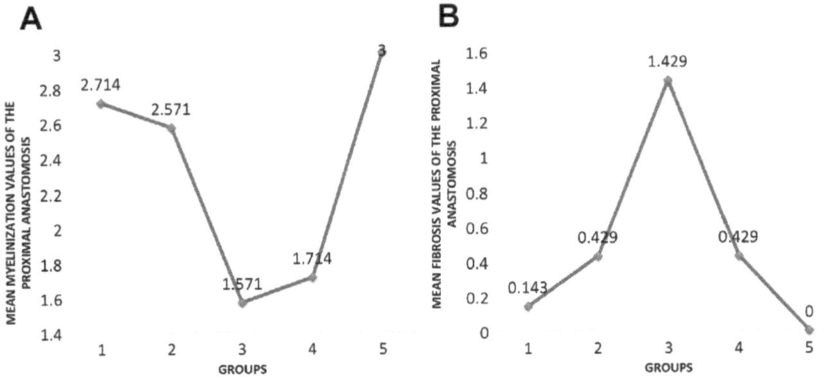

FIGURE 2.—A, B, Mean myelination and fibrosis values of proximal anastomoses. (Reprinted from Firat C, Geyik Y, Aytekin AH, et al. Comparison of nerve, vessel, and cartilage grafts in promoting peripheral nerve regeneration. *Ann Plast Surg*. 2014;73:54-61, with permission from Lippincott Williams & Wilkins.)

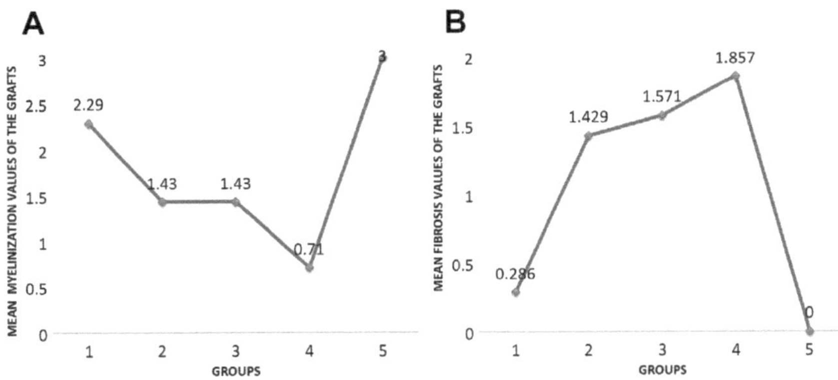

FIGURE 4.—A, B: Mean myelination and fibrosis values of grafts. (Reprinted from Firat C, Geyik Y, Aytekin AH, et al. Comparison of nerve, vessel, and cartilage grafts in promoting peripheral nerve regeneration. *Ann Plast Surg*. 2014;73:54-61, with permission from Lippincott Williams & Wilkins.)

tubularized cartilage graft. They used a standard rat model, and their results were best in the autograft group. Other groups did show mylenization across the proximal neurorrhaphy site and the entire graft, but there was also evidence of increased fibrosis (Figs 2 and 4).

The search for an alternative to autograft for nerve reconstruction remains elusive. Allograft nerve is promising but still does not seem to be equivalent to autograft, at least in motor recovery.[1] The lack of donor site morbidity is appealing, but for critical nerves, the compromise of recovery may be too great for many situations. Continued search for other materials is important to advance the science of nerve regeneration. Although cartilage autografts show some myelin across the graft site, there is also increased fibrosis. Further research is necessary to determine if this is a potential clinical alternative.

W. C. Hammert, MD

Reference

1. Giusti G, Willems WF, Kremer T, Friedrich PF, Bishop AT, Shin AY. Return of motor function after segmental nerve loss in a rat model: comparison of autogenousnerve graft, collagen conduit, and processed allograft (AxoGen). *J Bone Joint Surg Am.* 2012;94:410-417.

A quantitative study of vibration injury to peripheral nerves—introducing a new longitudinal section analysis

Davis J, Wang Z, Zhang LL, et al (Med College of Wisconsin, Milwaukee)
Hand 9:413-418, 2014

Purpose.—Long-term vibrations are known to cause neurovascular diseases, which are common in workers who operate handheld power tools or motor vehicles. Understanding the neuropathology of vibration-induced nerve injury is critical to its prevention and treatment. This study aims to evaluate whether light microscopy of longitudinal nerve sections can be used as a simple yet effective method for quantifying nerve injury.

Methods.—The rats were split into two groups that were subjected to vibration (4 h/day) for 7 or 14 days. They were then allowed to rest for varying periods of time. Longitudinal sections of the tail nerves were examined under light microscopy. Injuries to the nerves were classified into three types, counted, tallied, and then divided by the length of the nerve being studied.

Results.—Both 7 and 14 days of vibration showed significant damage when no recovery time was given. After 1 month of rest, the 7-day group began to show signs of recovery, but the 14-day group did not. After 2 months of rest, the 7 day vibration group showed almost complete recovery, while the 14-day vibration group still showed significant damage when compared to the sham control groups.

Conclusion.—The amount of damage to the myelin sheath directly correlated with vibration duration. When vibrated for longer than 7 days, nerve recovery was limited. This study also demonstrated that light microscopy of longitudinal slices is a simple yet effective method of quantifying the nerve damage (Figs 4 and 5).

▶ The strength of this study is that the authors created an experimental model that demonstrates a vibration injury to nerve fibers, which were assessed easily by light microscopic examination of longitudinal sections of each nerve specimen.

This study also has several weaknesses. The vibration-induced nerve injury was classified into 3 types according to the light microscopic appearance of the fibers but not by the severity of injury to the nerve fibers. The severity of nerve injury is often assessed using Seddon's classification (neurapraxia, axonotmesis, and neurotmesis).[1] If the injury only involves the myelin sheath and

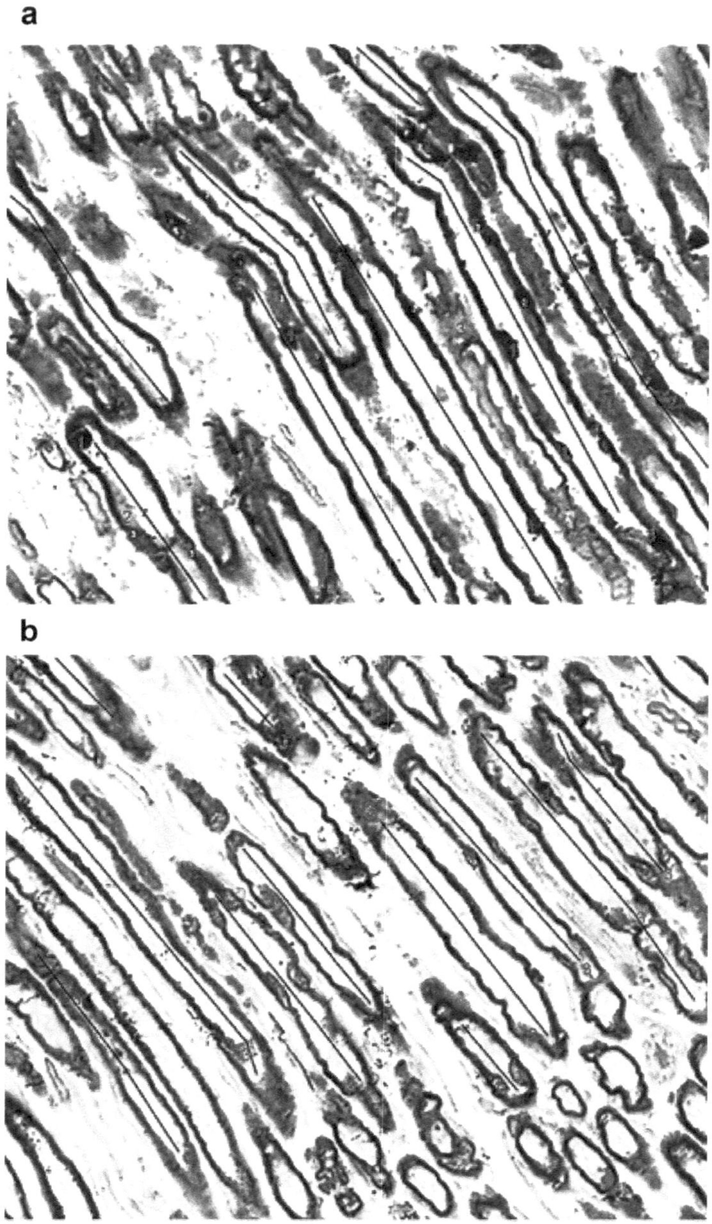

FIGURE 4.—14 day vibration harvest with Toluidine blue stain. **a** 30 days of recovery after 14 days of vibration experiments, the rat tail was harvested after 30 days. A photomicrograph of the rat tail nerve longitudinal cross section was captured. **b** 60 days of recovery after 14 days of vibration experiments, the rat was allowed to recover for 60 days prior to harvesting. A photomicrograph of the rat tail nerve longitudinal cross section was captured. All figures were captured at ×400 magnification. The three types of myelin abnormalities were labeled with *red numbers* as type 1, 2, or 3 (please refer to *Counting and Categorization of Axons* in the "Materials and Methods" section). The *black lines* indicate the center of the axons, from which length measurements were obtained. (With kind permission from Springer Science+Business Media: Davis J, Wang Z, Zhang LL, et al. A quantitative study of vibration injury to peripheral nerves—introducing a new longitudinal section analysis. *Hand.* 2014;9:413-418, with permission from American Association for Hand Surgery.)

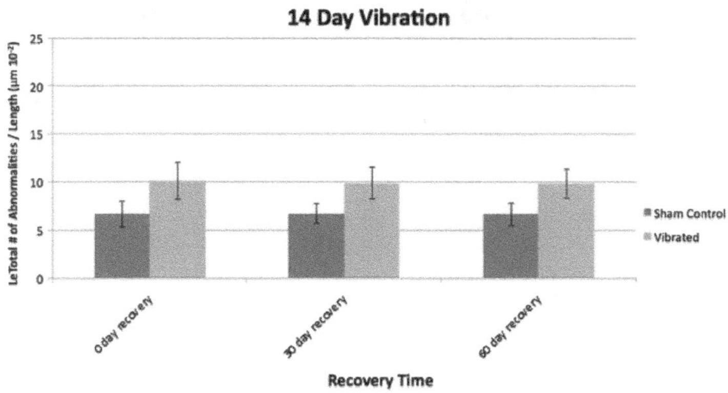

FIGURE 5.—14 day vibration. Results of total number of abnormalities/length (μm 10^{-2}) after 14 days of vibration with 0, 30, and 60 days of rest. All results of the 14 day rats that underwent vibration were statistically significant in terms of nerve recovery when compared to sham control ($P < 0.05$). (With kind permission from Springer Science+Business Media: Davis J, Wang Z, Zhang LL, et al. A quantitative study of vibration injury to peripheral nerves—introducing a new longitudinal section analysis. *Hand.* 2014;9:413-418, with permission from American Association for Hand Surgery.)

does not extend to the axon (neurapraxia), it can heal spontaneously and completely within several days and leave no structural abnormalities. However, injury involving the axons may not heal completely and can potentially leave permanent structural abnormalities within the nerve fibers (neurotmesis).

The number of nerve fiber injuries within the 7-day vibration group was significantly greater than that of the sham group immediately after applying the vibration. However, no significant differences were found 30 and 60 days after the vibration (Fig 4). The number of injuries within the 14-day vibration group was significantly greater than that of the sham group at all time points after the vibration (Fig 5). These findings can be interpreted as meaning that the vibration for 7 days generated neurapraxia, which was reversible, and the vibration for 14 days left irreversible changes to the axons (axonotmesis or neurotmesis). The outcomes of this study would have been more interesting if the study had been extended to an electromicroscopic investigation of the nerve fibers subjected to vibration for 7 and 14 days.

The symptoms produced by the vibration were not investigated in this study. The authors found that there were still nerve fiber injuries in the sham group. It is unknown whether the increased number of histologic nerve fiber injuries was actually related to the symptoms produced by vibration to the peripheral nerves.

R. Kakinoki, MD, PhD

Reference

1. Seddon HJ. *Surgical Disorders of the Peripheral Nerve.* Edinburgh, London, UK: Churchill Livingstone; 1972.

Evaluation of Sensory Recovery After Reconstruction of Digital Nerves of the Hand Using Muscle-in-vein Conduits in Comparison to Nerve Suture or Nerve Autografting

Manoli T, Schulz L, Stahl S, et al (Univ of Tuebingen, Germany)
Microsurgery 34:608-615, 2014

Background.—Muscle-in-vein conduits are a good alternative solution to nerve autografts for bridging peripheral nerve defects since enough graft material is available and no loss of sensation at the harvesting area is expected. The purpose of this study was to compare regeneration results after digital nerve reconstruction with muscle-in-vein conduits, nerve autografts, or direct suture.

Patients and Methods.—46 patients with 53 digital nerve injuries of the hand subjected to direct suture ($n = 22$) or reconstruction of 1-6cm long defects with either nerve autografts ($n = 14$) or muscle-in-vein conduits ($n = 17$) between 2008 and 2012, were examined using the two-point discrimination and Semmes-Weinstein Monofilaments.

Results.—The follow-up examinations took place 12 to 58 months after surgery. A median reduction of sensibility of 2 Semmes-Weinstein monofilaments compared with intact digits was observed after direct suture (DS) and of 2.5 and 2 Semmes-Weinstein monofilaments after reconstruction with autologous nerve grafts (ANG) and muscle-in-vein conduits (MVC), respectively. No statistically significant differences between all three groups could be found with a significance level set by a $P < 0.006$ ($P_{DS\text{-}ANG} = 0.24$, $P_{DS\text{-}MVC} = 0.03$, $P_{ANG\text{-}MVC} = 0.52$). After harvesting a nerve graft, reduction of sensibility at the donor site occurred in 10 of 14 cases but only in one case after harvesting a muscle-in-vein conduit.

Conclusions.—Muscle-in-vein conduits may be a good alternative solution to autografts for the reconstruction of digital nerves, since no significant differences could be demonstrated between the two methods.

▶ It is difficult to assess the sensory recovery of the fingers after digital nerve repair in the clinical setting because the outcomes can be influenced by many factors, including patient age, nerve gap length, condition of the nerve injury (sharp or crush), the time between the injury and surgery or between surgery and the assessment, location of the injury, nature of the wound involving the nerve injury, and the laterality of the injury (unilateral or bilateral digital nerve injury).

A significant overlap of the sensory innervation by both digital nerves of a finger is a well-known phenomenon and has important implications for interpretation of the results of digital nerve repair. The outcomes of sensory examinations of the fingers express the outcomes of the comprehensive sensation produced by the bilateral digital nerves of a finger. The outcomes of finger sensory examination after digital nerve repair depend on the sensory recovery of the repaired digital nerve and the overlapped sensation produced by the contralateral digital nerve of the finger.[1] In this study, finger digital nerves that had been injured under different conditions were treated using 3 different surgical procedures (direct suture, autogenous nerve grafting, and muscle-in-vein interposition). The results of this study may be influenced by the nerve regeneration resulting from the surgical procedures used for the digital nerve repair and from several other factors, including the above-mentioned conditions.

Because an autogenous nerve graft contains the basement membrane including several adherent molecules and Schwann cells (which are capable of producing several neurotrophic and neurotropic factors), the extension of nerve fibers is enhanced in the graft. However, in a muscle-in-vein conduit, there is a basement membrane of muscle fibers, which may be an alternative to a basement membrane of nerves.[2] However, the nonvascularized muscle within the vein conduit does not produce any neurotrophic or neurotropic factors. In addition, Schwann cells in nerves regenerated in the muscle-in-vein conduit move from the nerve stumps joined to either end of the conduit, whereas Schwann cells are already present in the nerve grafts. Considering the process of nerve regeneration through muscle-in-vein conduits and autogenous nerve grafts, it is difficult to believe that the recovery of nerves using muscle-in-vein conduits was comparable or sometimes superior to recovery using autogenous nerve grafts or direct nerve sutures.

R. Kakinoki, MD, PhD

References

1. Calder JS, McAllister RM. Interpreting the results of unilateral digital nerve repair. *J Hand Surg Br.* 1993;18:797-799.
2. Chen LE, Seaber AV, Urbaniak JR, Murrell GA. Denatured muscle as a nerve conduit: a functional, morphologic, and electrophysiologic evaluation. *J Reconstr Microsurg.* 1994;10:137-144.

A new device for nerve approximation in traumatic injuries of extremities

Forootan KS, Karimi H, Forootan N-sS (Iran Univ of Med Sciences, Tehran)

Eur J Plast Surg 37:497-502, 2014

Background.—Precise approximation of two nerve endings is a major determinant of outcomes following nerve repairs. Despite technical and instrumental advances, approximation of nerve endings remains a challenge in reconstructive surgeries. We designed a new nerve approximator device for precise approximation of nerve endings and evaluated its utility in surgeries of peripheral nerves.

Methods.—We conducted a longitudinal study comparing postoperative functional outcomes between patients with peripheral nerve injury undergoing surgical repair by the new approximator device and conventional technique.

Results.—A total of 204 nerve trunks were repaired by the new approximator device and 91 nerves by conventional technique. Patients were followed for a median of 30 months. Time required for nerve approximation was significantly reduced with the approximator device (4.5 min vs. 7 min, $p < 0.0001$). Nerve conduction velocity and tinel sign revealed similar results in both groups. However, grip, pinch and intrinsic muscle strength tests did not differ between the two groups.

Conclusions.—Our new nerve approximator device is feasible to use and reduces time of neurorrhaphy in microsurgical nerve repairs with sustained outcomes comparable to the conventional techniques.

Level of Evidence.—Level IV, therapeutic study.

▶ In fresh peripheral nerve injuries, transected nerve stumps are typically very mobile and may be approximated easily. Placing stitches in both nerve stumps can bring both stumps together. However, in chronic nerve injuries in which the interval between surgery and injury may be more than 2 or 3 weeks, the stumps tend to retract proximally and distally and have to be approximated by resisting the distraction force of the stumps. In surgery, the wrist and fingers should be put in a flexed position to reduce the distraction force of the stumps. The assistant usually keeps both stumps together, holding the tip of the epineurium of the stumps with microforceps, while the operating surgeon places stitches on the nerve stumps under microscopy. The assistant needs some microsurgical training to keep the approximated nerve stumps fixed under the microscope. The device described is capable of approximating the transected stumps and may allow the surgeon to perform nerve suturing safely, without the need for an assistant.

I am concerned about the possibility of injury to the perineurium and nerve fibers because the hooks of the device must be inserted into the nerve stumps through the perineurium to secure the transected nerve stumps when approximated.

R. Kakinoki, MD, PhD

Direct Radial to Ulnar Nerve Transfer to Restore Intrinsic Muscle Function in Combined Proximal Median and Ulnar Nerve Injury: Case Report and Surgical Technique

Phillips BZ, Franco MJ, Yee A, et al (Washington Univ School of Medicine, Saint Louis, MO)

J Hand Surg Am 39:1358-1362, 2014

A distal median to ulnar nerve transfer for timely restoration of critical intrinsic muscle function is possible in isolated ulnar nerve injuries but not for combined ulnar and median nerve injuries. We used a distal nerve transfer to restore ulnar intrinsic function in the case of a proximal combined median and ulnar nerve injury. Transfer of the nonessential radial nerve branches to the abductor pollicis longus, extensor pollicis brevis, and extensor indicis proprius to the motor branch of the ulnar nerve was performed in a direct end-to-end fashion via an interosseous tunnel.

This method safely and effectively restored intrinsic function before terminal muscle degeneration.

▶ In peripheral nerve transfer operations, several basic rules must be followed to achieve good outcomes. First, the distance between the site of neurorrhaphy and the target muscles (in motor reconstruction) or the skin receptors (in sensory reconstruction) should be as short as possible. The shorter the distance between the site of the neurorrhaphy and the target organs, the earlier nerve regeneration occurs. Second, donor nerves should be motor-fiber dominant for motor reconstruction and sensory-fiber dominant for sensory reconstruction. Third, the target muscles of nerve transfer should have synchronized functions with the muscles, which the donor nerves originally innervated, similar to the use of a tendon transfer in motor reconstruction. For example, it is known that elbow flexion is more easily separated from the motion for respiration after intercostal nerve transfer to the musculocutaneous nerves[1] than finger and wrist motion after partial ulnar nerve transfer to the musculocutaneous nerve.[2,3] Several previous researchers have described this phenomenon and have explained that the interneural cortical connection between the area administering the body trunk motions and that for elbow motion might be activated after intercostal nerve transfer.[4] We suspect that such an interneural connection would not exist between finger and wrist motion and elbow motion.

In a partial posterior interosseous nerve transfer (branches of the extensor pollicis brevis and abductor pollicis longus) to the motor branch of the ulnar nerve, the donor nerve is motor dominant and performs the functions of thumb abduction and extension, which are often synchronized with the proximal interphalangeal and distal interphalangeal joint extension of fingers (ulnar nerve function). However, because the site of the neurorrhaphy is at the midforearm level, the distances that the nerve fibers have to regenerate across are quite long. This operative procedure should be indicated for young people, and not for older people, because the potential for nerve regeneration is more active in younger patients. The outcomes of neurorrhaphy are influenced by many factors other than the distance between site of nerve repair and the target organs or patient age, including the operator's skill in performing neurorrhaphy and the condition of the repaired nerves. I prefer the use of muscle transfers (brachioradialis to flexor pollicis longus, extensor carpi radialis longus to flexor digitorum profundus) combined with Zancolli's metacarpophalangeal joint arthrodesis of the fingers over direct radial nerve transfer to the ulnar nerve to treat combined proximal median and ulnar nerve injury, because more stable outcomes can be achieved from the tendon transfer than the nerve transfer.

R. Kakinoki, MD, PhD

References

1. Tsuyama N, Hara T. Reconstructive surgery for traumatic brachial plexus injuries. *Clin Orthop.* 1968;3:675-687.
2. Oberlin C, Béal D, Leechavengvongs S, Salon A, Dauge MC, Sarcy JJ. Nerve transfer to biceps muscle using a part of ulnar nerve for C5-C6 avulsion of brachial plexus: anatomical study and report of four cases. *J Hand Surg Am.* 1994;19A: 232-237.

3. Kakinoki R, Ikeguchi R, Dunkan SF, et al. Comparison between partial ulnar and intercostal nerve transfers for reconstructing elbow flexion in patients with upper brachial plexus injuries. *J Brachial Plex Peripher Nerve Inj*. 2010;5:4.
4. Sokki AM, Bhat DI, Devi BI. Cortical reorganization following neurotization. A diffusion tensor image and functional magnetic resonance imaging study. *Neurosurgery*. 2012;70:1305-1311.

An anatomical study of transfer of the anterior interosseous nerve for the treatment of proximal ulnar nerve injuries

Sukegawa K, Kuniyoshi K, Suzuki T, et al (Chiba Univ, Chuo-ku, Japan)
Bone Joint J 96-B:789-794, 2014

We conducted an anatomical study to determine the best technique for transfer of the anterior interosseous nerve (AIN) for the treatment of proximal ulnar nerve injuries. The AIN, ulnar nerve, and associated branches were dissected in 24 cadaver arms. The number of branches of the AIN and length available for transfer were measured. The nerve was divided just proximal to its termination in pronator quadratus and transferred to the ulnar nerve through the shortest available route. Separation of the deep and superficial branches of the ulnar nerve by blunt dissection alone, was also assessed. The mean number of AIN branches was 4.8 (3 to 8) and the mean length of the nerve available for transfer was 72 mm (41 to 106). The transferred nerve reached the ulnar nerve most distally when placed dorsal to flexor digitorum profundus (FDP). We therefore conclude that the AIN should be passed dorsal to FDP, and that the deep and superficial branches of the ulnar nerve require approximately 30 mm of blunt dissection and 20 mm of sharp dissection from the point of bifurcation to the site of the anastomosis.

The use of this technique for transfer of the AIN should improve the outcome for patients with proximal ulnar nerve injuries.

► The authors present a thorough anatomic dissection of the anterior interosseous nerve (AIN) in a cadaveric model in an attempt to clarify a few points of the previously well-described AIN to ulnar nerve transfer. This procedure was developed by Dr Mackinnon and has been well described in the literature.[1] Although I have always found Dr Mackinnon's previous publications to be direct and well presented, this article attempts to clarify a few points and perhaps facilitate surgical technique. The authors found that passing the terminal branch of the AIN dorsal to the flexor digitorum profundus provided the longest segment and most tension-free repair. Additionally, the use of both blunt and sharp dissection provided optimal length of nerve transfer.

I have limited experience with this procedure, although from this and similar nerve cases, I can see the potential clinical relevance of integrating the AIN as distal as possibly along the ulnar nerve.

E. Lawler, MD

Reference

1. Brown JM, Yee A, Mackinnon SE. Distal median to ulnar nerve transfers to restore ulnar motor and sensory function within the hand: technical nuances. *Neurosurgery.* 2009;65:966-978.

An anatomical study of transfer of the anterior interosseous nerve for the treatment of proximal ulnar nerve injuries

Sukegawa K, Kuniyoshi K, Suzuki T, et al (Chiba Univ, Chuo-ku, Japan)
Bone Joint J 96-B:789-794, 2014

We conducted an anatomical study to determine the best technique for transfer of the anterior interosseous nerve (AIN) for the treatment of proximal ulnar nerve injuries. The AIN, ulnar nerve, and associated branches were dissected in 24 cadaver arms. The number of branches of the AIN and length available for transfer were measured. The nerve was divided just proximal to its termination in pronator quadratus and transferred to the ulnar nerve through the shortest available route. Separation of the deep and superficial branches of the ulnar nerve by blunt dissection alone, was also assessed. The mean number of AIN branches was 4.8 (3 to 8) and the mean length of the nerve available for transfer was 72 mm (41 to 106). The transferred nerve reached the ulnar nerve most distally when placed dorsal to flexor digitorum profundus (FDP). We therefore conclude that the AIN should be passed dorsal to FDP, and that the deep and superficial branches of the ulnar nerve require approximately 30 mm of blunt dissection and 20 mm of sharp dissection from the point of bifurcation to the site of the anastomosis.

The use of this technique for transfer of the AIN should improve the outcome for patients with proximal ulnar nerve injuries.

▶ The last decade has seen a paradigm shift toward nerve transfers and away from tendon transfers to address paralytic problems of the upper limb. Transfer of the nerve to the pronator quadratus anterior interosseous nerve to the motor fascicle of the ulnar nerve to restore some intrinsic muscle function was one of the earliest described. It has many potential advantages. Loss of pronator quadratus function seems little noticeable to patients, that is, there is no donor site morbidity. Good results using tendon transfers to restore intrinsic function are hard to come by. For these reasons, many surgeons have adopted this procedure in the circumstance of high ulnar nerve injuries. Others are applying this nerve transfer for patients with intrinsic atrophy secondary to long-standing cubital tunnel compression. One can choose an end-to-end or an end-to-side attachment. Although the anatomic details of this transfer have been previously well described, this article provides additional technical details that may simplify surgical decision making. Whether the unique findings that they demonstrate will result in improved outcomes is uncertain. My personal experience has been limited primarily to patients with long delays between injury and surgery.

The outcomes in these patients were not dramatic. For me, traditional muscle-tendon transfers for low ulnar nerve palsies offer more predictable outcomes.

V. R. Hentz, MD

Further Evidence for Treatment of Recalcitrant Neuropathy of the Upper Limb With Autologous Vein Wrapping

Mulgrew S, Kanabar GP, Papanastasiou S (The Lister Hosp, Stevenage, Hertfordshire, UK; Hertford County Hosp, Hertfordshire, UK)

Ann Plast Surg 69:288-291, 2012

The treatment of entrapment neuropathy in the upper extremity with surgical decompression has generally provided good results. Recurrence of symptoms, however, is not uncommon, and its management is both challenging and difficult. Autologous vein graft wrapping is an alternative technique, and it is recommended for the treatment of recalcitrant upper limb nerve compression in which 2 or more previous surgical procedures have failed to resolve the problem. Each patient underwent both subjective and objective evaluation. To our knowledge, this is the largest reported single series of vein wrapping cases in the upper limb outside the United States and the first to report results using the well-validated patient evaluation measure.

▶ This is a retrospective review of 20 patients treated for recalcitrant entrapment neuropathy with autogenous saphenous vein graft wrapping. The authors offer the largest case series of this technique outside the United States and sought to add to the existing literature on autogenous saphenous vein grafting as first reported by Xu et al.[1] In addition to reporting on the use of the technique on all 3 major upper-extremity peripheral nerves, the authors are the first to report the use of autogenous vein grafting for recalcitrant radial tunnel syndrome. Outcome measures were obtained using a comprehensive patient questionnaire (previously validated for scaphoid fractures and carpal tunnel syndrome) as well as subjective visual analog scales used to report pain and patient satisfaction. Another strength of the study is that 8 of the 10 limbs that had preoperative studies had postoperative nerve conduction studies, and the data suggest that the nerve conduction studies improved in most patients after autologous nerve wrapping (particularly carpal and cubital tunnel syndrome).

Of the reported cases, 5 involved the median nerve at the wrist, 3 involved the ulnar nerve at the cubital tunnel, and the remaining 2 cases involved the radial nerve at the radial tunnel. The cohort consisted of 9 men and 11 women with a mean age of 58 years. The mean number of previous procedures was 2.8, and the mean follow-up period was 37 months. The authors correctly point out the morbidity associated with autologous vein harvesting, which may include painful scar, neuroma, and aesthetic considerations (particularly in women).

The authors comment on other accepted surgical options including internal neurolysis only, regional or free flaps, silastic tubes/sheets, and porcine- or bovine-derived collagen tubes. With regard to technical pearls, the authors report their preference of using the entire length of the previous incision with proximal and distal dissection to find healthy appearing nerve. External neurolysis is performed, followed by harvest of the saphenous vein with a full-length incision (use of a vein-stripper is discouraged, based on the authors' preference to avoid intramural damage to the harvested vein), side branches of the vein are ligated, and a long segment of the vein is lastly harvested. Finally, the saphenous vein is split longitudinally, the endothelial surface of the vein is spiraled around the affected nerve, and each juncture is sealed with a 6-0 nylon suture at every turn.

Results from this study indicate that all patients reported subjective improvement that exceeded their preoperative expectations. In addition, the nerve study improved in all 5 carpal patients, motor conduction velocity improved across the elbow for the 2 cubital tunnel cases, and neurophysiological findings in the case of radial tunnel were within normal limits. There were 2 cases of donor-site swelling, 4 cases of aesthetic concerns related to the length of the scar, and 1 case of painful neuroma that required subsequent stump burial. Shortcomings of the study were appropriately addressed by the authors and include a lack of control group and the inherent limitations associated with the questionnaire.

In sum, the authors present a thoughtful review of autogenous saphenous nerve grafting that includes technique pearls and appropriate indications for this procedure. Methodology and data collection were appropriate, and the use of nerve studies lends credibility to objective evidence of procedure efficacy, particularly for revision carpal and cubital tunnel. Finally, the authors appropriately address the potential morbidity associated with donor site harvest as well the effectiveness of this technique for the relatively rare, but highly problematic, sequela of failed primary nerve decompressive surgery.

S. M. Jacoby, MD

Reference

1. Xu J, Varitimidis SE, Fisher KJ, Tomaino MM, Sotereanos DG. The effect of wrapping scarred nerves with autogenous vein graft to treat recurrent chronic nerve compression. *J Hand Surg Am.* 2000;25(1):93-103.

Functional and electrophysiological outcome after autogenous vein wrapping of primary repaired ulnar nerves

Sadek AF, Fouly EH, Hamdy M (El Minia Univ Hosp, Minya, Egypt)
Microsurgery 34:361-366, 2014

Purpose.—This study aimed at assessing the functional and electrophysiological recovery after vein wrapping of primary repaired ulnar nerves.

Methods.—From January 2010 till December 2012, 23 patients (diagnosed with distal ulnar nerve injury) were prospectively studied where they were divided into two groups; group one (11 patients) and group two (12 patients). The injury was sharp in all cases but for one. The first group was managed by primary epineurorraphy. The second group was managed by primary epineurorraphy and autogenous vein wrapping. Final outcome was based on sensory recovery, motor recovery, and the presence or absence of electrophysiological response.

Results.—Clinically, only one case in each group exhibited negative Tinel's sign. The second group achieved statistically significant superiority regarding motor recovery ($P = 0.018$), sensory recovery ($P = 0.042$) and electrophysiological recovery ($P = 0.044$). Group one showed two good, two satisfactory, six moderate, and one bad results while the second group showed five good, six satisfactory, one bad and no moderate results ($P = 0.026$). The first time to show clinical response in group one was the third month while in the second group it was at 1.5 month ($P < 0.001$). In addition, the first time to show electromyographic response in group one was at the sixth month while in group two it was at the third month.

Conclusions.—Vein wrapping is a simple technique that could be used reliably to augment primary neurorrhaphy particularly in cases with associated vascular or tendon injuries to prevent scarring and enhance functional and electrophysiological recovery.

▶ This randomized, prospective study sets out to critically assess the benefit of a greater saphenous vein wrap about the primary repair of distal ulnar nerve lacerations. The vein wrap has been postulated to reduce adhesions and protect the nerve at the repair site.

Unfortunately, this report did not include a discussion of a power analysis and the effect size. Ideally, both should be reported so that the reader has confidence that the study can detect a clinically relevant difference between the 2 groups. Another concern is that the study did not appear to have blinded postoperative evaluations. Although it would be difficult to blind the surgeon to the technique used, it would be preferable to have a blinded postoperative assessment to limit the possibility of bias in the motor and sensory examinations. Furthermore, information regarding the intervals at which the postoperative motor and sensory assessments were performed and a description of the rehabilitation protocol would be useful to the reader.

It is interesting to note that the reported range of room temperatures for the electrodiagnostic studies performed in this report was 13°C (21°-34°C). Motor and sensory nerve conduction velocities change with temperature fluctuations, and large variations in room temperature could potentially alter the reliability of nerve conduction velocity measurements in this study.

Finally, the absence of a discussion of postoperative complications in this report is a concern. Lower extremity complications after greater saphenous vein harvest are reported in the thoracic surgery literature and should be a consideration when electing to use this technique.[1,2] The difference in length of operating time between the 2 groups, even with a second team harvesting the graft, would also be relevant to a surgeon contemplating the use of a vein wrap to augment a nerve repair.

E. Kinnucan, MD

References

1. Rutkove SB. Effects of temperature on neuromuscular electrophysiology. *Muscle Nerve*. 2001;24:867-882.
2. Paletta CE, Huang DB, Fiore AC, Swartz MT, Rilloraza FL, Gardner JE. Major leg wound complications after saphenous vein harvest for coronary revascularization. *Ann Thorac Surg*. 2000;70:492-497.

Does the addition of a nerve wrap to a motor nerve repair affect motor outcomes?

Lee J-Y, Parisi TJ, Friedrich PF, et al (The Catholic Univ of Korea, Seoul; Mayo Clinic, Rochester, MN)

Microsurgery 34:562-567, 2014

The purpose of this study was to evaluate the effect of wrapping bioabsorbable nerve conduit around primary suture repair on motor nerve regeneration in a rat model. Forty rats were randomly divided into two experimental groups according to the type of repair of the rat sciatic nerve: group I had primary suture repair; group II had primary suture repair and bioabsorbable collagen nerve conduit (NeuraGen® 1.5 mm, Integra LifeSciences Corp., Plainsboro, NJ) wrapped around the repair. At 12 weeks, no significant differences in the percentage of recovery between the two groups were observed with respect to compound muscle action potentials, isometric muscle force, and muscle weight ($P = 0.816$, $P = 0.698$, $P = 0.861$, respectively). Histomorphometric analysis as compared to the non-operative sites was also not significantly different between the two groups in terms of number of myelinated axons, myelinated fiber area, and nerve fiber density ($P = 0.368$, $P = 0.968$, $P = 0.071$, respectively). Perineural scar tissue formation was greater in primary suture repair group (0.36 ± 0.15) than in primary repair plus conduit wrapping group (0.17 ± 0.08). This difference was statistically significant ($P < 0.001$). Wrapping bioabsorbable nerve conduit around primary nerve repair can decrease perineural scar tissue formation. Although the scar-decreasing effect of bioabsorbable nerve wrap does not translate into better motor nerve recovery in this study, it might have an effect on the functional outcome in humans where scar formation is much more evident than in rats.

► The authors present a well-designed experimental study on nerve regeneration in a rat model. They were evaluating the effect of wrapping a bioabsorbable nerve conduit around a coaptation area on motor regeneration. The end point was 12 weeks and then histomorphometric, nerve conduction, muscle weight, tetanic force, and ankle contracture studies were performed. Although they prove that epineural connective tissue formation was significantly greater in the suture repair group compared with the suture repair plus conduit-wrapped group, this scar-decreasing effect of bioabsorbable nerve wrap did not translate into better motor nerve recovery. This study is important because we still have problems with unsuccessful regeneration of motor function in our patients. Often nerve reconstruction is done in a posttraumatic area, an area susceptible for scar tissue formation, which diminishes the results.

From my personal experience in experimental studies on rats, their high potential of regeneration has to be taken into consideration when interpreting the results. So in those conditions, it can be hard to prove any gain from the nerve wrapping. Because humans are more sensitive for local healing conditions, we may take advantage from nerve wrapping support and protection from scarring of a regenerating nerve. In my practice, I don't use wrapping or nerve conduits. I am more devoted to gold standards with end-to-end or nerve grafting. In some salvage procedures I use vein bridging or end-to-side repair.

P. Czarnecki, MD, PhD

Direct Radial to Ulnar Nerve Transfer to Restore Intrinsic Muscle Function in Combined Proximal Median and Ulnar Nerve Injury: Case Report and Surgical Technique

Phillips BZ, Franco MJ, Yee A, et al (Washington Univ School of Medicine, Saint Louis, MO)

J Hand Surg Am 39:1358-1362, 2014

A distal median to ulnar nerve transfer for timely restoration of critical intrinsic muscle function is possible in isolated ulnar nerve injuries but not for combined ulnar and median nerve injuries. We used a distal nerve transfer to restore ulnar intrinsic function in the case of a proximal combined median and ulnar nerve injury. Transfer of the nonessential radial nerve branches to the abductor pollicis longus, extensor pollicis brevis, and extensor indicis proprius to the motor branch of the ulnar nerve was performed in a direct end-to-end fashion via an interosseous tunnel. This method safely and effectively restored intrinsic function before terminal muscle degeneration.

▶ A nerve transfer is an attractive alternative to tendon transfers in the setting of a proximal ulnar nerve injury. Typically, the branch of the anterior interosseous nerve supplying the pronator quadratus is transferred to the ulnar motor nerve to prevent irreversible loss of the ulnar-innervated intrinsic hand muscles. In this article, the authors tackle the difficult clinical problem of combined median and ulnar nerve injuries. This case report presents a technique for transferring branches of the posterior interosseous nerve to the motor branch of the ulnar nerve.

Several technical challenges exist in the described surgery. First, the individual terminal branches of the posterior interosseous nerve were identified and dissected distally to ensure adequate donor length. Second, internal neurolysis of the ulnar nerve motor branch was performed so that the nerve branch could be brought through the interosseous membrane without tensioning or tethering. Finally, to optimize the size match between donor and recipient nerves, the coaptation was performed between the ulnar nerve motor branch and 3 donor posterior interosseous nerve branches.

Because this is a case report, the ability to infer outcomes in other patients and with other surgeons is limited. Certainly, this report would suggest a guarded prognosis for recovery of hand function after this injury and surgery. At 1.5 years, the patient described in this article has continued ulnar motor dysfunction in the hand.

The surgical technique reported in this article reflects ongoing innovation and research in treating difficult nerve injuries in the upper extremity. As we continue to gain experience with the techniques used by these authors, the radial to ulnar nerve transfer may become part of our armamentarium for treating combined median and ulnar nerve injuries.

E. Kinnucan, MD

15 Microsurgery

Use of Integra Artificial Dermis to Reduce Donor Site Morbidity After Pedicle Flaps in Hand Surgery

Adani R, Rossati L, Tarallo L, et al (Univ Hosp of Verona, Italy; Univ of Modena and Reggio Emilia, Italy)

J Hand Surg Am 39:2228-2234, 2014

Purpose.—To assess the results obtained with Integra artificial dermis to cover donor site following the harvesting of pedicle flaps for hand reconstruction.

Methods.—Between April 2010 and August 2013, 11 patients (8 men and 3 women; mean age, 37 y) were treated with Integra Dermal Regeneration Template (Integra LifeSciences, Inc., Plainsboro, NY) to cover donor defects after raising pedicle flaps for hand and finger reconstruction: radial forearm flap (4 cases), ulnar artery perforator flap (2 cases), and heterodigital island flap (5 cases). After neodermis formation the silicone layer of the artificial dermis was removed (on average after 22 days) and a split- or full-thickness epidermal autograft placed.

Results.—No infections, hematoma, or bleeding were recorded during the entire phase in which the artificial skin was applied. Two patients experienced a partial skin graft loss. Median follow-up was 20 months, and results included an average Vancouver Scar Scale rating of 2.7 and an average DASH score of 39. There were no cases of graft adherence to the underlying tendons or muscles.

Conclusions.—Favorable cosmetic and functional outcomes were obtained using a dermal regeneration template for the treatment of donor site defects. Despite the drawback of an additional surgical procedure (secondary skin graft), the use of this artificial skin produced soft-tissue augmentation and graft-skin quality, reducing donor site morbidity.

Type of study/level of evidence.—Therapeutic IV.

▶ The authors report a case series of donor site coverage with Integra and a split-thickness skin graft after flap harvesting in 2 stages. Because there are already a couple of publications on the same topic,[1,2] I did not spot anything new or any refined data in this report. Even though the results presented here are pleasing both functionally and cosmetically, it is not my preference to use Integra, as the use of this dermal substitute necessitates a 2-stage approach, which renders wound coverage a prolonged procedure. Instead, I recommend the use of dermal substitutes, which can be covered with a split-thickness skin graft during the same procedure, such as Matriderm and Alloderm.[3,4]

M. Choi, MD

References

1. Gravvanis AI, Tsoutsos DA, Iconomou T, Gremoutis G. The use of integra artificial dermis to minimize donor-site morbidity after suprafascial dissection of the radial forearm flap. *Microsurgery.* 2007;27:583-587.
2. Murray RC, Gordin EA, Saigal K, Leventhal D, Krein H, Heffelfinger RN. Reconstruction of the radial forearm free flap donor site using integra artificial dermis. *Microsurgery.* 2011;31:104-108.
3. Haslik W, Kamolz LP, Manna F, Hladik M, Rath T, Frey M. Management of full-thickness skin defects in the hand and wrist region: first long-term experiences with the dermal matrix matriderm. *J Plast Reconstr Aesthet Surg.* 2010;63:360-364.
4. Wester JL, Pittman AL, Lindau RH, Wax MK. AlloDerm with split-thickness skin graft for coverage of the forearm free flap donor site. *Otolaryngol Head Neck Surg.* 2014;150:47-52.

Microsurgical Pedicle Lengthening for Pedicled Thoracodorsal Artery Perforator Flap Transfer

Park BY, Seo SW, Mun G-H (Sungkyunkwan Univ School of Medicine, Seoul, South Korea)
Ann Plast Surg 73:174-176, 2014

The pedicled thoracodorsal artery perforator flap has been shown to be an effective option for reconstruction of various regions, including the breast, axilla, upper arm, lateral chest, and shoulder area. However, the original length of the pedicle limits the flap's reach to remote locations. We devised a technique that involves microsurgical lengthening of the pedicle to extend the arc of rotation of the pedicled perforator flap. After exposure of the subscapular vascular tree, we divided the thoracodorsal vessel at the point of bifurcation to the serratus branch and then the pedicle was reconnected to the distal end of the serratus branch. Here, we present 2 cases in which this technique was effectively applied to reconstruct a defect of the elbow using a thoracodorsal artery perforator flap with a pedicle lengthening procedure.

► The authors present a 2-patient case series in which they describe a technique for lengthening the pedicle of a pedicled thoracodorsal artery perforator flap via a microsurgical anastomosis with the distal end of the branch to serratus, which did have a size discrepancy with the thoracodorsal pedicle. The additional lengths of pedicle they were able to obtain were 5.5 and 6 cm, respectively, for the 2 cases presented. The extended length of the pedicle allowed for the flap to be tunneled in a subcutaneous pocket from the donor site through and axillary incision and along a subcutaneous tunnel down to the elbow. The donor site was closed primarily in each case, and there was adequate tissue coverage for the defects.

This technique provides an additional tool for the microsurgeon who is faced with complex elbow wounds, particularly in the setting of minimal recipient vessels at the site of the defect, by demonstrating the use of a recipient vessel that is out of the zone of injury.

C. Heinrich, MD

Use of a Distal Ulnar Artery Perforator—Based Bilobed Free Flap for Repairing Complex Digital Defects

Zheng D-W, Li Z-C, Sun F, et al (Xuzhou Renci Hosp, People's Republic of China; Wuxi Hand Surgery Hosp, People's Republic of China)
J Hand Surg Am 39:2235-2242, 2014

Purpose.—To retrospectively evaluate the effectiveness and safety of using a distal ulnar artery perforator (DUAP)-based bilobed free flap (BFF) for the repair of complex digital defects in the hand.

Methods.—We retrospectively studied 15 patients who sustained traumatic digital defects with complicating tendon and phalanx exposure and were hospitalized for repair using a DUAP-based BFF. Main outcome measures included patients' self-assessed physical appearance, total active motion, and 2-point discrimination.

Results.—The flaps survived and the wounds healed with primary intention in all patients except one who experienced partial flap necrosis of the distal margin and required treatment with a second skin graft. Patients were observed for a mean of 13 months. The physical appearance and texture of the repaired fingers were assessed as good with minimal scarring. Total active motion and 2-point discrimination were 113° to 255° (contralateral, 255° to 275°) and 6 to 11 mm (contralateral, 5 to 8 mm), respectively.

Conclusions.—Use of the DUAP-based BFF is a feasible, effective, and safe treatment alternative for repairing complex digital defects with favorable aesthetic and sensorimotor outcomes.

Type of Study/Level of Evidence.—Therapeutic IV (Figs 2 and 3, Table 1).

► This introduces a thin chimeric flap based on the distal perforator of the ulnar artery. Because it is thin and hairless, it can be an elegant solution for the coverage of 2 separate but adjacent defects on one hand. Another advantage is that the ulnar artery can be spared during flap harvest.

Because the comitant veins are very thin (0.8 mm), it is better to use the subcutaneous veins, which are much larger in caliber. The diameter of the artery is 1.3 mm. The pedicle length is 1.2 cm, which makes the use of this flap limited.

From the patient photograph in the report (Fig 2G) and also from my experience with scars in this region, I assume that the donor site scar will be quite conspicuous.

Even though I agree with the authors that the distal ulnar artery perforator (DUAP) flap is relatively thin, the normal skin of the finger dorsum is even

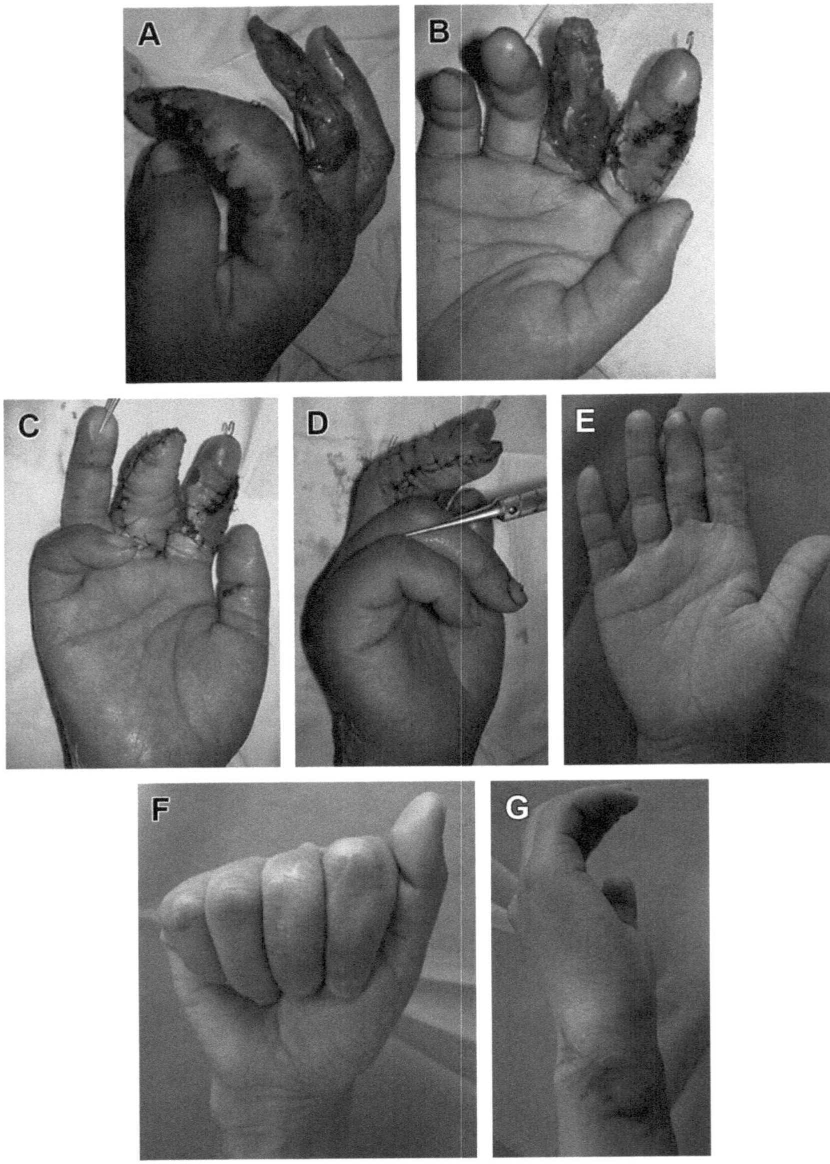

FIGURE 2.—Case 1 (patient 3). Complex soft tissue degloving defect of the middle finger: **A** dorsal and **B** palmar views; appearance of repaired finger **C, D** after surgery and **E** at the follow-up visit; **F** active movement (clenching) of the repaired finger; and **G** appearance of the donor site. (Reprinted from The Journal of Hand Surgery. Zheng D-W, Li Z-C, Sun F, et al. Use of a distal ulnar artery perforator—based bilobed free flap for repairing complex digital defects. *J Hand Surg Am*. 2014;39:2235-2242, Copyright 2014, with permission from the American Society for Surgery of the Hand.)

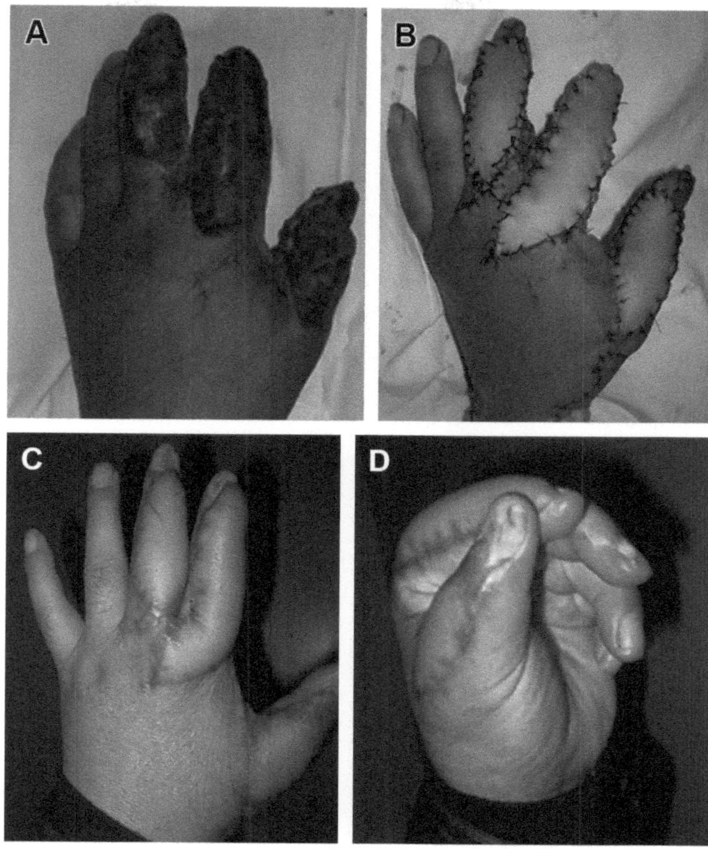

FIGURE 3.—Case 2 (patient 11). Complex soft tissue defect of 3 adjacent fingers (thumb, index, and middle): **A** dorsal view; appearance of the repaired fingers **B** after surgery and **C** at the follow-up visit; **D** active movement (digital opposition) of the repaired fingers. (Reprinted from The Journal of Hand Surgery. Zheng D-W, Li Z-C, Sun F, et al. Use of a distal ulnar artery perforator—based bilobed free flap for repairing complex digital defects. *J Hand Surg Am.* 2014;39:2235-2242, Copyright 2014, with permission from the American Society for Surgery of the Hand.)

thinner. For this reason, a secondary defatting procedure will be necessary in many cases.

Looking at Fig 3 of this article, a question came into my mind, which is still left unanswered. The pictures show a left hand of a patient (patient 11) with deep soft-tissue defects on the dorsal side of the thumb, the index finger, and the middle finger. The postoperative photos show all 3 lesions covered. The figure legend, however, fails to explain, how the third defect was covered. Table 1 with patient data does not provide any information either. It can only be guessed that the surgeon used a bilobed DUAP flap as described in this study for the index and the middle fingers and that he or she used a second free flap for the closure of the thumb, which he or she failed to mention.

TABLE 1.—Clinical Data

No.	Age, y/Sex	Cause of Injury	Affected Digit(s)	Location of Defect(s)	Size of Defect(s), cm^2	Upper Lobe Size, cm^2	Lower Lobe Size, cm^2	Anastomosed Artery, Vein, and Nerve
1	22/F	Crushing	Right index	Middle and distal segments	6.4 × 5.0	3.5 × 5.5	3.5 × 5.5	PDA, DDV/SSV, and PDN
2	55/M	Electrical sawing	Left middle	Palmar and dorsal sides	2.5 × 3.0, 2.8 × 4.5	3.0 × 3.4	3.6 × 5.0	PDA, DDV/SSV, and PDN
3	29/F	Motor vehicle accident	Right index	Distal to middle proximal segment	6.0 × 7.0	3.2 × 7.2	3.1 × 7.2	PDA, DDV/SSV, and PDN
4	35/M	Electrical sawing	Left index	Radial and proximal dorsal sides	2.5 × 6.0, 2.0 × 3.0	3.0 × 6.2	2.5 × 3.5	PDA, DDV/SSV, and PDN
5	24/M	Electrical sawing	Right ring	Full length	6.5 × 9.0	4.0 × 10.0	3.5 × 9.0	PDA, DDV/SSV, and PDN
6	45/M	Motor vehicle accident	Right index	Middle and distal segments	6.0 × 5.5	3.5 × 6.0	3.3 × 5.5	PDA, DDV/SSV, and PDN
7	19/M	Crushing	Left middle	Middle and distal segments	6.9 × 4.8	4.5 × 5.5	3.4 × 5.5	PDA, DDV/SSV, and PDN
8	37/F	Motor vehicle accident	Right middle/ring	Proximal segment	2.6 × 3.5, 2.0 × 2.5	3.0 × 4.0	2.5 × 3.0	CDA, DMV/SSV, and RNSB
9	43/F	Crushing	Right ring	Middle and distal segments	5.8 × 4.8	3.2 × 5.5	3.4 × 5.5	PDA, DDV/SSV, and PDN
10	31/M	Crushing	Right middle	Full length	6.7 × 6.8	3.8 × 8.0	3.5 × 7.5	PDA, DDV/SSV, and PDN
11	57/M	Electrical sawing	Left index/middle	Proximal and middle segments	2.9 × 5.7, 2.5 × 4.0	3.3 × 6.5	3.0 × 4.5	CDA, DMV/SSV, and RNSB
12	34/F	Crushing	Left index/middle	Proximal and middle segments	3.4 × 6.1, 3.0 × 5.2	4.0 × 7.0	3.5 × 6.0	CDA, DMV/SSV, and RNSB
13	20/F	Crushing	Right index	Middle and distal segments	2.8 × 5.2	3.4 × 6.0	3.2 × 5.8	PDA, DDV/SSV, and PDN
14	22/F	Crushing	Left ring	Middle and distal segments	2.8 × 4.8	3.4 × 5.5	3.3 × 5.5	PDA, DDV/SSV, and PDN
15	44/M	Crushing	Right index/middle	Proximal segment	2.6 × 4.8, 2.6 × 4.5	3.0 × 5.5	3.0 × 5.0	CDA, DMV/SSV, and RNSB

PDA, proper digital artery; DDV, deep digital vein; SSV, subcutaneous superficial vein; PDN, proper digital nerve; CDA, common digital artery; DMV, deep metacarpal vein; RNSB, radial nerve superficial branch.

Reprinted from The Journal of Hand Surgery. Zheng D-W, Li Z-C, Sun F, et al. Use of a distal ulnar artery perforatordbased bilobed free flap for repairing complex digital defects. J Hand Surg Am. 2014;39:2235-2242, Copyright 2014, with permission from the American Society for Surgery of the Hand.

Despite the limitations of this DUAP flap, it adds a flap to the microsurgical armamentarium for the coverage of digital defects.

M. Choi, MD

Tamai zone I fingertip replantation: Is external bleeding obligatory for survival of artery anastomosis-only replanted digits?

Chen K-K, Hsieh T-Y, Chang K-P (Kaohsiung Med Univ Hosp, Taiwan)

Microsurgery 34:535-539, 2014

Background.—Distal fingertip replantation is associated with good functional and aesthetic results. Venous anastomosis is the most challenging procedure. For replantation with an artery anastomosis-only procedure (no venous anastomosis), some protocols have been designed to relieve venous congestion involve anticoagulation and the creation of wounds for persistent bleeding. This report presents the authors' experience of fingertip survival after artery anastomosis-only replantation with no persistent external bleeding.

Methods.—Twelve Tamai zone I fingertip total amputation patients who underwent artery anastomosis-only replantations were recruited from February 2009 to June 2012. Nerve repair was performed if identified. The patients were not subjected to conventional external bleeding methods. Both the blood color on pinprick and fingertip temperature difference between the replanted and uninjured digits were used as indicators of deteriorated venous congestion.

Results.—The replanted digits of 11 patients survived. The only failed replant exhibited an average temperature difference of more than 6°C compared with the uninjured digits and consistently exhibited darker blood during the pinprick test. All other replants exhibited average temperature differences of less than 6°C.

Conclusions.—In these Tamai zone I artery anastomosis-only replantations, fingertips survived without the use of external bleeding method, indicating that external bleeding is probably not obligatory for survival of artery anastomosis-only replanted digits distal to Tamai zone I. An increasing temperature difference between the replanted and uninjured digits and darker blood on pinprick may be used as indicators of deteriorating congestion signs.

▶ Survival after fingertip replantation without venous anastomosis commonly relies on external bleeding, which relieves venous congestion transiently until spontaneous venous connections develop in the skin. External bleeding, however, is not only bothersome because of frequent dressing changes and being hygienically undesirable, but it can also necessitate blood transfusions because of significant blood loss in severe cases.

In this article, replantations in Tamai zone I survive in 93.8% of cases without any intentionally made external bleeding source. The authors assume that the bone marrow canal can serve as another source of venous recanalization, which is sufficient to support survival of a replanted fingertip.

The significance of circulation in the bone marrow has been known for a long time. Tanaka et al[1] showed in an experimental study that reestablishment of venous connections in the bone marrow, together with marginal bleeding from the skin edges, may actually be sufficient to allow for replant survival.

In light of this new finding, hand surgeons should try to realign the bone surfaces as closely as possible to allow for a faster reconnection of venous reflow in the future.

The authors point out that the bone marrow may not be a sufficient source of venous return for replantations at a more proximal level, as these have more soft tissue mass.

M. Choi, MD

Reference

1. Tanaka K, Kobayashi K, Murakami R, et al. Venous drainage through bone marrow after replantation: an experimental study. *Br J Plast Surg*. 1998;51:629-632.

Functional Free Muscle Transfer for Upper Extremity Reconstruction

Stevanovic M, Sharpe F (Univ of Southern California Keck School of Medicine, Los Angeles, CA)

Plast Reconstr Surg 134:257e-274e, 2014

Background.—Functional losses in the upper extremity that cannot be restored by nerve or tendon transfer present a treatment dilemma to the reconstructive surgeon. Common indications for functional free muscle transfer include late reconstruction of brachial plexus injuries, traumatic muscle loss, Volkmann ischemic contracture, loss resulting from oncologic resection, and congenital absence of motor function as seen in arthrogryposis.

Methods.—This article reviews the authors' experience in upper extremity reconstruction using functional free muscle transfer. The indications and technique for functional free muscle transfer in the upper extremity are reviewed. Surgical details for sites of reconstruction and the nuances of harvesting the main donor muscles are presented.

Results.—Specific cases and outcome reviews for several series of functional free muscle transfers are presented.

Conclusion.—Functional free muscle transfer is the best and final option for restoring function in an otherwise nonreconstructible limb.

► This review covers the gamut of current techniques for free functioning muscle transfer in upper limb reconstruction. Strevanovic and Sharpe provide an excellent illustration of how the free gracilis, latissimus, and serratus muscles can be used to restore shoulder, elbow, and digital motion after deficits caused by brachial plexus injury, tumor resection, Volkman's ischemic contracture, and other trauma conditions. Particularly helpful are tables that help organize the choices available for specific defects requiring free muscle transfer, including important technical considerations. Absent in the outcomes sections are the reported outcomes or the authors' experiences with use of free muscle transfer for the restoration of shoulder animation. Overall, this is an excellent summary of the current available options for free functioning muscle transfer for upper extremity reconstruction.

P. Murray, MD

16 Trauma

CT scan-evaluated outcome of pulsed electromagnetic fields in the treatment of acute scaphoid fractures: a randomised, multicentre, double-blind, placebo-controlled trial

Hannemann PFW, van Wezenbeek MR, Kolkman KA, et al (Maastricht Univ Med Centre, The Netherlands; Rijnstate Hosp Arnhem, The Netherlands; et al)
Bone Joint J 96-B:1070-1076, 2014

We hypothesised that the use of pulsed electromagnetic field (PEMF) bone growth stimulation in acute scaphoid fractures would significantly shorten the time to union and reduce the number of nonunions in a randomised, double-blind, placebo-controlled multicentre trial. A total of 102 patients (78 male, 24 female; mean age 35 years (18 to 77)) from five different medical centres with a unilateral undisplaced acute scaphoid fracture were randomly allocated to PEMF (n = 51) or placebo (n = 51) and assessed with regard to functional and radiological outcomes (multiplanar reconstructed CT scans) at 6, 9, 12, 24 and 52 weeks. The overall time to clinical and radiological healing did not differ significantly between the active PEMF group and the placebo group. We concluded that the addition of PEMF bone growth stimulation to the conservative treatment of acute scaphoid fractures does not accelerate bone healing.

▶ The authors conducted a randomized double-blind, placebo-controlled trial to investigate the effect of pulsed electromagnetic field (PEMF) exposure on the healing time of acute scaphoid fractures. They found no differences between the 2 study groups.

The authors of this study have to be commended for their thorough study design and execution. The routine of CT scans to assess osseous union seems especially valuable. In our practice, we use PEMF treatments only in selected cases of scaphoid fractures and delayed unions. It should be acknowledged that treatments like PEMF may be a valuable adjunct but do not solve problems relating to poor indications or a sloppy operative technique. Although basic research has found increased cell metabolism and a positive effect on inflammatory cytokines for PEMF treatments, one probably should not overestimate the potency of these treatments in a clinical setting, as this study beautifully illustrates.

K. Megerle, MD

Scapholunate Ligament Reconstruction Using a Flexor Carpi Radialis Tendon Graft

Sousa M, Aido R, Freitas D, et al (Centro Hospitalar Do Porto, Portugal)
J Hand Surg Am 39:1512-1516, 2014

Purpose.—To review the results of scapholunate ligament reconstruction using a flexor carpi radialis tendon graft.

Methods.—We performed a retrospective review of 22 patients with post-traumatic scapholunate instability who were treated with a modification of the Brunelli, a flexor carpi radialis tendon graft.

Results.—The mean follow-up was 61 months. The average age was 40 years. The average loss of flexion was 23° and of extension was 22° compared with the contralateral side. Grip strength averaged 67% of the nonoperated side. All patients except 2 returned to work. Degenerative changes were seen in 3 patients at the time of revision. Complications occurred in 2 patients and included avascular necrosis of the scaphoid.

Conclusions.—Perfect biomechanical reconstruction might not be possible for scapholunate dissociation. Our results show, however, that ligament reconstruction led to satisfactory results from the patient's point of view.

Type of Study/Level of Evidence.—Therapeutic IV.

▶ The authors report their long-term results after reconstruction of chronic scapholunate instabilities using a modified Brunelli procedure. They found good functional results after a mean follow-up of 61 months.

Despite their rather favorable results, I fully agree with the authors that perfect biomechanical reconstruction might not be possible for chronic scapholunate instability at this point. None of the many options currently available really restores carpal stability and kinematics.

Although I also think that the flexor carpi radialis tenodesis is probably one of the better options for scapholunate reconstruction, this publication is limited by some weaknesses in methodology. Most importantly, the follow-up is rather short by most patients. Also, the authors do not really state how many patients were operated on and lost to follow-up in the study period.

Because none of the reconstructive options for scapholunate instability adequately restores original kinematics, but all inevitably reduce range of motion, it must be assured that patients are really aware of the big picture. The postoperative result of most procedures may be due to reduction of the range of motion and denervation effects. Therefore, the most important aspect in choosing the correct treatment is the preoperative clinical situation (eg, age, chronicity of the injury, activity level, presence of degenerative change) of the patient. If the patient can cope with his or her current symptoms, even a watch-and-wait strategy may be considered.

K. Megerle, MD

Reduction and Association of the Scaphoid and Lunate Procedure: Short-Term Clinical and Radiographic Outcomes

Larson TB, Stern PJ (Univ of Cincinnati College of Medicine, OH)

J Hand Surg Am 39:2168-2174, 2014

Purpose.—To evaluate the success of reduction and association of the scaphoid and lunate with a fibrous union in an effort to evaluate the technique's validity and reproducibility.

Methods.—A retrospective review was performed on 7 patients (8 wrists) with an average follow-up of 38 months. Static and grip radiographs were examined in the preoperative, immediate postoperative, and final follow-up settings to evaluate scapholunate (SL) diastasis, SL angle, hardware position, and complications. At final follow-up, grip strength and wrist range of motion were recorded, and patients completed the Disabilities of the Arm, Shoulder, and Hand and the Patient-Rated Wrist Evaluation outcome questionnaires.

Results.—Radiographic success, defined by maintenance of corrected SL diastasis, absence of dorsal intercalated segmental instability, and no progression of SL advanced collapse was achieved in 3 of the 8 wrists. One wrist developed radioscaphoid arthritis. No patients required a salvage procedure. Despite the loss of reduction that occurred in all patients, the patients' disability remained minimal as detected by the scores on the outcome measures.

Conclusions.—The procedure was ineffective in providing stability about the SL interval. With a majority of patients experiencing early radiographic failure of the procedure in the short term, our experience suggests that the reduction and association of the scaphoid and lunate procedure should be abandoned despite the relatively low outcomes measures scores, which may be reflective of the short follow-up duration for this series.

Type of Study/Level of Evidence.—Therapeutic IV.

▶ The results of the reduction and association of the scaphoid and lunate (RASL) appear to be operator dependent. Favorable results may be difficult to achieve if the technical points described by Rosenwasser et al[1] are not strictly adhered to. Aviles et al[2] achieved good pain relief in 6 of 7 patients using an arthroscopic RASL (ARASL) technique. The mean scapholunate (SL) gap was reduced from 4.2 to 1.75 at an average 19-month follow-up. They stressed that even the slightest malposition of the screw led to failure. Although Caloia et al[3] reported good results in 8 of 9 patients, 3 patients required screw removal secondary to loosening, and Cognet et al[4] had to remove the screws in all 7 patients treated with an ARASL due to partial destruction of the lunate and/or scaphoid.

A limitation of this study is the narrow radiographic outcome criteria of an SL diastasis <3 mm and SL angle of 30 to 70 degrees. Three of 7 patients were immediate failures on this basis. The average Disabilities of the Arm, Shoulder and Hand of 15 and Patient Rated Wrist Evaluation of 26 are generally considered good outcome scores, but there was no statistical analysis and therefore no demonstrable significant differences between those with and without a radiographic failure. The results of a preoperative and postoperative Watson test were not specified, which makes it difficult to determine whether the SL joint was a pain generator.

The lack of a critical analysis of the screw position is a major omission. The screw should enter low on the scaphoid, which is facilitated by a radial styloidectomy, pass through the center of the scaphoid and lunate in both the coronal and sagittal planes, and engage the proximal medial corner of the lunate. One patient had immediate backing out of the screw, and 4 of 5 screws were removed for progressive lucency, which suggest poor screw position. Fig 3 in the original article shows a screw that enters too distally on the scaphoid, is too short, and does not engage the proximal medial lunate. The authors used a 3-mm Synthes HCS vs the 4.0 mm cannulated Herbert screw, which may be a crucial difference. Rosenwasser et al used a dorsal radiocarpal ligament sparing capsulotomy. They did not completely dechondrify the SL joint surfaces.

An arthroscopic staging using the Geissler classification[5] was not performed, which makes it difficult to assess the competence of the secondary SL joint stabilizers. The type of work was not specified. Pomerance[6] reviewed 17 patients at 66 months after an SL ligament repair and dorsal capsulodesis. The SL gap for a strenuous job was 4 mm static and 6 mm with stress, whereas for a nonstrenuous job, the SL gap was 2 mm static and 3 mm with stress.

In my experience, this procedure should be reserved for patients with a chronic Geissler 2. The results of a RASL with a Geissler 3 or 4 are unpredictable. A static carpal instability is a contraindication in my view. This procedure should be approached with caution in the manual laborer.

D. Slutsky, MD

References

1. Rosenwasser MP, Miyasaki KC, Strauch RJ. The RASL procedure: reduction and association of the scaphoid and lunate using the Herbert screw. *Tech Hand Up Extrem Surg*. 1997;1:263-272.
2. Aviles AJ, Lee SK, Hausman MR. Arthroscopic reduction associationof the scapholunate. *Arthroscopy*. 2007;23:101.e1-101.e5.
3. Caloia M, Caloia H, Pereira E. Arthroscopic scapholunate joint reduction Is an effective treatment for irreparable scapholunate ligament tears? *Clin Orthop Relat Res*. 2007;470:972-978.
4. Cognet JM, Levadoux M, Martinache X. The use of screws in the treatment of scapholunate instability. *J Hand Surg Eur*. 2011;36:690-693.
5. Pomerance J. Outcome after repair of the scapholunate interosseous ligament and dorsal capsulodesis for dynamic scapholunate instability due to trauma. *J Hand Surg Am*. 2006;31:1380-1386.
6. Geissler WB, Freeland AE, Savoie FH, McIntyre LW, Whipple TL. Intracarpal soft-tissue lesions associated with an intra-articular fracture of the distal end of the radius. *J Bone Joint Surg Am*. 1996;78:357-365.

Clinical Diagnostic Evaluation for Scaphoid Fractures: A Systematic Review and Meta-Analysis

Mallee WH, Henny EP, van Dijk CN, et al (Univ of Amsterdam, the Netherlands)

J Hand Surg Am 39:1683-1691, 2014

Purpose.—To provide an overview of available clinical evaluation tests for scaphoid fractures and to compare their diagnostic accuracies.

Methods.—PWe performed a systematic review of all studies assessing diagnostic characteristics of clinical evaluation in scaphoid fractures by searching MEDLINE, EMBASE, Cochrane, and CINAHL databases. Only studies on clinical testing prior to radiographic evaluation and with acceptable reference standard for occult fractures were included. Thirteen relevant articles were analyzed that described a total of 25 tests. Diagnostic characteristics of the tests were used to construct contingency tables. If possible, data were pooled and summary receiver operating characteristic curves were fitted.

Results.—Anatomic snuff-box tenderness (ASB, 8 studies, 1,164 patients) and longitudinal thumb compression (LTC, 8 studies, 961 patients) had sufficient data for statistical analyses. Sensitivity for ASB ranged from 0.87 to 1.00; for LTC, 0.48 to 1.00. Specificity of ASB ranged from 0.03 to 0.98; for LTC, 0.22 to 0.97. Owing to considerable heterogeneity, pooled estimate points were not calculated. Other high-sensitivity tests were scaphoid tubercle tenderness, with sensitivity and specificity ranging from 0.82 to 1.00 and 0.17 to 0.57, respectively, and painful ulnar deviation, ranging from 0.67 to 1.00 and 0.17 to 0.60, respectively. Three studies showed that combining tests increased the specificity and post-test fracture probability while maintaining high sensitivity. Quality assessment showed high or unclear risk of bias and applicability concerns in reference standard and patient selection. Twelve study designs were prospective, and 1 was retrospective.

Conclusions.—Anatomical snuff box tenderness was the most sensitive clinical test. The low specificity of the clinical tests may result in a considerable number of overtreated patients. Combining tests improved the post-test fracture probability. This can be used to limit unnecessary immobilization, number of hospital visits, and use of imaging. The data presented herein may help to develop clinical prediction rules that could increase specificity without reducing sensitivity.

Type of Study/Level of Evidence.—Diagnostic II.

▶ The authors aim to provide an overview of available evidence supporting various clinical tests for the evaluation of scaphoid fractures and compare their diagnostic accuracies. They performed a comprehensive review of the available literature, screening more than 2000 articles. Limitations of this study are inherent to the weaknesses of the included studies and the heterogeneity of the results, making it difficult to calculate pooled estimates. Despite this, the authors were able to make some recommendations; they report that anatomic snuffbox tenderness had the highest sensitivity and that the most realistic option was a combination of tests that would help rule in or rule out the presence of a scaphoid fracture, similar to the Ottawa Ankle Rules. More work is needed to establish the ideal method of evaluating for the presence of a scaphoid fracture. However, because the consequences of a missed scaphoid fracture are significant, I believe imaging will always be an important part of the diagnostic evaluation. However, refining the use of first-line and advanced imaging-based on the results of a clinical prediction rule will be helpful in containing costs associated with unnecessary imaging, but the disability costs associated with missing a scaphoid fracture must also be considered.

R. Grewal, MD

Scaphoid Nonunions Treated With 2 Headless Compression Screws and Bone Grafting

Garcia RM, Leversedge FJ, Aldridge JM, et al (Duke Univ Med Ctr, Durham, NC; Triangle Orthopedic Associates, Durham, NC)
J Hand Surg Am 39:1301-1307, 2014

Purpose.—To evaluate union and complication rates associated with the use of 2 headless compression screws and bone grafting for the treatment of scaphoid nonunions.

Methods.—A total of 19 patients (18 male and 1 female) at an average age of 21 years were treated with open reduction and internal fixation with 2 cannulated, headless, compression screws for scaphoid nonunions. Bone grafting techniques included corticocancellous autograft from the iliac crest in 14 patients, capsular-based vascularized distal radius graft in 3, and medial femoral condyle free vascularized bone graft in 2. Patients were treated an average 19 months after the injury. Fracture nonunions were at the waist (n = 12), proximal third (n = 5), or distal third (n = 2) of the scaphoid. Dorsal (n = 7) and volar (n = 12) surgical approaches were used.

Results.—All fractures had clinical and radiographic evidence of bone union at an average of 3.6 months. Postoperative computed tomography scans were available in 13 patients and showed union without evidence of screw penetration of the scaphoid cortex. No complications occurred in this series, and no revision procedures have been necessary.

Conclusions.—Our results indicate that the use of 2 headless compression screws for the treatment of scaphoid nonunions is safe and effective. A variety of bone grafting techniques can be used with this technique. The use of 2 compression screws may provide superior biomechanical stability and ultimately improve outcomes measured with future long-term comparative studies.

Type of Study/Level of Evidence.—Therapeutic IV.

▶ This article describes an interesting technique for the fixation of scaphoid fractures. Although it makes sense intuitively that the use of 2 screws would provide more stability, there is little evidence presented in the article to support the use of the second screw.

The collection of scaphoid fractures presented is too heterogeneous a group to draw any meaningful conclusions. The location of the fractures, the approaches, and the types of bone graft were all highly variable. In a series of only 19 patients, this is concerning. Also, the use of both vascularized and nonvascularized grafts leads to more questions than answers.

Also concerning was the absence of postoperative CT scans in approximately one-third of the cases. The inadvertent penetration of a cortex with the screw would be one of the most demanding technical aspects of the treatments described. In patients in whom this might be suspected based on the radiographs, the surgeon might be hesitant to obtain the CT scan. Therefore, the conclusion that this technique can be done safely is not confirmed by the data presented.

It is unfortunate that the authors did not have motion data to present. It could be surmised that greater stability allowed for earlier motion, and therefore better final motion. Also, the use of structural graft seems somewhat excessive, and technically demanding, with the use of 2 screws.

I do agree with the premise of this study that stability is the key to union in most cases (those with avascular necrosis and collapse excluded). Therefore, the use of a second screw is intriguing because it provides significantly more torsional strength than most other techniques. There is a scaphoid plate available, which might also provide this torsional stability without the technical skill needed to place 2 screws, although I have no clinical experience with this device.

T. Hughes, MD

Intraobserver and Interobserver Variability in Diagnosing Scapholunate Dissociation by Cineradiography

Sulkers GSI, Schep NWL, Maas M, et al (Academic Med Ctr, Amsterdam, The Netherlands)

J Hand Surg Am 39:1050-1054.e3, 2014

Purpose.—To evaluate the intraobserver and interobserver variability in diagnosing scapholunate dissociation (SLD) by wrist cineradiography.

Methods.—A musculoskeletal radiologist, hand surgeon, and trauma surgeon assessed the records of 50 consecutive wrist cineradiographies performed in 25 patients. Fluoroscopy was performed on the unaffected and affected wrist and consisted of radiographer-controlled passive flexion-extension and passive radial-ulnar deviation in both posteroanterior and lateral projections. To determine the intraobserver variability, the 3 reviewers reassessed all wrist cineradiographies 6 months after their first assessment. The kappa coefficient for interobserver agreement was calculated using the jackknife method. The Cohen kappa was used to assess intraobserver variability.

Results.—The interobserver variability for diagnosing SLD by cineradiography was excellent ($\kappa = 0.84$). The intraobserver variability for the hand surgeon was excellent ($\kappa = 0.80$), and was good for the radiologist ($\kappa = 0.72$) and the trauma surgeon ($\kappa = 0.76$).

Conclusions.—Cineradiography is a promising and helpful, noninvasive tool for diagnosing SLD. It is widely available and has relatively low costs. Conventional radiographs remain essential in the primary workup for suspected SLD. However, we recommend cineradiography when an SLD is clinically suspected.

Type of Study/Level of Evidence.—Diagnostic III.

▶ The authors present a well-designed study about the intra- and interobserver variability in diagnosing scapholunate dissociation (SLD) by wrist cineradiography between a musculoskeletal radiologist, a hand surgeon, and a trauma surgeon. They found that the interobserver variability was excellent and that the intraobserver variability was excellent to good among the 3 physicians.

The strength of this study is that 2 of the observers were very experienced and that the protocol was strict and reproducible.

The weaknesses of this study are a relatively small number of patients, the lack of detailed definition of the diagnostic subcategorization of the SLD according to the characteristics of the patients, the delay between trauma and examination, and other factors such as general laxity of each individual.

Cineradiography is not a new way to diagnose and evaluate SLD. It has been shown by many studies that arthro-CT, MRI studies, and especially arthroscopy may provide a detailed and accurate characterization of SLD, allowing optimization of the treatment. Although the authors have elegantly shown that cineradiography can be useful, I do not use it routinely at the diagnosis stage of SLD because I do not have such a dedicated radiological team available. I still prefer to rely on arthroscopic findings.

G. Herzberg, MD

Load Transfer at the Distal Ulna Following Simulated Distal Radius Fracture Malalignment

Ferreira LM, Greeley GS, Johnson JA, et al (Lawson Health Research Inst, London, Ontario, Canada; Western Univ, London, Ontario, Canada)

J Hand Surg Am 40:217-223, 2015

Purpose.—To measure the effects of distal radius malalignment on loading at the distal ulna.

Methods.—Using an adjustable mechanism to simulate angulated and translated malalignments, clinically relevant distal radius deformities were simulated in a cadaveric model. A custom-built load cell was inserted just proximal to the native ulna head to measure the resultant force and torque in the distal ulna. Loads were measured before and after transecting the triangular fibrocartilage complex (TFCC).

Results.—There was an increase in distal ulna load and torque with increasing dorsal translation and angulation. Combined conditions of angulation and translation increased force and torque in the distal ulna to a greater extent than with either condition in isolation. Transecting the TFCC resulted in a reduction in distal ulna load and torque.

Conclusions.—A progressive increase in load at the distal ulna was observed with increasing severity of malalignment, which may be an important contributor to residual ulnar wrist pain and dysfunction. However, no clear-cut threshold of malalignment of a dorsally angulated and translated distal radius fracture was identified. These observations suggest that radius deformities cause articular incongruity, which increases TFCC tension and distal radioulnar joint load. Cutting of the TFCC decreased distal ulna loading, likely by releasing the articular constraining effect of the TFCC on the distal radioulnar joint, allowing the radius to rotate more freely with respect to the ulna.

Clinical Relevance.—Anatomical reduction of a distal radius fracture minimizes the forces in the distal ulna and may reduce residual ulnar wrist pain and dysfunction.

▶ This interesting article investigates the effects of simulated distal radius fracture malunion on load transmission at the wrist. Eight cadaver forearms underwent creation of simulated distal radius fracture malunions, with testing conditions simulating (independently and in combination) dorsal angulation of 0°, 10°, 20°, and 30°; and 0, 5, and 10 mm of dorsal translation. In each case, an implanted force sensor at the ulna measured load transmission across the ulna under simulated pronation and supination. The testing conditions were done with the triangular fibrocartilage complex (TFCC) intact and subsequently following TFCC detachment from the ulna. Ulnar load and torque were greater with increasing dorsal translation and angulation, and combined angulation and translation resulted in significantly greater ulna load and torque than either in isolation. There was a decrease in ulna load (not statistically significant) and torque (significant) after transection of the TFCC, simulating the loss of the constraint of the TFCC and reduction in joint loading that occurs in the presence of a distal radius fracture with associated ligament rupture or basal styloid fracture. These findings may help explain the pain associated with distal radius deformities and better define indications for surgery as the multiplanar deformities are investigated by this study.

J. E. Adams, MD

The Role of Prophylactic Ulnar Nerve Release During Elbow Contracture Release

Chen NC, Liu A (Thomas Jefferson Univ Hosp, Philadelphia, PA)
J Hand Surg Am 39:1837-1839, 2014

Background.—When patients undergo release for posttraumatic elbow stiffness, some will also benefit from ulnar nerve release. This is certainly true when there is ulnar neuropathy preoperatively, but the case is not as clear for patients who exhibit no ulnar nerve symptoms. A case and a discussion of the current evidence were presented.

> *Case Report.*—Man, 40, was seen for a 50° flexion contracture and 80° flexion 1 year after open reduction and plate fixation of an olecranon fracture. He experienced no tingling or numbness of the fingers, had a negative Tinel's sign over the ulnar nerve at the elbow, had normal sensation, and showed no signs of atrophy. Radiographs revealed complete olecranon fracture healing, congruent ulnohumeral joint, and no errant or loose implants of the posterior plate. The patient was interested in surgery to address his elbow stiffness.

Analysis of Evidence.—When surgery for primary osteoarthritis is done, prophylactic ulnar nerve decompression may help if the patient has less than 90° or 100° of flexion preoperatively or can be expected to have a gain in the range of motion exceeding 30° to 40°. However, preoperative flexion and postoperative ulnar neuropathy are not necessarily linked, so the risks and benefits of prophylactic ulnar nerve release must be evaluated on an individual basis. The incidence of ulnar neuropathy defined using electromyographic or nerve conduction velocity studies in patients with stiff elbows is unknown but has been shown to vary from 0% to 38%. The evidence indicates that ulnar neuropathy is often diagnosed based on symptoms and signs rather than objective testing. As a result, the decision to release the ulnar nerve can be subjective. Some patients who are asymptomatic may have abnormal neurodiagnostic test results and could benefit from the ulnar nerve release. Because many factors contribute to posttraumatic elbow stiffness, it may be difficult to establish an independent relationship between statistical tests and conclusions.

Future research should evaluate routine electrodiagnostic tests of patients with elbow stiffness to determine the incidence and natural history of ulnar neuropathy after trauma and how the neuropathy relates to the stiffness. Better analysis of adverse events associated with prophylactic ulnar nerve release would also help to guide the decision to perform this procedure.

Conclusions.—Each patient should have a careful evaluation of the ulnar nerve and be offered the release procedure if abnormal results are obtained on electrodiagnostic testing and a substantial lack of flexion is present. If the test results are normal, the patient should be given the option after a careful presentation of the benefits and risks of prophylactic ulnar nerve release.

▶ Elbow stiffness after trauma of the upper extremity is a relatively common entity. Few patients require surgical release but those that do often have severe functional limitations. This article reviews the most recent evidence about ulnar nerve decompression at the elbow in patients with elbow contractures. The article asks a clinically relevant question and reviews the appropriate evidence to help determine whether prophylactic nerve decompression is warranted. The article has no true limitations, as it is a review of the literature. It effectively reviews the current literature and has salient points with regard to each study mentioned. For the commentator, this is an intriguing topic that warrants further investigation. It is clear that patients with ulnar nerve symptoms before surgery warrant decompression of the nerve at the time of their contracture release. What is not clear is how to decide which patients without nerve symptoms would benefit from decompression. In the commentator's experience, the major risk factors for developing ulnar neuropathy after contracture release include severe limited flexion before surgery, substantial recovery of flexion after surgery, and significant scarring of the neural bed from the initial trauma. These 3 entities affect the inherent gliding mechanism of the nerve and likely place patients at high risk of incurring symptoms. Results of electrodiagnostic studies for the ulnar nerve can often be normal. These results may be owing to how the nerve is tested, as many patients will not have their arm in a provocative position at the time of testing. If there are any concerns for ulnar nerve irritation or the probability of substantial increase of flexion, it is prudent to prophylactically release the ulnar nerve before contracture release. As with any surgical procedure, it is important to inform the patient that they may need further surgery for nerve decompression at a later date, as surgical expectations often dictate patients' perceived outcomes.

M. B. Gottschalk, MD
J. T. Capo, MD

Soft-Tissue Mallet Injuries: A Comparison of Early and Delayed Treatment

Altan E, Alp NB, Baser R, et al (Selcuk Univ, Konya, Turkey; Agri State Hosp, Turkey; the Manus Hand Surgery Ctr, Istanbul, Turkey; et al)
J Hand Surg Am 39:1982-1985, 2014

Purpose.—To compare the results of early and delayed extension orthosis fabrication in closed tendinous mallet injuries.

Methods.—Between March 1992 and May 2011, 45 patients with isolated closed tendinous mallet finger injuries were treated with orthosis fabrication. The patients were classified into 2 different groups based on their date of presentation. Group 1 consisted of 28 patients who presented within 2 weeks of sustaining the trauma, and group 2 consisted of 17 patients who received treatment beginning between 2 and 4 weeks after sustaining the trauma. During the final assessments, the patients were assessed clinically using the Crawford classification scale and satisfaction ratings.

Results.—The mean delay between initial injury and presentation to our center was 3 days (range, 1–14 d) in group 1 and 19 days (range, 15–30 d) in group 2. There were no significant differences between the groups regarding their ages, initial extension lag, and arc of flexion. According to the Crawford classification criteria, 72% of the patients in group 1 had excellent results, and 59% of the patients in group 2 had excellent results. There was no significant difference between the groups.

Conclusions.—The treatment results of patients with different presentation times have been reported for heterogeneous groups of osseous and nonosseous mallet finger injuries. Our results suggest that conservative management of tendinous mallet finger injuries that have been neglected for 2 to 4 weeks can be treated as well as those injuries in patients presenting within the first 2 weeks of injury with low long-term complication rates.

Type of Study/Level of Evidence.—Therapeutic III.

▶ This report aims to clarify if there is a difference in functional outcomes depending on early or late initiation of splint therapy for a soft tissue mallet injury. After comparing 2 groups (group 1, splinting within 2 weeks; group 2, splinting between 2 and 4 weeks), the authors found no significant differences in final outcome.

Even though some aspects about the treatment of mallet fingers are still debated, most surgeons agree on splinting as the best treatment option, especially if there is no bone involvement. The strength of this work is that the investigators compared the onset of conservative therapy as a single variable. The preexisting studies comparing early and late initiation of splinting had the limitation that they compared the time variable with inhomogeneous patient groups, as they did not compare tendinous mallet lesions alone, but tendinous and bony mallet injuries mixed together.

According to the authors' findings, there is no difference in functional outcome between early and late splinting of soft tissue mallet injuries.

A typical method of managing tendinous (soft tissue) mallet fingers is to splint the distal interphalangeal joint in full extension for 8 weeks, regardless of the chronicity of the injury.

M. Choi, MD

Cortical comminution in distal radial fractures can predict the radiological outcome: a cohort multicentre study

Wadsten MÅ, Sayed-Noor AS, Englund E, et al (Umeå Univ, Sweden; Sundsvall Hosp, Sweden)

Bone Joint J 96-B:978-983, 2014

This paper investigates whether cortical comminution and intra-articular involvement can predict displacement in distal radius fractures by using a classification that includes volar comminution as a separate parameter.

A prospective multicentre study involving non-operative treatment of distal radius fractures in 387 patients aged between 15 and 74 years (398 fractures) was conducted. The presence of cortical comminution and intra-articular involvement according to the Buttazzoni classification is described. Minimally displaced fractures were treated with immobilisation in a cast while displaced fractures underwent closed reduction with subsequent immobilisation. Radiographs were obtained after reduction, at 10 to 14 days and after union. The outcome measure was re-displacement or union.

In fractures with volar comminution (Buttazzoni type 4), 96% (53 of 55) displaced. In intra-articular fractures without volar comminution (Buttazzoni 3), 72% (84 of 117) displaced. In extra-articular fractures with isolated dorsal comminution (Buttazzoni 2), 73% (106 of 145) displaced while in non-comminuted fractures (Buttazzoni 1), 16% (13 of 81) displaced.

A total of 32% (53 of 165) of initially minimally displaced fractures later displaced. All of the initially displaced volarly comminuted fractures re-displaced. Displacement occurred in 31% (63 of 205) of fractures that were still in good alignment after 10 to 14 days.

Regression analysis showed that volar and dorsal comminution predicted later displacement, while intra-articular involvement did not predict displacement. Volar comminution was the strongest predictor of displacement.

▶ The authors present a well-designed prospective multicenter radiologic study of a significant number of distal radius fractures (DRFs; 398 after exclusions). They investigated whether dorsal or volar comminution and/or intraarticular involvement could predict secondary displacement after initial closed management. They showed that dorsal and volar comminution predicted secondary displacement, whereas intraarticular involvement did not. Volar comminution was found to be the strongest predictor in this cohort of patients, which is the main message of this article.

This study has several strengths. It is prospective, it includes 2 teaching hospitals, and the number of patients is substantial. Among the many interesting findings of this article, it is the first study to highlight the association between dorsal comminution and secondary displacement not only in displaced but also in minimally displaced DRF. The weaknesses of this study are outlined in the Discussion. Combined injuries of the ulna and/or carpus, combined ligamentous distal radial ulnar joint and intracarpal injuries were not analyzed. It is rare in our practice to see such a large number of DRFs (20%) without dorsal comminution. This raises the question of the definition of dorsal comminution used in this study. The age distribution of this series ranges from 15 years to 74-year-old patients, who obviously have very different structural bony characteristics, making comparisons difficult. It seems unlikely that a uniform initial management could be the best way to go in such different populations. The use of the Buttazzoni classification is questionable because the use of the B letter for all types of fractures is confusing considering the widely used AO classification system, which uses B only for partial articular fractures.

This carefully done study questions the use of initial closed management for most displaced or minimally displaced DRF. In our practice, we use a different paradigm, which is actually supported by this study. Given the large number of

DRFs we also attend to, we manage to make the final therapeutic decision at the acute stage, not waiting for secondary displacement to occur after an initial closed management. We rely on a 1-page chart[1] that comprises many factors, including the volar or circumferential comminution highlighted in this study. We defined extra- and intraarticular displacement indices including "tolerable zones." The decision to treat a patient with or without surgery at the acute stage is primarily based on patients' characteristics (health status, functional expectations) and displacement indices when they exceed "tolerable zones" of displacement.

G. Herzberg, MD, PhD

Reference

1. Herzberg G. Acute distal radius fractures: PAF analysis. *J Wrist Surg*. 2012;1:81-82.

Interobserver Variability in the Treatment of Little Finger Metacarpal Neck Fractures

Tosti R, Science of Variation Group (Temple Univ School of Medicine, Philadelphia, PA; et al)

J Hand Surg Am 39:1722-1727, 2014

Purpose.—To address the null hypothesis that surgeons shown radiographs of little finger metacarpal neck fractures with measured fracture angulation would recommend surgery as often as surgeons shown unmarked radiographs.

Methods.—Members of the Science of Variation Group, an international collaboration of fully trained orthopedic and trauma surgeons, were asked to review 20 little finger metacarpal neck fracture cases, which included a vignette and 3 high-quality radiographs. Members were then randomized to review radiographs with or without measured fracture angulation on the lateral view and select operative or nonoperative management.

Results.—Surgeons shown radiographs with measured angulation were more likely to recommend surgery, and there was less variability among these surgeons, particularly for fractures with less angular deformity.

Conclusions.—Measured fracture angulation has a small but significant influence on treatment recommendations for little finger metacarpal neck fractures.

Type of Study/Level of Evidence.—Diagnostic III.

▶ Little finger metacarpal neck fractures are common. Despite this, and in the presence of the increasing trend of evidence-based treatment of medical conditions, the fifth metacarpal neck fracture is still a condition for which there is marked variability in treatment recommendations. Common variables that influence the treatment are clinical findings such as malrotation, pseudo-clawing, and radiological parameters such as the degree of angulation of the fracture.

In the abstract, the primary hypothesis was that surgeons shown measured fracture angulation would recommend surgery at the same rate as surgeons shown unmarked radiographs. The finding that measured angulations slightly increased the likelihood of recommending surgery is intriguing. In their discussion, the authors note that the surgeons may have incorrectly estimated the true angulation as a result of errors in the marked radiographs or wrong assessment by the observers in those unmarked ones. This is consistent with previous work showing that interobserver reliability in measuring metacarpal neck fracture angles was only fair.[1]

In both measured and unmeasured cases, there was much variation in the choice of treatment. With increasing angulation, there was increased surgery recommended, but, at the same time, agreement decreased.

Clearly, decision making was influenced by more than just angulation. Training and the surgeon's own clinical experience are likely factors that influence the choice of recommendation.

Surgeon recommendation plays one of the biggest parts in patient decision making. In many cases, the surgeon recommendation, either explicit or implicit, determines the patient's final choice. Understanding what affects surgeon decision and variability is an important but understudied aspect of medical care. This study helps shed some light on the topic of metacarpal fractures.

A. Chong, MD

Reference

1. Leung YL, Beredjiklian PK, Monaghan BA, Bozentka DJ. Radiographic assessment of small finger metacarpal neck fractures. *J Hand Surg Am*. 2002;27: 443-448.

The Impact of Three-Dimensional CT Imaging on Intraobserver and Interobserver Reliability of Proximal Humeral Fracture Classifications and Treatment Recommendations

Berkes MB, Dines JS, Little MTM, et al (Hosp for Special Surgery, NY)
J Bone Joint Surg Am 96:1281-1286, 2014

Background.—The classification systems for fractures of the proximal part of the humerus provide low interobserver and intraobserver reliability when radiographs or two-dimensional computed tomography scans are used. The purpose of this investigation was to determine whether the use of three-dimensional computed tomography scans could improve interobserver and intraobserver reliability of AO/OTA (Arbeitsgemeinschaft für Osteosynthesefragen/Orthopaedic Trauma Association) and Neer classifications and treatment recommendations.

Methods.—Two trauma surgeons, one shoulder surgeon, two senior orthopaedic residents, and two junior orthopaedic residents reviewed the radiographs and two and three-dimensional computed tomography scans of forty fractures of the proximal part of the humerus. Each imaging modality was reviewed in isolation, and fractures were classified according to the Neer and AO/OTA classifications and treatment recommendations were provided. This process was repeated for intraobserver analysis. Interobserver agreement was calculated within and between levels of training for each classification and treatment recommendation with respect to radiographs and two and three-dimensional computed tomography scans.

Results.—Among attending orthopaedic surgeons and senior residents, the use of three-dimensional computed tomography did not improve agreement compared with the use of two-dimensional computed tomography for the Neer classification based on planes, the AO/OTA classification, or the treatment recommendation, but it did improve agreement among junior residents. Comparing between levels of training, three-dimensional computed tomography increased agreement only between junior residents and more experienced reviewers for the Neer classification based on planes and for the AO/OTA classification but not for the treatment recommendation. Intraobserver agreement for each reviewer for classification and treatment ranged from slight to fair and was not improved through the use of three-dimensional computed tomography.

Conclusions.—In this investigation, the use of three-dimensional computed tomography imaging did not offer improved interobserver and intraobserver agreement compared with the use of two-dimensional computed tomography imaging with regard to classification and treatment of fractures of the proximal part of the humerus, except among reviewers with limited clinical experience.

Level of Evidence.—Diagnostic Level III. See Instructions for Authors for a complete description of levels of evidence.

▶ As much as 3-dimensional reconstructions may improve an individual's understanding of a fracture, they do not improve the ability of experienced surgeons to agree on classification of complex proximal humerus fractures. At initial presentation, this may seem counterintuitive. A surgeon considers many parameters when attempting to place a fracture that truly sits on a continuum of pathology into a rigid and limited classification system.

With the difficulty noted in multiple publications when attempting to gain consensus on classification of proximal humerus fractures, it makes one wonder if it's time for a different system.

R. Papandrea, MD

Upright Versus Supine Radiographs of Clavicle Fractures: Does Positioning Matter?

Backus JD, Merriman DJ, McAndrew CM, et al (Washington Univ in St Louis, MO; Mercy Clinic Orthopedic Trauma - Surgery Ctr, Springfield, MO)

J Orthop Trauma 28:636-641, 2014

Objectives.—To determine whether clavicle fracture displacement and shortening are different between upright and supine radiographic examinations.

Design.—Combined retrospective and prospective comparative study.

Setting.—Level I Trauma Center.

Patients.—Forty-six patients (mean age, 49 years; range, 24–89 years) with an acute clavicle fracture were evaluated.

Intervention.—Standardized clavicle radiographs were obtained in both supine and upright positions for each patient. Displacement and shortening were measured and compared between the 2 positions.

Main Outcomes Measurements.—One resident and 3 traumatologists classified the fractures and measured displacement and shortening. Data were aggregated and compared to ensure reliability with a 2-way mixed intraclass correlation.

Results.—Fracture displacement was significantly greater when measured from upright radiographs (15.9 ± 8.9 mm) than from supine radiographs (8.4 ± 6.6 mm, $P < 0.001$), representing an 89% increase in displacement with upright positioning. Forty-one percent of patients had greater than 100% displacement on upright but not on supine radiographs. Compared with the uninjured side, 3.0 ± 10.7 mm of shortening was noted on upright radiographs and 1.3 ± 9.5 mm of lengthening on supine radiographs ($P < 0.001$). The intraclass correlation was 0.82 [95% confidence interval (CI), 0.73–0.89] for OTA fracture classification, 0.81 (95% CI, 0.75–0.87) for vertical displacement, and 0.92 (95% CI, 0.88–0.95) for injured clavicle length, demonstrating very high agreement among evaluators.

Conclusions.—Increased fracture displacement and shortening was observed on upright compared with supine radiographs. This suggests that upright radiographs may better demonstrate clavicle displacement and predict the position at healing if nonoperative treatment is selected.

▶ In this article, the authors review both upright and supine radiographs in 46 adult patients presenting with acute clavicle fractures. They noted an 89% increase in displacement when the patient was standing for the X-ray compared to laying supine. The authors also note that the popularity of clavicle open reduction internal fixation is increasing, yet it is difficult to be critical of proposed surgical indications because the radiographic technique has not been standardized.

Frankly, I was quite surprised by this article. I have always obtained standing bilateral radiographs of the clavicles ... at least I think they are standing? I had wrongly assumed that this topic had been already proven in the literature years ago. After I reviewed the literature, I found only a passing mention of the benefit of the upright views, the 2 most readily evident sources being in a poster abstract from Erich Gauger and colleagues[1] at the 2013 American Academy of Orthopaedic Surgeons meeting in Chicago and an article by Harris et al[2] in *International Journal of Shoulder Surgery*. In the poster abstract, the authors mention that the upright gravity view highlights displacement, and they recommend a change in protocol to include the upright view. In the Harris article, the authors state that upright views are taken if possible because the supine view "alters the effect of gravity."

I think that this is an eloquent and important study that gives scientific validation to a radiographic technique that many of us may have already been doing.

N. A. Hoekzema, MD

References

1. Gauger EM, Jacobson A, Will R, Cole P. Progressive displacement after clavicle fracture; an observational study. Poster presentation. January 14, 2013. American Academy of Orthopaedic Surgeons meeting. Chicago, IL.
2. Harris JD, Latshaw JC. Improved clinical utility in clavicle fracture decision-making with true orthogonal radiographs. *Int J Shoulder Surg*. 2012;6:130-134.

Factors Predicting Complication and Reoperation Rates Following Surgical Fixation of Proximal Humeral Fractures

Petrigliano FA, Bezrukov N, Gamradt SC, et al (Univ of California at Los Angeles; et al)
J Bone Joint Surg Am 96:1544-1551, 2014

Background.—The purpose of this study was to report complication and reoperation rates following non-arthroplasty fixation of shoulder fractures determined on the basis of observational, population-based data from all inpatient admissions in California over an eleven-year period.

Methods.—Records from all inpatient hospital discharges and subsequent readmissions related to operative non-arthroplasty treatment of proximal humeral fractures were obtained for patients in California from December 1994 through December 2005. These admissions were evaluated to identify patient and hospital characteristics associated with short and intermediate-term complications (within and after ninety days, respectively) as well as reoperation rates. Procedures performed included open reduction and internal fixation in 9254 patients, closed reduction and internal fixation in 1903 patients, and internal fixation without reduction in 302 patients.

Results.—The short-term complications included mortality in 401 patients (3.5%), which was associated with a higher Charlson comorbidity index (odds ratio [OR] = 1.5, $p < 0.001$) and male sex (OR = 1.7, $p < 0.001$); and pulmonary embolism in sixty patients (0.5%), which was associated with male sex (OR = 2.2, $p = 0.007$) and patient age of seventy-five years or older (OR = 3.6, $p = 0.001$). Intermediate-term reoperations included conversion to hemiarthroplasty in 174 patients (1.5%); and conversion to total shoulder arthroplasty in eight patients (0.07%), which was associated with an age of fifty to sixty-four years (hazard ratio = 2.8, $p = 0.007$). Overall, an age of sixty-five years or older, male sex, residence in an area with an income in the lowest two quintiles, and the presence of preexisting comorbidities were associated with elevated risks of short-term complications but not of intermediate-term conversion to arthroplasty. The ninety-day revision rate was 5.3%.

Conclusions.—Surgical fixation of proximal humeral fractures has a low complication and mortality profile. The data provided in this study can serve in counseling patients about risks associated with operative fixation of displaced proximal humeral fractures.

▶ This is a level 4 study that reported on both short-term (< 90 days) and intermediate-term (> 90 days) complications and reoperation rates after surgical fixation of proximal humerus fractures. The authors use a database and records from the state of California from 1994 through 2005. Procedures performed included open reduction and internal fixation (ORIF) (9254 patients), closed reduction internal fixation (1903 patients), and internal fixation without reduction (302 patients).

A strength of this study is the large patient population to identify both short- and intermediate-term complications and reoperations. Overall complications were low; however, there were specific findings worth noting. For instance, male patients older than 65 who resided in an area in the lowest 2 quintiles with comorbid conditions were associated with elevated risks of short-term complications including pulmonary embolism and mortality. Intermediate complications including conversion to hemiarthroplasty or total shoulder arthroplasty were associated with an age of 50 to 64. These findings suggest that the overall revision rate of proximal humerus fixation is low at 5.3%, and even lower in patients treated initially with ORIF at 4.9%.

There are some weaknesses worth mentioning. First, fracture patterns were not stratified (ie, 2-part vs 3- and 4-part fractures). Type of fixation was also not considered (locking vs nonlocking plates). Finally, only serious complications requiring readmission were considered, thereby precluding the capture of infectious cases or patients who required removal of hardware.

This is a useful study that reports on short- and intermediate-term results after fixation of proximal humerus fractures. Complications are relatively low; however, mortality was found to be greater after fracture fixation compared with after elective total shoulder arthroplasty. Based on the data offered in this study, older patients with coexisiting morbidities are at higher risk of perioperative complications and should be counseled accordingly, and, in certain circumstances, nonoperative treatment may be preferred given these risk factors for adverse consequences in this select group.

S. M. Jacoby, MD

A comparison of suprascapular nerve block and procedural sedation analgesia in shoulder dislocation reduction

Tezel O, Kaldirim U, Bilgic S, et al (Gulhane Military Med Academy, Ankara, Turkey; Haydarpasa Educational Hosp, Istanbul, Turkey; et al)

Am J Emerg Med 32:549-552, 2014

Objectives.—Dislocation of the shoulder joint is one of the most common dislocations. The reduction procedure is a painful procedure. In this study, 2 different treatment groups were compared for pain control during shoulder dislocation reduction. It was aimed to evaluate the differences between the groups in reduction, success, length of hospital stay, complications, side effects, patient-physician satisfaction, and ease of application.

Methods.—The study was planned to be prospective and randomized. As procedural sedation analgesia (SA), titration of ketamine 1 to 2 mg/kg was administered intravenously to group 1. Suprascapular nerve block (SNB) was applied under ultrasound guidance (USG) to group 2. Conformity to normal distribution of variables was examined with the Kolmogorov-Smirnov test. The χ^2 test and Fisher test were used to evaluate differences between the groups in categorical variables and the Mann-Whitney *U* test, and a value of $P < .05$ was accepted as statistically significant.

Results.—The study comprised a total of 41 patients; 20 in the group 1 and 21 in the group 2. No statistically significant difference was determined between the groups in terms of age ($P = .916$), sex ($P = .972$), reduction success ($P = .540$), and patient-physician satisfaction ($P = .198$). The time spent in the emergency department (ED) by patients in the SA group was signficantly longer compared with the SNB group. No side effects were observed in the SNB group.

Conclusions.—Suprascapular nerve block, which can be easily applied under USG in the ED, can be evaluated as a good alternative to SA in the reduction of shoulder dislocations.

▶ This prospective study compared suprascapular nerve block with procedural sedation for emergency department reductions of glenohumeral dislocations. This submission found no difference in success of reduction or physician satisfaction. The authors were able to show a reduction in the time spent in the emergency department from the start of the procedure to discharge (125 minutes in the nerve block group vs 25 minutes in the sedation group). This finding was significantly different and no complications occurred in the nerve block group, whereas complications in the sedation group included agitation when awakening, nausea, and hypoxia requiring supplemental oxygen administration. It should be noted that suprascapular nerve blocks were performed under ultrasound guidance, and this technique requires access to an ultrasound machine and familiarity with this particular technique. The authors conclude that suprascapular nerve block was safe and effective and allowed for a faster rate of discharge from the emergency department compared with procedural sedation.

J. Macalena, MD

The Influence of Local Bone Density on the Outcome of One Hundred and Fifty Proximal Humeral Fractures Treated with a Locking Plate

Kralinger F, Blauth M, Goldhahn J, et al (Med Univ Innsbruck, Austria; Inst for Biomechanics, Zürich, Switzerland; et al)
J Bone Joint Surg Am 96:1026-1032, 2014

Background.—There is biomechanical evidence that bone density predicts the mechanical failure of implants. The aim of this prospective study was to evaluate the influence of local bone mineral density on the rate of mechanical failure after locking plate fixation of proximal humeral fractures.

Methods.—We enrolled 150 patients who were from fifty to ninety years old with a closed, displaced proximal humeral fracture fixed with use of a locking plate from July 2007 to April 2010. There were 118 women and thirty-two men who had a mean age of sixty-nine years. Preoperative computed tomography (CT) scans were done to assess bone mineral density of the contralateral humerus, and dual x-ray absorptiometry of the distal end of the radius of the unaffected arm was conducted within the first six weeks postoperatively. At follow-up evaluations at six weeks, three months, and one year postoperatively, pain, shoulder mobility, strength, and multiple functional and quality-of-life outcome measures (Disabilities of the Arm, Shoulder and Hand [DASH] questionnaire; Shoulder Pain and Disability Index [SPADI]; Constant score; and EuroQuol-5D [EQ-5D]) were done and standard radiographs were made. We defined mechanical failure as all complications related to bone quality experienced within one year.

Results.—After locking plate fixation, fifty-three (35%) of 150 patients had mechanical failure; loss of reduction and secondary screw loosening with perforation were common. CT assessments of local bone mineral density showed no difference between patients with and without mechanical failure (89.82 versus 91.51 mg/cm^3, respectively; $p = 0.670$). One-year DASH, SPADI, and Constant scores were significantly better for patients without mechanical failure ($p \leq 0.05$).

Conclusions.—We did not find evidence of an association between bone mineral density and the rate of mechanical failures, which may suggest that patients with normal bone mineral density are less prone to sustain a proximal humeral fracture. Future studies should target other discriminating factors between patients with and without mechanical failure.

Level of Evidence.—Prognostic Level III. See Instructions for Authors for a complete description of levels of evidence.

▶ This article investigates whether bone mineral density (BMD), and various other factors, affects the outcome of proximal humerus fractures. The study has sound methods, good outcome measurements, appropriate clinical follow-up, and relevant variables. The largest limitation of the study is that the effect size may be smaller than the study is able to detect given that most patients with proximal humerus fractures already have poor bone mineral density. The study did not show any difference in BMD between the nonfailure and failure groups, but both groups had low BMD. Certainly, another consideration of the study should be that the Neer fracture classification has relatively poor intra- and interobserver reliability and often fails to characterize the fracture appropriately. Interestingly, there was also no difference in mechanical failure considering the factors of suture augmentation of the rotator cuff, type of plate used, or the experience of the surgeon.

For the commentator, the article adds only a few points to what is already known about proximal humerus fractures. In the commentator's practice, bone mineral density is measured via the method from Tingart et al,[1] and the fracture pattern is assessed using the criteria from Hertel et al.[2] The combination of these 2 methods allows a surgeon to determine whether mechanical failure is likely to occur. Based on the findings from these 2 methods, one must plan ahead and have the following available if needed: proximal humeral locking plates, braided reinforced suture, fibular strut allografts, bone fillers, and salvage implants (eg, reverse shoulder arthroplasty). Only some cases in this study used allograft; thus, the effect of this technique cannot be fully assessed. Although the advent of the proximal humerus locking plate has assisted greatly with the treatment of proximal humerus fractures, this fixation method is not without complications, and the actual surgical technique and placement of screws is critical for success.

M. B. Gottschalk, MD
J. T. Capo, MD

References

1. Tingart MS, Apprelexa M, von Stechow D, Zurakowski D, Warner JJ. The cortical thickness of the proximal humeral diaphysis predicts bone mineral density of the proximal humerus. *J Bone Joint Surg Br.* 2003;85:611-617.
2. Hertel R, Hempfing A, Stiehler M, Leunig M. Predictors of humeral head ischemia after intracapsular fracture of the proximal humerus. *J Shoulder Elbow Surg.* 2000;13:427-433.

The outcome of proximal humeral fractures in the elderly: predictors of mortality and function

Clement ND, Duckworth AD, McQueen MM, et al (Royal Infirmary of Edinburgh, UK)
Bone Joint J 96-B:970-977, 2014

This study describes the epidemiology and outcome of 637 proximal humeral fractures in 629 elderly (≥65 years old) patients. Most were either minimally displaced (n = 278, 44%) or two-part fractures (n = 250, 39%) that predominantly occurred in women (n = 525, 82%) after a simple fall (n = 604, 95%), who lived independently in their own home (n = 560, 88%), and one in ten sustained a concomitant fracture (n = 76, 11.9%). The rate of mortality at one year was 10%, with the only independent predictor of survival being whether the patient lived in their own home ($p = 0.025$). Many factors associated with the patient's social independence significantly influenced the age and gender adjusted Constant score one year after the fracture. More than a quarter of the patients had a poor functional outcome, with those patients not living in their own home ($p = 0.04$), participating in recreational activities ($p = 0.01$), able to perform their own shopping ($p < 0.001$), or able to dress themselves ($p = 0.02$) being at a significantly increased risk of a poor outcome, which was independent of the severity of the fracture ($p = 0.001$).

A poor functional outcome after a proximal humeral fracture is not independently influenced by age in the elderly, and factors associated with social independence are more predictive of outcome.

▶ Proximal humerus fractures in the elderly are common and increasing in number as our population ages. In this case, a quarter of the patients studied had a poor functional outcome, which greatly affects their quality of life.

The population studied is an urban population primarily referred to a single institution for the region in the United Kingdom. Disabilities of the Arm, Shoulder and Hand scores were available for 76% of patients at 1 year, with only 6 patients refusing to participate, 10% mortality rate, and the others being too frail to return to clinic, which is valuable information. Additionally, the authors were able to evaluate many social factors, such as driving, independent living, and dressing oneself, that would typically be difficult to gather and report. The authors should be commended for these significant strengths in their work.

One of the limitations of this study is that patients in this institution were treated operatively (N = 50) or nonoperatively (N = 587) based on the recommendations of the consultant caring for the patient. The criteria for the patients treated operatively are not discussed. It is, therefore, difficult to draw conclusions based on operative treatment and their outcome.

The primary determinants of outcomes were nonmodifiable at the time of presentation and independent of fracture severity, which is traditionally used as important criteria for intervention. This leaves us searching for ways to improve outcomes for our patients.

This study overall reinforces social themes that run true for other fractures in the elderly. It is increasingly clear that preinjury functional status is one of the strongest predictors of outcome and mortality, independent of the fracture severity or the actual age of the patient. Aims at reducing morbidity for these patients may well need to occur in the community, prior to fracture, with an emphasis on prevention.

J. Geissler, MD

A new morphological classification for greater tuberosity fractures of the proximal humerus: validation and clinical implications

Mutch J, Laflamme GY, Hagemeister N, et al (Hopital Sacre-Coeur de Montréal, Québec, Canada)

Bone Joint J 96-B:646-651, 2014

In this study, we describe a morphological classification for greater tuberosity fractures of the proximal humerus. We divided these fractures into three types: avulsion, split and depression. We retrospectively reviewed all shoulder radiographs showing isolated greater tuberosity fractures in a Level I trauma centre between July 2007 and July 2012.

We identified 199 cases where records and radiographs were reviewed and included 79 men and 120 women with a mean age of 58 years (23 to 96). The morphological classification was applied to the first 139 cases by three reviewers on two occasions using the Kappa statistic and compared with the AO and Neer classifications. The inter- and intra-observer reliability of the morphological classification was 0.73 to 0.77 and 0.69 to 0.86, respectively. This was superior to the Neer (0.31 to 0.35/0.54 to 0.63) and AO (0.30 to 0.32/0.59 to 0.65) classifications. The distribution of avulsion, split and depression type fractures was 39%, 41%, and 20%, respectively. This classification of greater tuberosity fractures is more reliable than the Neer or AO classifications. These distinct fracture morphologies are likely to have implications in terms of pathophysiology and surgical technique.

▶ This study presents an insightful new classification for isolated greater tuberosity fractures of the proximal humerus. Based on radiographic morphology, fractures are classified as impacted, split, or avulsed. Depressed fractures had a history of dislocation twice as frequently as those with a split or avulsed morphology. The authors report higher reliability of the proposed fracture classification compared with the Neer and AO classifications. However, it is unclear as to how the latter classifications were applied. With greater tuberosity fractures presenting as either displaced or nondisplaced fractures, the included fractures would be classified as either Neer 1 or 2 part fractures. Moreover, as per AO classification, the included fractures could only be catalogued as 11A1 fractures (unifocal extra-articular greater tuberosity fractures). The low reliability values for these classifications, therefore, do not seem intuitive.

Although the authors suggest that this classification may be of value with regard to surgical treatment, this is not further studied. Future studies may apply this classification to validate its utility in clinical and surgical decision making.

P. Streubel, MD

17 Pediatric/Congenital

Hand Function in Adults with Radial Longitudinal Deficiency

Ekblom AG, Dahlin LB, Rosberg H-E, et al (Karolinska Institutet, Stockholm, Sweden; Lund Univ, Malmö, Sweden; et al)

J Bone Joint Surg Am 96:1178-1184, 2014

Background.—Functional impairment in individuals with radial longitudinal deficiency can be influenced by several factors, including a short and bowed forearm, radial deviation of the wrist, a non-functional or absent thumb, limited finger motion, and impaired grip strength, but their relationship with activity and participation in adults with radial deficiency is not known.

Methods.—Twenty individuals, eighteen to sixty years of age, who had Bayne type-II to V radial longitudinal deficiency, were examined in the context of the International Classification of Functioning, Disability and Health. Body function and structure were evaluated by measures of range of motion, grip strength, key pinch, sensibility, and radiographic parameters. Activity was evaluated by the Box and Block Test and the Sollerman test, and participation was evaluated by QuickDASH (the short form of the Disabilities of Arm, Shoulder and Hand outcome measure) and by the Medical Outcomes Study 12-Item Short Form Health Survey. Statistical correlations among assessments of body function and structure, activity, and participation were examined.

Results.—The mean total active motion of the wrist (43°) and mean total active motion of the digits (377°) were less than the norms. The mean radial deviation of the wrist was 31°. The mean grip strength (4.0 kg), key pinch (1.4 kg), and scores for the Box and Block Test (55 blocks per minute) and the Sollerman test on hand function (56 points) were considerably lower than the norms. The mean scores were 18 points for QuickDASH, 51 points for Short Form-12 physical component summary, and 53 points for Short Form-12 mental component summary. Significant relationships were found between the Box and Block Test and grip strength ($p = 0.012$), key pinch ($p < 0.001$), and total active motion of digits ($p < 0.001$); between the Sollerman test and the total active motion of elbow ($p < 0.001$) and the total active motion of digits ($p < 0.001$); between the QuickDASH and forearm length ($p < 0.001$), the total active motion of elbow ($p = 0.001$), and the total active motion of digits ($p < 0.001$); between the Short Form-12 physical component summary and grip strength ($p = 0.016$), forearm length ($p < 0.001$), total active elbow motion ($p < 0.001$), and total active digit motion ($p < 0.001$); and between the Short-Form-12 mental component summary and radial deviation of the wrist ($p = 0.019$). No significant correlations were found between the radiographic measurement of the radial deviation of the wrist (total forearm angle) and the Box and Block Test ($p = 0.244$), the Sollerman test ($p = 0.775$), QuickDASH ($p = 0.156$), Short Form-12 physical component summary ($p = 0.107$), or Short Form-12 mental component summary ($p = 0.129$).

Conclusions.—In individuals with radial longitudinal deficiency, grip strength, key pinch, forearm length, and elbow and digital motion seem to be more important for the individual's activity and participation than the radial angulation of the wrist.

Level of Evidence.—Prognostic Level IV. See Instructions for Authors for a complete description of levels of evidence.

▶ This study evaluates radial longitudinal deficiency of adults and how functional impairment determines participation in life experiences. Although relatively rare, or .20 to .05 per live 10 000 births, congenital radial longitudinal deficiency does occur bilaterally in half of the cases and is most severe asymmetrically. This study is admittedly limited by size, yet this subject of functional impairment has not been well addressed in adults in other reviews or research. Consideration for children and its future impact is relevant to determine outcomes for parents of children with radial longitudinal deficiency. The methodology of the objective measurements and subjective questionnaires are familiar and can be easily replicated in future studies. Surgical corrections, including centralization procedure, bone lengthening, and pollicization and vascular bone grafts have been used. In studying children, authors mention that a recent study of children with similar radial longitudinal deficiency indicates the radial angulation of the wrist is the most important factor for activity and self-perceived disability. In an attempt to study this in adults, the authors' findings indicated the wrist angulation was not the primary determinant for activity limitation. Thus, the wrist angulation was less of a factor than the grip, pinch strength, and elbow motion in the outcome of activity participation. Overall, the article brings up the need to reevaluate surgical considerations in correcting radial longitudinal deficiency. From this article, the readers have a view point that radial longitudinal deficiency affecting wrist angulation does not necessarily restrict activity participation in adult life. Yet, additional studies should be considered to address if better preservation of elbow, wrist and digit motion, and grip and pinch strength will improve functional outcome of the radial longitudinal deficiency.

S. Kranz, CHT

Hand Surgery for Dystrophic Epidermolysis Bullosa

Luria S, Radwan S, Zinger G, et al (Univ Med Ctr, Jerusalem, Israel; et al)

J Pediatr Orthop 34:710-714, 2014

Background.—Epidermolysis bullosa (EB) is a group of inherited, mechanobullous disorders caused by mutations in various structural proteins in the skin. The manifestation of these disorders in the hand is of digital contractures and pseudosyndactyly or "cocoon hands," causing

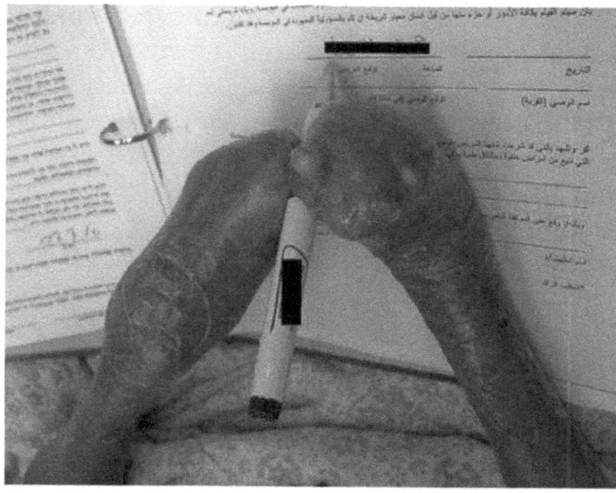

FIGURE 1.—An 18-year-old male signing the surgery consent form bimanually. (Reprinted from Luria S, Radwan S, Zinger G, et al. Hand surgery for dystrophic epidermolysis bullosa. *J Pediatr Orthop*. 2014;34:710-714, with permission from Lippincott Williams & Wilkins.)

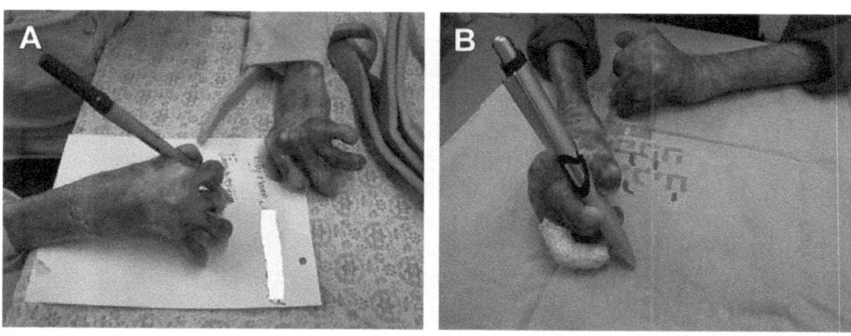

FIGURE 4.—A 16-year-old female. A, 3 months postoperatively. B, 3.5 years postoperatively. (Reprinted from Luria S, Radwan S, Zinger G, et al. Hand surgery for dystrophic epidermolysis bullosa. *J Pediatr Orthop*. 2014;34:710-714, with permission from Lippincott Williams & Wilkins.)

significant functional impairment. Our preferred surgical treatment of these patients involves separation of the digits from the palm by releasing the finger flexion contractures and separating them, primarily the adducted thumb. However, recurrence is common. Our hypothesis was that functional improvement is gained irrespective of recurrence of contractures.

Methods.—We retrospectively evaluated 4 patients, 2 male and 2 female, whose average age was 11 years, treated surgically by the separation of all their digits and by coverage with skin grafts. The follow-up period was between 1 and 3½ years.

Results.—Partial recurrence of the deformity was observed in all patients. Recurrence was more pronounced in the nondominant hand, especially between the digits and of flexion contractures, but did not preclude the use of precision or oppositional pinch at final follow-up. The patient with the longest follow-up has been referred for revision surgery to gain further release of contractures. Significant rehabilitation goals were achieved in all 4 patients after surgery. After 6 months, both of the younger patients were measured for finger dexterity, which showed lower scores than the norm, although this was felt to be dependent on which daily manual activities they were more familiar with. These tests could not have been performed before surgery.

Conclusions.—All patients and families felt the effort was worthy. Separating the thumb and straightening the digits was found to be significant, yet the indication for separating all the digits is debatable. The need for revision surgery, to maintain the digit function, is clear.

Level of Evidence.—Level 4, case series. (Figs 1 and 4).

▶ This article reviews surgery for more complex patients with (recessive) dystrophic epidermolysis bullosa (RDEB), a rare but devastating genetic disorder. There is nothing new in this article, but it is worth review (Figs 1 and 4), especially for colleagues who might come across patients with RDEB and wish to shore a team and jump in (I encourage you). The hand surgeon plays a critical role as team leader, and it takes a dedicated team, if my 25-year history serves.[1-3] My experiences may be summed up as follows, many of which are highlighted in this article. The most important is working with a team both knowledgeable and willing to support care of these children. The surgery to release contractures is not at all difficult; most can be done with an arm or wrist block with intravenous sedation. They do not, unlike this article states, require transfusions, tourniquets, skin grafts, or hospitalization. Adequate analgesia, if necessary working with a pain management team, is helpful, as extensive blistering (the inevitability of surgery) is extremely painful. Recurrence is inevitable. But the surgery and the caregiving is worth it, especially when older kids, teens, and adults come back regaling with their altered keyboard skills, smartphone capabilities, driving, and school accomplishments—all evidence of the more important connection of a powerful brain when the hand has limited resources.

A. Ladd, MD

References

1. Ladd AL, Kibele A, Gibbons S. Surgical treatment and postoperative splinting for recessive dystrophic epidermolysis bullosa. *J Hand Surg Am.* 1996;21:888-897.
2. Ladd AL, Eggleston JM III. Hand management for patients with epidermolysis bullosa. In: Mathes SJ, Hentz VR, eds. *Plastic Surgery.* New York: WB Saunders Co; 2005.
3. Ladd AL, Diaz R, Chan J. Epidermolysis bullosa. In: Laub D Jr., ed. *Congenital Anomalies of the Upper Extremity.* Springer; 2014.

Developing a Pollicization Outcomes Measure

Zlotolow DA, Tosti R, Ashworth S, et al (Shriners Hosps for Children, Philadelphia, PA; Temple Univ School of Medicine, Philadelphia, PA, Univ of Maryland Med Ctr, Baltimore)

J Hand Surg Am 39:1784-1791, 2014

Purpose.—To evaluate which objective criteria correlated with subjective impressions of outcome following index finger pollicization for thumb hypoplasia.

Methods.—Forty-two pollicizations in 35 patients were assessed by a comprehensive subjective and objective measurement analysis. In the subjective measures, the surgeon, therapist, and caregiver rated how the pollicized digit "looks like a thumb" and "works like a thumb." The caregiver also completed a subjective questionnaire. For objective results, we measured appearance, strength, range of motion, stability, and ability to pick up objects. The subjective results were then correlated with objective data via a linear regression analysis.

Results.—When combining the total subjective score for "looks like a thumb," "works like a thumb," and the caregiver questionnaire, we found significant correlation scores for palmar abduction, lateral pinch, tip pinch, and picking up a bead, a die, and a table tennis ball. The strongest correlations were found with composite flexion, metacarpophalangeal (MCP) joint range of motion, interphalangeal (IP) joint range of motion, and the sticker test. Three of these 4 items (sticker test and MCP joint and IP arcs of motion) also correlated best with children who preferred using their thumbs for small object acquisition instead of scissor pinch.

Conclusions.—Composite flexion, MCP and IP joint arcs of motion, and the sticker test correlated the strongest with the subjective criteria. These parameters appear to be the most critical measures that impress a good outcome following pollicization.

Type of Study/Level of Evidence.—Prognostic IV (Figs 1 and 2).

► The authors describe the development of an outcomes measure for patients who have undergone a pollicization to hopefully provide a method to compare surgical techniques. A retrospective review was performed to evaluate charts for various subjective and objective data. A total of 42 patients were included in the analysis, and evaluations were made by a surgeon, a therapist, and a caregiver. Figs 1 and 2 provide objective criteria to use when assessing the outcomes of a pollicization, including a pictogram (Fig 1). Additional assessments can be made by having the patient perform activities, such as peeling a sticker or acquiring a die. The authors concluded that the ability to peel a sticker was significantly correlated with the "works like a thumb" subjective assessment. Therefore, having pollicization patients peel a sticker postoperatively may be a good test to see the functional utilization of the thumb postoperatively. Although a definitive outcome tool was not able to be developed from this study, assessment of the sticker test and range of motion including composite flexion and metacarpophalangeal and interphalangeal arcs of motion may be

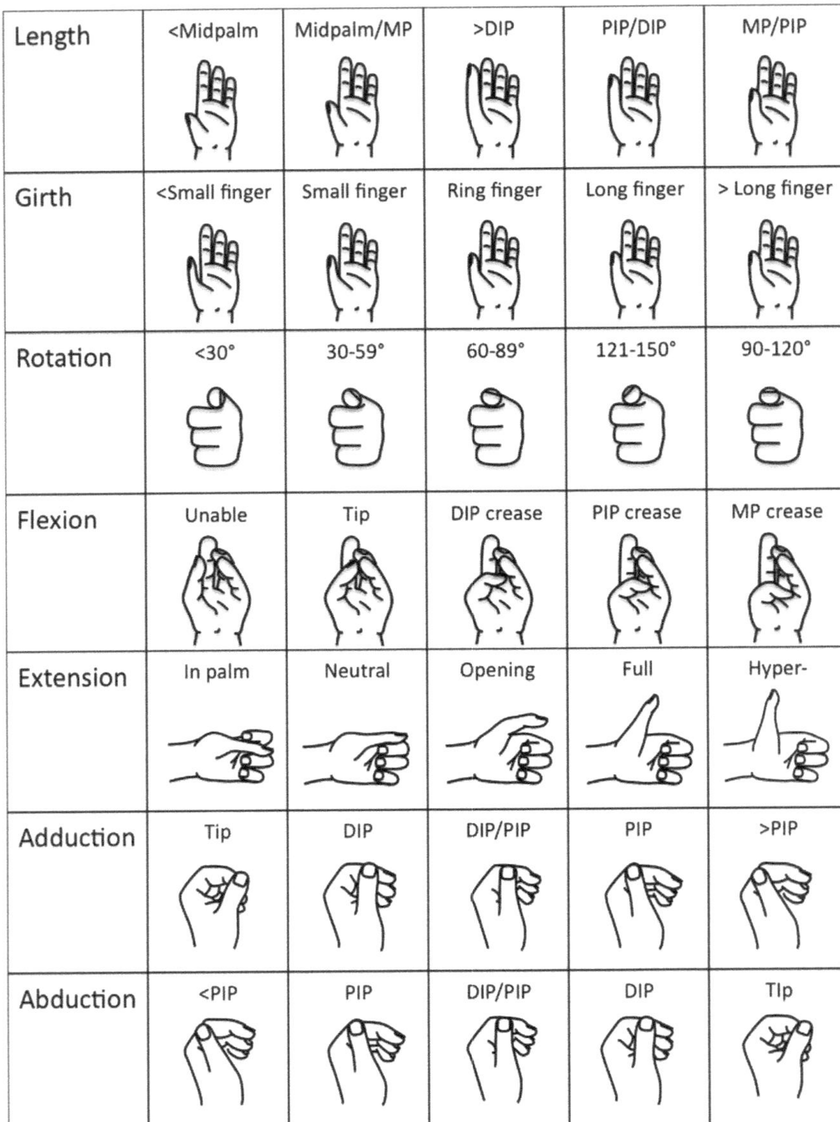

FIGURE 1.—A Likert scale pictogram was developed to simplify as many objective criteria as could be adapted to graphic form. (Courtesy of Shriners Hospital for Children Philadelphia.) (Reprinted from The Journal of Hand Surgery. Zlotolow DA, Tosti R, Ashworth S, et al. Developing a pollicization outcomes measure. *J Hand Surg Am.* 2014;39:1784-1791, Copyright 2014, with permission American Society for Surgery of the Hand.)

ACTIVE MOTION	0	1	2	3	4
IP arc	0-15°	16-30°	31-45°	46-60°	>60°
MCP arc	0-15°	16-30°	31-45°	46-60°	>60°
ACQUISITION					
Bead	Ulnar sided	Very difficult	Difficult	Easy	Normal
Die	Ulnar sided	Very difficult	Difficult	Easy	Normal
Table tennis ball	Ulnar sided	Very difficult	Difficult	Easy	Normal
Sticker test	Ulnar sided	Very difficult	Difficult	Easy	Normal

STRENGTH		1st attempt	2nd attempt	3rd attempt	Average
Lateral pinch	Unable	kg	kg	kg	kg
Tip pinch	Unable	kg	kg	kg	kg

EXAMINATION	0	1	2	3	4
Palmar Abduction	0-10°	11-20°	21-30°	31-40°	>40°
Radial Abduction	0-10°	11-20°	21-30°	31-40°	>40°
CMC stability	Dislocatable	≥50% subluxation	<50% subluxation	Varus/valgus instability	Stable
CMC hyperextension	≥90°	60-89°	30-59°	>0-29°	Neutral

FIGURE 2.—The objective criteria that were more easily represented in text form comprised the second page of the outcomes measure. (Courtesy of Shriners Hospital for Children Philadelphia.) (Reprinted from The Journal of Hand Surgery. Zlotolow DA, Tosti R, Ashworth S, et al. Developing a pollicization outcomes measure. *J Hand Surg Am.* 2014;39:1784-1791, Copyright 2014, with permission American Society for Surgery of the Hand.)

the best indicators of subjective outcomes. Therefore, I have incorporated the assessment of these objective findings into my practice, and they are performed on all postoperative pollicization patients.

J. Abzug, MD

Long-Finger Pollicization for Macrodactyly of the Thumb and Index Finger

Donohue KW, Zlotolow DA, Kozin SH (Shriners Hosps for Children, Philadelphia, PA)

J Pediatr Orthop 34:e50-e53, 2014

Pollicization of the long finger is rarely performed, and previously described for treating traumatic thumb and index finger loss. Because the long finger lacks the independence of motion and muscular attachments of the index finger, pollicization of the long finger requires modifications of the technique. We present the case of a 3-year-old girl with progressive macrodactyly of the thumb and index finger associated with a lipofibromatous hamartoma of the median nerve. The involved digits were severely enlarged, stiff, and nonfunctional. The child was treated with first and second ray resection followed by long-finger pollicization. Surgical pearls and pitfalls are discussed (Figs 4 and 5b).

▶ Pollicization of the index finger has become the most accepted treatment for thumb hypoplasia. Toe-to-thumb procedures, while not common, do have some advantages in traumatic loss and symbrachydactyly. This case report uses a more controversial strategy for the treatment of thumb and index reconstruction after resection. Because the index was not available, the long finger was pollicized instead. Functional outcomes of nonindex pollicizations have not been as good as index pollicizations, most likely because of the lack of independent motors. There is only one extrinsic extensor to the long finger, and the profundus is much less likely to be independent than in the index finger. The argument could be made for a toe-to-thumb transfer in this case, as the extrinsic tendons were salvageable. This procedure would have left the child with 4

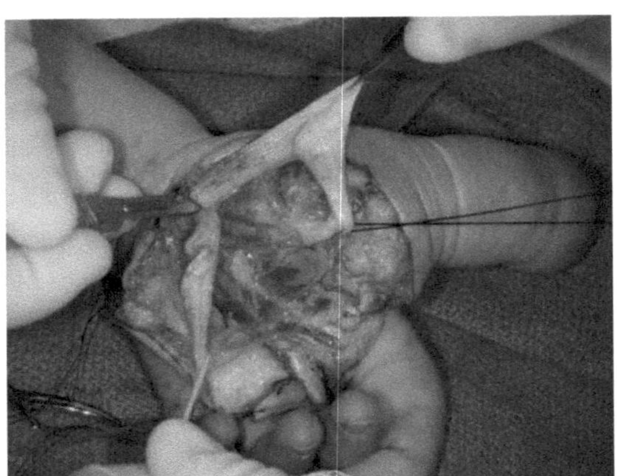

FIGURE 4.—The involved segment of the median nerve was resected from the uninvolved nerve using sharp dissection. Blunt dissection attempts proved futile. Courtesy of Shriners Hospital for Children, Philadelphia. (Reprinted from Donohue KW, Zlotolow DA, Kozin SH. Long-finger pollicization for macrodactyly of the thumb and index finger. *J Pediatr Orthop*. 2014;34:e50-e53, with permission from Lippincott Williams & Wilkins.)

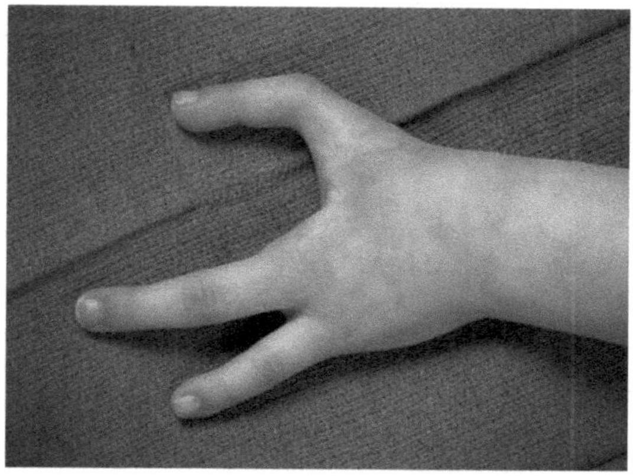

FIGURE 5.—After surgery, her function and clinical appearance were improved compared with before surgery. Courtesy of Shriners Hospital for Children, Philadelphia. (Reprinted from Donohue KW, Zlotolow DA, Kozin SH. Long-finger pollicization for macrodactyly of the thumb and index finger. *J Pediatr Orthop*. 2014;34:e50-e53, with permission from Lippincott Williams & Wilkins.)

digits instead of 3. However, the toe transfer would have added more complication risks and a separate site of morbidity. It is unclear if there would have been any functional difference between the 2 reconstructive schemes.

D. A. Zlotolow, MD

Long-Term Outcomes Following Radial Polydactyly Reconstruction

Stutz C, Mills J, Wheeler L, et al (Texas Scottish Rite Hosp for Children, Dallas)
J Hand Surg Am 39:1549-1552, 2014

Purpose.—To report long-term outcomes (> 10 y) after radial polydactyly reconstruction.

Methods.—We evaluated 43 surgically reconstructed thumbs in 41 patients with radial polydactyly whom we had observed for more than 10 years. The study group included 12 Flatt type II, 8 type III, 17 type IV, and 6 type V. The average age of surgery was 1 year and mean follow-up was 17 years. Objective outcome values and validated patient-oriented outcome evaluations were obtained.

Results.—No early postsurgical complications were encountered. Eight patients had 10 revision procedures at an average of 8 years after the initial procedure. Five patients had interphalangeal joint arthrodesis, all for angulation with accompanying pain. The average Tada score was 4.1. Lateral, tripod, and tip pinch strengths were 96%, 86%, and 92%, respectively, of the unaffected side. As a group, the treated thumbs had significantly weaker tip and tripod pinch strengths than the untreated thumbs. The average Disabilities of the Arm, Shoulder, and Hand score was 4.5 and the average Pediatric Quality of Life Inventory score was 87 when administered to both the patient and the parent.

Conclusions.—Long-term results after surgical reconstruction for radial polydactyly were excellent but the revision rate trended upward over time despite maintenance of favorable scores on the objective outcome measures used.

Type of Study/Level of Evidence.—Therapeutic IV.

▶ The authors present 10-year follow-up data on 41 of 46 patients after split thumb reconstruction. The high rate of follow-up inclusion and the length of follow-up make this a noteworthy study. The authors' revision rate was lower than previously reported at nearly 20%, and revisions tended to occur late, about 8 years after the index procedure. Revision procedures were most commonly either interphalangeal fusions for pain and/or instability or tendon realignments for a zigzag deformity. All tendon realignments were in Wassel type IV thumbs. One patient did develop complex regional pain syndrome, but no other complications were reported. This study further validates previous studies and the prevailing wisdom that thumb duplication surgery is not as simple as it might seem. Although the revision rate was 1 in 5, this does not account for the many more patients who live with a painless thumb deformity or a functionally deficient thumb without opting for a revision.

D. A. Zlotolow, MD

Chronic Anterior Monteggia Lesions in Children: Report of 4 Cases Treated With Closed Reduction by Ulnar Osteotomy and External Fixation

Bor N, Rubin G, Rozen N, et al (Haemek Med Ctr, Afula, Israel; et al)

J Pediatr Orthop 35:7-10, 2015

Background.—Chronic, subacute, and chronic Monteggia fracture dislocations of the elbow are challenging problems. The literature generally recommends complex open reconstructive procedures. We present an alternative, minimally invasive, percutaneous method with external fixation.

Methods.—This was a retrospective review of 4 cases presenting with chronic Monteggia lesions with anterior dislocation of the radial head.

Results.—Reduction of the radiocapitellar joint was successfully achieved in all patients after ulnar osteotomy and gradual correction using the Ilizarov external fixation. Open reduction or reconstruction of the radio-ulnar-capitellar joint and/or ligament was not undertaken. The patients were between 9 and 11 years of age at the time of injury. The time from injury to treatment was between 3 and 56 months. At follow-up of an average of 3.5 years (range, 2 to 6 y), all patients had full movement of the elbow and normal function of the forearm. Radiographically, all radial heads were well reduced and the ulnar osteotomy showed remodeling.

Conclusions.—The technique is relatively simple and avoids the risks and technical challenges of open osteotomies, open reduction, and ligament reconstruction. Gradual reduction of the radial head with the aid of an external fixation is a safe and effective method of treatment for chronic Monteggia lesions.

▶ Missed Monteggia fracture dislocations in children pose a treatment challenge for pediatric and upper extremity orthopedic surgeons. Myriad surgical approaches have been proposed including open vs closed reduction, annular ligament repair or reconstruction, and osteotomy of the ulna, radius, or both. The authors present a new surgical technique to address chronic Monteggia fracture dislocations in children. Their retrospective case series included 4 children more than 3 months out from a missed anterior radial head dislocation (Bado Type 1). All 4 patients underwent open ulnar osteotomy through a limited incision with application of a single half-ring-hinged Ilizarov external fixator. The external fixator was in place for 3.5 months on average, and ulnar length and angulation were corrected. Elbow range of motion was improved at final follow-up, most notably in flexion. The only noted complication was a pin tract infection requiring intravenous antibiotics. All 4 radial heads remained reduced at 3.75 years of follow-up.

The authors correctly identify the advantages and disadvantages of this surgical technique. Although this procedure eliminates the need for an open radial head reduction and theoretically decreases the likelihood for delayed ulnar union, the drawbacks include the social implications and technical skill required to apply and manage the Ilizarov fixator. Regardless, the authors add another option to the surgical armamentarium in treating chronic radial head dislocations in children.

Perhaps the most important reminder for all orthopedic surgeons is to obtain orthogonal radiographs of the elbow in any child with an ulnar fracture or plastic deformation of the ulna. I would prefer to treat an acute Monteggia fracture dislocation, and I am sure many surgeons would agree.

A. T. Moeller, MD

Capitellar Fractures—Is Open Reduction and Internal Fixation Necessary?

Cutbush K, Andrews S, Siddiqui N, et al (Brisbane Hand and Upper Limb Res Inst, Queensland, Australia)

J Orthop Trauma 29:50-53, 2015

Objective.—The purpose of this retrospective study was to evaluate the medium-term to longer-term results of type 1 displaced capitellar fractures treated with closed reduction.

Design.—Retrospective case series.

Patients.—Eight consecutive cases (7 adults; 1 child) with type 1 capitellar fractures.

Intervention.—Closed reduction of type 1 capitellar fractures and 4 weeks of postreduction immobilization.

Outcome Measures.—Complications (including radiographic), Disabilities of the Arm, Shoulder, and Hand Score, and active elbow range of motion.

Results.—Average follow-up was 41.6 months (range, 18–77 months). All 8 fractures were united. The patients obtained near full return of the range of motion when compared with the uninjured contralateral side. Mean average Disabilities of the Arm, Shoulder, and Hand Score scores were 4.36 (SD, 2.68; Range, 0–9). No complications were observed.

Conclusions.—This study demonstrated that type 1 capitellar fractures can be treated successfully with closed reduction and cast immobilization.

Level of Evidence.—Therapeutic Level IV. See Instructions for Authors for a complete description of levels of evidence.

▶ The authors present a retrospective consecutive case series of type I capitellar fractures treated with closed reduction and 4 weeks of immobilization. Seven adults and 1 child were treated with this technique with an average follow-up of approximately 3.5 years (41.6 months). They report acceptable clinical outcomes with minimal side-to-side differences in elbow range of motion and an average Disabilities of the Arm, Shoulder, and Hand Score of 4.36. Radiographs were obtained at variable time points throughout the treatment period and at final follow-up. Interestingly, CT imaging was performed at the time of injury but was not repeated at any time point subsequently. At final follow-up, all fractures were united without evidence for avascular necrosis or early osteoarthritic changes. There is no assessment regarding the accuracy of capitellar reduction. However, the authors conclude that closed reduction can achieve anatomic reduction of type I capitellar fractures. Drawing this conclusion is dangerous in light of the study design, small sample size, and retrospective nature. I would also argue that follow-up of 3.5 years does not constitute medium-term to long-term follow-up for true assessment of arthritic changes in a non-weight-bearing joint, such as the elbow. Although closed reduction of type 1 capitellar fractures may prove to be an acceptable treatment method, further prospective, randomized studies that include radiographic assessment of reduction and patient outcomes are necessary to determine the appropriateness of closed treatment.

A. T. Moeller, MD

Closed Reduction and K-Wiring With the Kapandji Technique for Completely Displaced Pediatric Distal Radial Fractures

Satish BRJ, Vinodkumar M, Suresh M, et al (BRJ Orthocentre, Coimbatore, India; Ganganagar Orthocentre, Bangalore, India; et al)

Orthopedics 37:e810-e816, 2014

In completely displaced pediatric distal radial fractures, achieving satisfactory reduction with closed manipulation and maintenance of reduction with casting is difficult. Although the Kapandji technique of K-wiring is widely practiced for distal radial fracture fixation in adults, it is rarely used in pediatric acute fractures. Forty-six completely displaced distal radial fractures in children 7 to 14 years old were treated with closed reduction and K-wire fixation. One or 2 intrafocal K-wires were used to lever out and reduce the distal fragment's posterior and radial translation. One or 2 extrafocal K-wires were used to augment intrafocal fixation. Postoperative immobilization was enforced for 3 to 6 weeks (with a short arm plaster of Paris cast for the first half of the time and a removable wrist splint for the second half), after which time the K-wires were removed. Patients were followed for a minimum of 4 months. Mean patient age was 9.5 years. Near-anatomical reduction was achieved easily with the intrafocal leverage technique in all fractures. Mean procedure time for K-wiring was 7 minutes. On follow-up, there was no loss of reduction; remanipulation was not performed in any case. There were no pin-related complications. All fractures healed, and full function of the wrist and forearm was achieved in every case. The Kapandji K-wire technique consistently achieves easy and near-anatomical closed reduction by a leverage reduction method in completely displaced pediatric distal radial fractures. Reduction is maintained throughout the fracture-healing period. The casting duration can be reduced without loss of reduction, and good functional results can be obtained (Fig 4).

▶ The authors detail their experience with Kapandji pinning of extraphyseal, extra-articular fractures of the pediatric distal radius in 46 patients. The

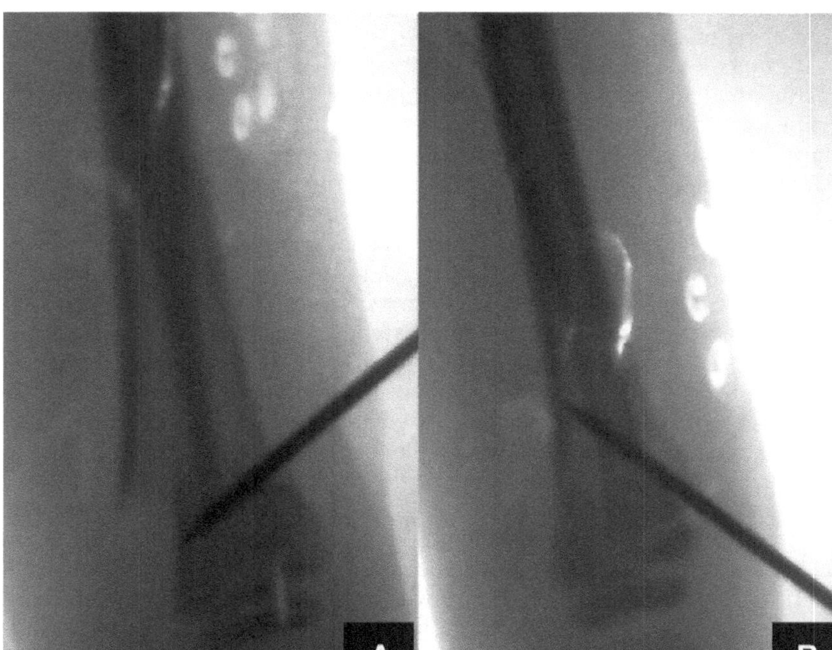

FIGURE 4.—Fluoroscopic lateral views showing levering out of the proximal fragment (A) and reduction to the distal fragment (B) by intrafocal K-wire. (Reprinted with permission from SLACK Incorporated: Satish BRJ, Vinodkumar M, Suresh M, et al. Closed reduction and K-wiring with the Kapandji technique for completely displaced pediatric distal radial fractures. *Orthopedics*. 2014;37:e810-e816.)

technique is well described, and their examples are showpieces of how to perform the technique well. Several points should be noted that contribute to their success: (1) the smallest pins used were 1.5 mm (approximately 0.054 inches), (2) larger children were treated with 2-mm pins, (3) a minimum of 2 orthogonal pins were used (1 dorsal and 1 radial), (4) all pins were placed in the metaphysis with pins not crossing the physis whenever possible, (5) dorsal translation was corrected first followed by radial translation if necessary, and (6) the pins were not buried and were bent for easier removal. The most common mistake that adult hand surgeons make is using small pins for small bones. As Scott Kozin says, "Big pins for big people, big pins for little people."

D. A. Zlotolow, MD

Supracondylar Humeral Fractures with Isolated Anterior Interosseous Nerve Injuries: Is Urgent Treatment Necessary?

Barrett KK, Skaggs DL, Sawyer JR, et al (Children's Hosp Los Angeles, CA; Univ of Tennessee-Campbell Clinic, Memphis; et al)
J Bone Joint Surg Am 96:1793-1797, 2014

Background.—It is unclear if pediatric patients with a supracondylar humeral fracture and isolated anterior interossous nerve injury require urgent treatment.

Methods.—A retrospective, multicenter study of 4409 patients with operatively treated supracondylar humeral fractures was conducted. Exclusion criteria were additional nerve injuries other than the anterior interosseous nerve, any sensory changes, pulselessness, ipsilateral forearm fractures, open fractures, less than two months of follow-up, or pathological fractures.

Results.—Thirty-five of 4409 patients met inclusion criteria. The average time to surgery was 14.6 hours (range, two to thirty-six hours). No patient developed compartment syndrome. There was no significant difference in time to return of anterior interosseous nerve function relative to the time to surgical reduction and fixation ($p = 0.668$). A complete return of anterior interosseous nerve function occurred in all patients with an average time of forty-nine days (range, two to 224 days). Ninety percent of patients recovered anterior interosseous nerve function by 149 days.

Conclusions.—To our knowledge, this is the largest series to date of supracondylar humeral fractures with anterior interosseous nerve injuries. There is no evidence that a supracondylar humeral fracture with an isolated anterior interosseous nerve injury requires urgent treatment. A delay in treatment up to twenty-four hours was not associated with an increased time of nerve recovery or other complications. This series excluded patients with sensory nerve injuries, pulselessness, and ipsilateral forearm fractures, which all may require urgent surgery. Barring other clinical indications for urgent treatment of a supracondylar humeral fracture, an isolated anterior interosseous nerve injury (no sensory changes) may not by itself be an indication for urgent surgery. The anterior interosseous nerve injuries in this series showed complete recovery at a mean time of forty-nine days.

▶ The authors present a retrospective multicenter study of 4409 patients with operative supracondylar humerus fractures and review the outcomes of 35 patients with isolated anterior interosseous nerve injuries. Complete recovery of anterior interosseous nerve (AIN) function occurred in all patients at an average of 49 days, with 90% recovering by 149 days. The average time to surgery was 14.6 hours, and a delay of up to 24 hours was not associated with delayed nerve recovery or other complications. The majority of patients (80%) received no treatment for the nerve injury other than observation, whereas the other 20% received therapy. This is the largest reported series of AIN injuries in association with supracondylar humerus fractures. Based on the data, isolated AIN injuries in this population do not require urgent treatment. Patients and their families can also be reassured that these nerve injuries will recover spontaneously, usually by 5 months, and do well with observation alone. However, supracondylar humerus fractures with multiple nerve injuries or pulselessness on examination do require urgent treatment.

J. I. Huang, MD

Iatrogenic Nerve Injuries in the Treatment of Supracondylar Humerus Fractures: Are We Really Just Missing Nerve Injuries on Preoperative Examination?

Joiner ERA, Skaggs DL, Arkader A, et al (Children's Hosp Los Angeles, CA)
J Pediatr Orthop 34:388-392, 2014

Background.—Recent studies report the rate of iatrogenic nerve injury in operatively treated supracondylar humerus (SCH) fractures is 3% to 4%. A reliable neurological examination can be difficult to obtain in a young child in pain. We hypothesized that nerve injuries may be missed preoperatively, later noted postoperatively in a more compliant patient, and then falsely considered an iatrogenic injury.

Methods.—A prospective study was conducted on patients who presented between April 2011 and April 2013 with an extension-type SCH fracture that was managed surgically. A neurological examination was performed preoperatively, postoperatively, and at follow-up visits by a fellowship-trained attending pediatric orthopaedic surgeon. Only patients in whom the attending surgeon felt a reliable neurovascular examination was obtained were included in this study.

Results.—Of the 100 patients, 16% had a nerve injury recognized on preoperative examination and 3% had a new nerve injury on postoperative examination (1 anterior interosseous, 1 median sensory, and 1 radial motor). The Gartland type ($P = 0.421$), type of reduction (open vs. closed; $P = 0.720$), and number of lateral-entry ($P = 0.898$) or medial-entry ($P = 0.938$) pins used were not associated with patients who had a new nerve injury found postoperatively. A trend was seen between fracture severity and rate of a preoperative nerve injury: type II 7% (2/28), type III 19% (9/58), and type IV 36% (5/14) ($P = 0.058$). Preoperatively, nerve injuries were noted at the following rates: median 12% (12/100) (including 8 anterior interosseous nerve injuries), radial 8% (8/100), ulnar 3% (3/100).

Conclusions.—In this prospective study, in patients who were able to comply with a preoperative neurological examination done by an attending pediatric orthopaedic surgeon, the rate of iatrogenic nerve injury after operative treatment of SCH fractures is 3%. We conclude that this finding is true, and not a result of inadequate preoperative neurological examinations.

Level of Evidence.—Level I prognostic study.

▶ The authors present a prospective study of 100 patients with extension-type pediatric supracondylar fractures that were treated operatively and had a thorough preoperative neurologic examination performed by an attending pediatric orthopedic surgeon. Sixteen patients were noted to have a preoperative neurologic deficit, and only 3 patients were noted to have a new nerve injury postoperatively. This likely represents the ability of a thorough preoperative examination performed by an attending physician to detect a neurologic injury preoperatively. Previous studies may have overreported iatrogenic injuries because of the lack of an adequate preoperative examination. Furthermore, it is possible that some nerve injuries are progressive in nature, and therefore the injury may not be apparent preoperatively but become evident postoperatively. In my institution, all pediatric supracondylar fractures undergo a thorough preoperative neurovascular examination by an attending physician to assess for the presence of any neurologic injury or vascular compromise. Specifically, the anterior interosseous, median, radial, and ulnar nerves are assessed as well as the radial pulse. This also aids the attending physician in determining which patients may be at higher risk for developing an impending compartment syndrome postoperatively and which ones may require additional observation time postoperatively.

J. Abzug, MD

Observation and surgery are associated with low risk of amputation for blunt brachial artery injury in pediatric patients

Tan T-W, Rybin D, Doros G, et al (Louisiana State Univ Health Shreveport; Boston Univ School of Public Health, MA; et al)

J Vasc Surg 60:443-447, 2014

Background.—The ideal treatment for blunt brachial artery (BBA) injury in pediatric patients is controversial. We compared outcomes of surgical and nonsurgical management of BBA injury using the National Trauma Data Bank.

Methods.—All patients younger than 18 years who had suffered BBA injury were identified in the pediatric National Trauma Data Bank

(2002-2010) by Current Procedural Terminology code. Patients with a penetrating mechanism of injury were excluded. By the International Classification of Diseases, Ninth Revision procedure codes, patients were stratified on the basis of treatment modality: observation vs arterial surgery. Outcomes including upper extremity amputation, mortality, and intensive care unit length of stay were compared between the two groups by two-sample *t*-test or χ^2 test as appropriate.

Results.—Among 119 patients with BBA injury, 49 patients (41.2%) underwent arterial surgery and 70 patients (58.8%) were observed. Patients treated with observation were significantly younger, whereas other characteristics including gender and Injury Severity Score were similar. There was no difference in the type of hospital (academic vs nonacademic) or trauma center category between the groups. Two amputations were identified in the database, and both were in the 13- to 17-year age group of the observation cohort (vs arterial surgery; $P = .22$). There were eight fasciotomies identified; five were in the arterial surgery group (10.2% vs observation, 4.3%; $P = .20$). No amputation or fasciotomy was required in the 0- to 6-year age group. Length of stay was similar between groups.

Conclusions.—Despite slightly lower adverse outcomes, arterial surgery does not appear to confer a significant advantage over nonoperative treatment in pediatric patients with BBA injury. In patients younger than 6 years, both modalities appear to be equality effective.

▶ This is a comparative study of outcomes of pediatric patients with blunt brachial artery injury following supracondylar fracture of the humerus and a pink but pulseless hand who underwent either surgical exploration or observation. Patients were accrued through a large national trauma database, the pediatric National Trauma Data Bank. Multivariable analysis was performed, which showed no significant differences in intensive care unit and total hospital length of stay between groups. Also, preoperative outcomes, including mortality, amputation, and fasciotomy, were similar between patients who underwent arterial surgery and those observed. Strengths of the study include a large number of patients accrued through a national trauma database. Weaknesses include a heterogenous patient population of varying ages and different surgical interventions in the group that underwent surgical exploration. In addition, this was a retrospective review, not a prospective study or randomized controlled trial. This study reviews only short-term perioperative outcomes and not the more important long-term functional outcomes in the injured hand or the incidence of complications such as Volkmann ischemic contracture. Overall, this study supports nonoperative treatment in pediatric patients with blunt brachial artery injury. However, more studies are needed to determine the optimal management strategy.

H. Chim, MD

18 Rehabilitation

Sex Differences in Dynamic Closed Kinetic Chain Upper Quarter Function in Collegiate Swimmers

Butler R, Arms J, Reiman M, et al (Duke Univ, Durham, NC; Appalachian State Univ, Boone, NC; et al)

J Athl Train 49:442-446, 2014

Context.—Upper quarter injuries have a higher incidence in female swimmers; however, to date, there are few ways to assess the basic functional ability of this region. The upper quarter Y balance test (YBT-UQ) may assist in this process because it was developed to provide a fundamental assessment of dynamic upper quarter ability at the limit of stability.

Objective.—To examine how sex affects performance on the YBT-UQ in swimmers.

Design.—Cohort study.

Patients or Other Participants.—Forty-three male and 54 female National Collegiate Athletic Association Division I college swimmers were recruited preseason.

Main Outcome Measure(s).—We measured YBT-UQ performance for the left and right limbs in the medial, inferolateral, and superolateral directions. The maximum score for each direction was normalized to upper extremity length. The average of the greatest normalized reach scores in each reach direction was used to develop a composite score (average distance in 3 directions/limb length [LL] × 100). To examine reach symmetry between sexes, the difference in centimeters between the left and right sides was calculated for each reach direction prior to normalization. Statistical analysis was conducted using an independent-samples t test ($P < .05$).

Results.—Average scores in the medial (women: 92.5 ± 7.4% LL, men: 100.0 ± 8.7% LL; $P < .01$) and inferolateral (women: 85.6 ± 10.3% LL, men: 89.8 ± 10.8% LL; $P = .05$) directions and composite score (women: 83.4 ± 8.3% LL, men: 88.3 ± 8.9% LL; $P < .01$) were higher in men than in women. No differences were observed for reach symmetry in any direction.

Conclusions.—Performance on several YBT-UQ indices was worse for female than male collegiate swimmers. These results may have implications for the use of preseason and return-to-sport testing in swimmers as a measurement of upper quarter function and symmetry.

▶ The upper quadrant is reported to be the most commonly injured region among collegiate swimmers. The rate of injury, although high across both genders, is particularly high among women. Reduced core, periscapular, and glenohumeral strength and endurance are predictive of increased risk for upper quadrant injury. Relatedly, there is also some, although minimal, evidence to support that improved closed kinetic chain function is associated with heightened performance and reduced risk of injury among collegiate swimmers.

Leisure swimming is presumably an open chain exercise, as the limbs meet limited resistance; however, competitive swimmers experience greater resistance to limb movement; thus, in that context, swimming could be considered closed chain. For this reason, measures of closed-chain upper quadrant function would appear to have ecologic validly in this population.

Given (1) the association between upper quadrant closed-chain function and upper quadrant injury and (2) the predictive nature of gender on injury among collegiate swimmers, the authors of this study sought to explore if gender differences in closed-chain upper limb function exist within this population. The Upper Quarter Y Balance Test, a reliable measure of dynamic unilateral upper limb reach from a stable quadruped position, was used to measure right and left upper quadrant closed-chain function across 3 movement patterns in 43 male and 54 female noninjured collegiate swimmers.

The results showed that the reach distances used during 2 of the movement patterns (ie, away from midline and diagonally toward the contralateral hip), even when normalized by anthropometrics, were significantly less in women. This was also the trend when composite scores across all 3 patterns were calculated. Within-subject bilateral reach asymmetries, however, were no greater in women than they were in men.

This study's findings support that gender differences in upper quadrant closed-chain performance in this at-risk population do exist. Further study is required to explore how this difference (1) is explained by the performance of select muscle groups or training type and (2) predicts athletic performance and the onset of an upper limb disorder. After predictive validity is established, this tool might serve as a threshold biomarker for off-season training and, in the event that rehabilitation is needed, might provide an indicator of how much improvement is needed for enhanced swimming performance (ie, MCID). Additionally, this tool may have utility in the study of other overhead sports.

The authors suggest that the reach values per limb and across patterns could be used as gender-specific, but not age-specific, reference values. Surgeons and therapists should be familiar with this tool and consider administering to patients who are swimmers with upper quadrant injuries to determine if their values fall outside of what is normal. These findings might aid in planning treatment and discontinuation of services. However, given that the use of this tool in this population requires additional study, careful clinical reasoning must be used when interpreting and applying the findings to the treatment of collegiate swimmers with upper quarter injuries.

C. McGee, PhD, OTR/L, CHT

A custom bicycle handlebar adaptation for children with below elbow amputations

Baker SA, Calhoun VD (Shriners Hosps for Children, St Louis, MO)
J Hand Ther 27:258-260, 2014

As hand therapists, we are always using our creativity to help our patients participate in functional, desired activities. These authors share their expertise in adapting bicycles for children with below elbow amputations.

▶ The authors devised a simple, inexpensive, and effective adaptation for children who have below-elbow amputation or limb discrepancy in order to ride a bicycle. The option of using an upper limb prosthetic, along with the adaptation of bicycles or tricycles that includes knee brakes or custom handle bars, are cited to be costly and often not acceptable to the user. In this article, the bicycle adaptation for grasp of the handlebar is made of thermoplastic material and hose clamps. This adaptation represents an easy means to adapt grasp to control the bicycle handlebar to get on and off and to steer. This article discusses the younger child with increased interest in the activity and the emphasis of keeping up with developmental motor skills concordant with other children. A substantial segment of the article was devoted to the actual supplies and technical aspects of the process to produce the adaptation. The visual illustrations and detailed directions on use of the materials allow the therapist to replicate the adaptations for his or her clients. I believe this handlebar adaptation for children can be also applicable for adults with upper limb discrepancy, making it worthwhile in the clinical practice when working on functional independence.

S. Kranz, OT, CHT

The push-off test: Development of a simple, reliable test of upper extremity weight-bearing capability

Vincent JI, MacDermid JC, Michlovitz SL, et al (Univ of Western Ontario, London, Ontario, Canada; McMaster Univ, Hamilton, Ontario, Canada; et al)
J Hand Ther 27:185-191, 2014

Study Design.—Longitudinal clinical measurement study.

Introduction.—The push-off test (POT) is a novel and simple measure of upper extremity weight-bearing that can be measured with a grip dynamometer. There are no published studies on the validity and reliability of the POT. The relationship between upper extremity self-report activity/participation and impairment measures remain an unexplored realm.

Purpose.—The primary purpose of this study is to estimate the intra and inter-rater reliability and construct validity of the POT. The secondary purpose is to estimate the relationship between upper extremity self-report activity/participation questionnaires and impairment measures.

Methods.—A convenience sample of 22 patients with wrist or elbow injuries were tested for POT, wrist/elbow range of motion (ROM), isometric wrist extension strength (WES) and grip strength; and completed two self-report activity/participation questionnaires: Disability of the Arm, Shoulder and the Hand (DASH) and Work Limitations Questionnaire (WLQ-26). POT's inter and intra-rater reliability and construct validity was tested. Pearson's correlations were run between the impairment measures and self-report questionnaires to look into the relationship amongst them.

Results.—The POT demonstrated high inter-rater reliability (ICC affected = 0.97; 95% C.I. 0.93–0.99; ICC unaffected = 0.85; 95% C.I. 0.68–0.94) and intra-rater reliability (ICC affected = 0.96; 95% C.I. 0.92–0.97; ICC unaffected = 0.92; 95% C.I. 0.85–0.97). The POT was correlated moderately with the DASH ($r = -0.47$; $p = 0.03$). While examining the relationship between upper extremity self-reported activity/participation questionnaires and impairment measures the strongest correlation was between the DASH and the POT ($r = -0.47$; $p = 0.03$) and none of the correlations with the other physical impairment measures reached significance. At-work disability demonstrated insignificant correlations with physical impairments.

Conclusion.—The POT test provides a reliable and easily administered quantitative measure of ability to bear the load through an injured arm. Preliminary evidence supports a moderate relationship between loading bearing measured by the POT and upper extremity function measured by the DASH.

Level of Evidence.—1b.

▶ This study tests the inter- and intrarater reliability and the construct validity of a novel clinic measurement for weight bearing for the upper extremity, with a secondary purpose to estimate the relationship to a self-report activity/participation questionnaire and impairment measures of the Disabilities of the Arm, Shoulder and Hand (DASH)[1] and the Work Limitations Questionnaire (WLQ-26).[2] Those tested in this study were adults with wrist or elbow pain with an average postinjury date of 32 weeks.

The Push-off Test (POT) is described using the readily available grip dynamometer in most clinics. The testing position is the person standing at a table with the buttocks leaning against the table but not sitting on the table. The test arm is positioned in 10° to 40° shoulder extension, and 10° to 40° of elbow flexion. Hand and wrist position is determined by the person in a comfortable position. The dynamometer is placed with the table with the handle in the second stop position (standard position for gripping), the convexity of the handle facing the ceiling. To prevent slippage of the device, the dynamometer is placed on a nonskid surface of the table and further stabilized by the testing therapist.

The test is made to align with the standard gripping procedure of Mathiowetz et al.[3] The verbiage change is from "grip" to "push" using the standard 3 trials. The authors use a 30-second rest between trials.

Impairment tests also used were active range of motion of the wrist and elbow and standard static grip strength. The self-report tests were the DASH and the WLQ-26.

Results of the study found high inter- and intrarater reliability in both the affected and unaffected limbs. The construct validity found a significantly moderate correlation to the DASH but not with the WLQ-26. Also between the DASH and WLQ-26, no significant correlations were found in the subscales. As well, the only impairment measure that correlated to the DASH was the POT.

The authors completed a well-designed clinical measurement study for measurement of weight bearing of the upper limb, using readily available equipment for the physician and the therapist. This early study of the psychometrics will add to the evidence of the rehabilitation progression for wrist and elbow conditions. Further research is, of course, warranted and outlined by the authors.

V. H. O'Brien, OTD, OTR/L, CHT

References

1. Beaton DE, Katz JN, Fossel AH, Wright JG, Tarasuk V, Bombardier C. Measuring the whole or the parts? validity, reliability, and responsiveness of the disabilities of the arm, shoulder and hand outcome measure in different regions of the upper extremity. *J Hand Ther.* 2001;14:128-146.
2. Lerner D, Amick BC 3rd, Rogers WH, Malspeis S, Bungay K, Cynn D. The work limitations questionnaire. *Med Care.* 2001;39:72-85.
3. Mathiowetz V. Effects of three trials on grip and pinch strength measurements. *J Hand Ther.* 1990;3:195-198.

Differences in response rates between mail, e-mail, and telephone follow-up in hand surgery research

Nota SPFT, Strooker JA, Ring D (Massachusetts General Hosp, Boston)
Hand 9:504-510, 2014

Background.—There is a need to determine the difference in response to mail, email, and phone in clinical research surveys.

Methods.—We enrolled 150 new and follow-up patients presenting to our hand and upper extremity department. Patients were assigned to complete a survey by mail, email, or phone 3 months after enrollment, altering the follow-up method every 5 patients, until we had 3 groups of 50 patients. At initial enrollment and at 3 month follow-up (range 2–5 months), patients completed the short version of the Disabilities of the Arm, Shoulder, and Hand questionnaire (QuickDASH), the short version of the Patient Health Questionnaire (PHQ2), the Pain Self-Efficacy Questionnaire (PSEQ), and rated their pain intensity.

Results.—The percent of patients that completed the survey was 34% for mail, 24% for email, and 80% for phone. Factors associated with responding to the survey were older age, nonsmoking, and lower pain intensity. Working fulltime was associated with not responding.

Conclusions.—The response rate to survey by phone is significantly higher than by mail or email. Younger age, smoking, higher pain intensity, and working fulltime are associated with not responding.

Type of Study/Level of Evidence.—Prognostic I.

▶ This study looked at response rates to surveys using 3 different methods: mail, email, and phone. The results showed that phone call surveys had a much higher response rate (80%) compared with the other 2: mail 34% and email 24%. There were some weaknesses of this study: They excluded patients who used the Internet less than once a week and contacted the email/mail participants only once (which has been found to result in a lower response rate). Yet, the results confirm what is well known to those who perform survey work—that direct phone calls result in the best response rate, and email surveys result in the lowest. These results present a dilemma for researchers designing a study: how to balance cost and results. The higher the response rate, the less likely that the sample will be missing a group with important results. However, techniques such as direct participant phone calls, which have the best response rate, are more costly and often not feasible. Thus, much effort has been spent on how to increase response rate for mailed surveys, which are less costly. Some techniques to increase response rate to mailed surveys include increasing number of contacts, hand writing envelopes, and using stamps for postage. Including a small incentive with the survey has been found to increase response rate, appealing to a sense of obligation (whereas a gift after survey completion tends not to increase response rate). Appealing to participants' senses of social responsibility can also improve response rate. Using phrases such as "your participation will really help us out" can improve response rate. A nice review of these techniques is in the "Survey Kit" by Arlene Fink.[1] However, the role of mailed surveys is becoming less clear, as paper mail is used less and less in the digital age. This leaves future researchers in a difficult position because electronic surveys have repeatedly performed poorly. Future efforts will need to study methods to improve response rates using electronic methods.

C. Curtin, MD

Reference

1. Fink A. *The Survey Kit*. 2nd ed. Thousand Oaks, CA: Sage publications; 2003.

Elbow Joint Fatigue and Bench-Press Training

Huang Y-P, Chou Y-L, Chen F-C, et al (Cheng-Kung Univ, Tainan, Taiwan; et al)
J Athl Train 49:317-321, 2014

Context.—Bench-press exercises are among the most common form of training exercise for the upper extremity because they yield a notable improvement in both muscle strength and muscle endurance. The literature contains various investigations into the effects of different bench-press positions on the degree of muscle activation. However, the effects of fatigue on the muscular performance and kinetics of the elbow joint are not understood fully.

Objective.—To investigate the effects of fatigue on the kinetics and myodynamic performance of the elbow joint in bench-press training.

Design.—Controlled laboratory study.

Setting.—Motion research laboratory.

Patients or Other Participants.—A total of 18 physically healthy male students (age = 19.6 ± 0.8 years, height = 168.7 ± 5.5 cm, mass = 69.6 ± 8.6 kg) participated in the investigation. All participants were right-hand dominant, and none had a history of upper extremity injuries or disorders.

Intervention(s).—Participants performed bench-press training until fatigued.

Main Outcome Measure(s).—Maximal possible number of repetitions, cycle time, myodynamic decline rate, elbow-joint force, and elbow-joint moment.

Results.—We observed a difference in cycle time in the initial (2.1 ± 0.42 seconds) and fatigue (2.58 ± 0.46 seconds) stages of the bench-press exercise ($P = .04$). As the participants fatigued, we observed an increase in the medial-lateral force ($P = .03$) and internal-external moment ($P \leq .04$) acting on the elbow joint. Moreover, a reduction in the elbow muscle strength was observed in the elbow extension-flexion ($P \leq .003$) and forearm supination-pronation ($P \leq .001$) conditions.

Conclusions.—The results suggest that performing bench-press exercises to the point of fatigue increases elbow-joint loading and may further increase the risk of injury. Therefore, when clinicians design bench-press exercise regimens for general athletic training, muscle strengthening, or physical rehabilitation, they should control carefully the maximal number of repetitions.

▶ Rehabilitation is a crucial part of recovery for shoulder and elbow injuries. The exact protocol that should be used remains ambiguous, but strengthening regimens become important after the initial healing phase for most injuries. It is important that patients safely and effectively rehabilitate. The current study evaluates muscle fatigue while bench pressing and its effects on the elbow joint. The study is well designed and incorporates complex video motion analysis. The data clearly show that when an individual bench press exercises to the point of fatigue, the elbow kinematics is altered, and there is a risk of injury. Some of the limitations of the study include the number of assumptions needed to do the analysis, the potential error from the equipment itself, and the variation in placement of the skin markers. The clinical applicability remains to be seen. For this commentator, the study underscores the importance of involving a certified therapist in the rehabilitation of postsurgical patients to minimize associated injuries. It is up to the physician to decide which patient needs extra guidance and who is safe for unguided therapy. As with all rehabilitation, form should be emphasized over weight, and patients should be encouraged to stop once fatigued. The future of rehabilitation medicine may include muscle strength and fatigue testing to determine whether patients are able to return to activities of daily living, driving, or work.

M. B. Gottschalk, MD
J. T. Capo, MD

Evaluation of the PROMIS Physical Function Computer Adaptive Test in the Upper Extremity

Tyser AR, Beckmann J, Franklin JD, et al (Univ of Utah, Salt Lake City)
J Hand Surg Am 39:2047-2051, 2014

Purpose.—To compare psychometric and responder burden characteristics between the Patient-Reported Outcomes Measurement Information System Physical Function Computer Adaptive Test (PF CAT) and the Disabilities of Arm, Shoulder, and Hand (DASH) instruments in a tertiary hand and upper extremity practice.

Methods.—Adult patients who presented to the clinic of 2 hand and upper extremity surgeons in a university-based tertiary care center were enrolled in this study. Participants received the DASH and PF CAT administered via tablet computer. Time to completion was recorded for both the DASH and PF CAT. We conducted statistical analyses to calculate Pearson correlation coefficients between the 2 instruments and performed a Rasch item response theory analysis to determine dimensionality, reliability, ceiling and floor effects, and item bias for each instrument.

Results.—A total of 134 patients were included. Time to completion for the DASH was 262 seconds, and for the PF CAT 57 seconds. The instruments had strong correlation ($r = 0.726$). The item and Pearson reliability were 0.97 and 0.94, respectively, for the DASH and 0.99 and 0.96 for the PF CAT. The DASH and PF CAT had 5% and 5% of unexplained variance, respectively. The DASH exhibited 5% of ceiling effect and 1% floor effect whereas the PF CAT had no ceiling or floor effects.

Conclusions.—The psychometric characteristics of the Patient-Reported Outcomes Measurement Information System PF CAT instrument compared favorably with the DASH in a tertiary upper extremity practice. Patient time burden was significantly reduced with the PF CAT compared with the DASH.

Type of Study/Level of Evidence.—Diagnostic III.

▶ The Patient Reported Outcomes Measurement Information System Physical Function Computer Adaptive Test (PROMIS PF CAT) is a validated patient self-assessment outcomes measurement tool that has the advantage of brevity and nominal cost. The authors of this study sought to compare the utility of this tool with that of the Disabilities of Arm, Shoulder, and Hand (DASH) outcomes measurement tool within the context of a hand and upper extremity practice at a large tertiary care university medical center. The authors found that time to completion of the PROMIS questionnaire was significantly less and that there was strong correlation in terms of reliability between the PROMIS questionnaire and the DASH. One uncontrolled variable in the study was the inclusion of all diagnoses of new patients and return patients to each group, whereby some element of selection bias could have influenced the results of the study. Nonetheless, the PROMIS PF CAT has applicability to hand and upper extremity surgery. Studies concerning specific conditions would be helpful in further defining the usefulness of this measurement tool.

P. Murray, MD

19 Miscellaneous

Primary Tuberculosis of the Clavicle

Prakash J, Aggarwal S, Mehtani A (Lady Hardinge Med College, New Delhi, India)

Orthopedics 37:e879-e884, 2014

Tuberculosis of the clavicle is a rare lesion, accounting for less than 1% of all osteoarticular tuberculosis. The lesion has been described in a few case reports. The lesion can have a varied presentation, ranging from dull, aching pain to bony swelling and a draining sinus. The rarity of the lesion, its nonspecific symptoms, and its striking resemblance to common cystic conditions such as bone tumors and metabolic conditions such as rickets make diagnosis difficult. The authors describe a series of 17 patients with primary tuberculosis of the clavicle. Radiographs and magnetic resonance images were obtained for all patients, and a preliminary diagnosis was made on the basis of clinical features and the results of erythrocyte sedimentation rate, C-reactive protein, and Mantoux tests. Erythrocyte sedimentation rate was uniformly elevated. Radiographs showed diffused thickening and honeycombing, eccentric expansile lytic lesions with surrounding osteopenia, or sequestration not unlike pyogenic infection. Magnetic resonance imaging is useful for determining the extent of the lesion and soft tissue involvement. The radiological and laboratory findings provided complementary information. The diagnosis was confirmed on biopsy material that was analyzed with histopathology, pus culture and sensitivities, gram stain, acid-fast stain, and cultures on Löwenstein-Jensen medium. Patients were treated with multidrug antitubercular chemotherapy for 18 months and were assessed on pre- and post-treatment radiology, erythrocyte sedimentation rate, and University of California, Los Angeles (UCLA) shoulder rating scale. The results of conservative management of tubercular osteomyelitis were uniformly good, and all patients recovered well.

▶ In this article, the New Delhi-based authors describe a prospective case series of patients who were treated for isolated tuberculosis infection of the clavicle. The tuberculosis was diagnosed with biopsy, MRI, radiographs, serum laboratory values, and Mantoux skin testing. All patients were treated with medication only; no surgical debridement was performed. All patients had complete resolution of their infection without relapse.

This is an article that I initially dismissed as being irrelevant to my daily practice. However, after reviewing the article and casually observing my patients, I changed my mind. We live in a modern, global community in which patients' lives are not confined to tidy national and geographic boarders. Patients can be exposed to tuberculosis from a variety of sources. Visiting foreign family members, personal travel, immigration from other countries, and even occupational contacts can be a source of tuberculosis infection.

I feel the article is pertinent and that there are 3 salient points worth remembering: (1) osseous clavicular tuberculosis infection is rare but yet a possible presentation, (2) the disease may be manifest without clinical evidence of pulmonary involvement, and (3) surgical debridement is not necessary for a cure.

N. A. Hoekzema, MD

Surgical Trends in the Treatment of Superior Labrum Anterior and Posterior Lesions of the Shoulder: Analysis of Data From the American Board of Orthopaedic Surgery Certification Examination Database

Patterson BM, Creighton RA, Spang JT, et al (Univ of North Carolina at Chapel Hill; et al)

Am J Sports Med 42:1904-1910, 2014

Background.—After failure of nonoperative treatment, repair has long been the primary treatment option for symptomatic superior labrum anterior and posterior (SLAP) lesions of the shoulder. There is growing evidence to support both biceps tenotomy and tenodesis as effective alternative treatments for SLAP lesions.

Hypotheses.—For patients with isolated SLAP lesions, the frequency of SLAP repair has decreased, while treatment with biceps tenodesis and tenotomy has increased. Similar trends are expected in patients with SLAP lesions undergoing concomitant rotator cuff repair.

Study Design.—Cohort study; Level of evidence, 3.

Methods.—A query of the American Board of Orthopaedic Surgery part II database was performed from 2002 to 2011. The database was searched for patients with isolated SLAP lesions undergoing SLAP repair, open biceps tenodesis, arthroscopic biceps tenodesis, or biceps tenotomy. The database was then queried a second time for patients undergoing arthroscopic rotator cuff repair with concomitant SLAP repair, biceps tenodesis, or biceps tenotomy.

Results.—From 2002 to 2011, there were 8963 cases reported for the treatment of an isolated SLAP lesion and 1540 cases reported for the treatment of SLAP lesions with concomitant rotator cuff repair. For patients with isolated SLAP lesions, the proportion of SLAP repairs decreased from 69.3% to 44.8% ($P < .0001$), while biceps tenodesis increased from 1.9% to 18.8% ($P < .0001$), and biceps tenotomy increased from 0.4% to 1.7% ($P = .018$). For patients undergoing concomitant rotator cuff repair, SLAP repair decreased from 60.2% to 15.3% ($P < .0001$), while biceps tenodesis or tenotomy increased from 6.0% to 28.0% ($P < .0001$). There was a significant difference in the mean age of patients undergoing SLAP repair (37.1 years) versus biceps tenodesis (47.2 years) versus biceps tenotomy (55.7 years) ($P < .0001$).

Conclusion.—Practice trends for orthopaedic board candidates indicate that the proportion of SLAP repairs has decreased over time, with an increase in biceps tenodesis and tenotomy. Increased patient age correlates with the likelihood of treatment with biceps tenodesis or tenotomy versus SLAP repair.

▶ The authors queried the database from American Board of Orthopaedic Surgery part II test takers to ascertain the changes in treatment of superior labrum anterior and posterior (SLAP) tears over time. An increase in use of biceps tenodesis and tenotomy over SLAP repair was seen, particularly in those test takers who had subspecialty training in shoulder and elbow surgery. The changes likely reflect recent changes in the understanding of treatment of SLAP tears and suggest that those with subspecialty training may be at the forefront of the shift in treatment strategies. These data remind us that surgical trends and our understanding of the optimal treatment strategies for certain conditions are subject to changes over time.

J. E. Adams, MD

Comparison of 3-Dimensional Shoulder Complex Kinematics in Individuals With and Without Shoulder Pain, Part 2: Glenohumeral Joint

Lawrence RL, Braman JP, Staker JL, et al (Univ of Minnesota, Minneapolis; et al)

J Orthop Sports Phys Ther 44:646-655, 2014

Study Design.—Cross-sectional.

Objectives.—To compare differences in glenohumeral joint angular motion and linear translations between symptomatic and asymptomatic individuals during shoulder motion performed in 3 planes of humerothoracic elevation.

Background.—Numerous clinical theories have linked abnormal glenohumeral kinematics, including decreased glenohumeral external rotation and increased superior translation, to individuals with shoulder pain and impingement diagnoses. However, relatively few studies have investigated glenohumeral joint angular motion and linear translations in this population.

Methods.—Transcortical bone pins were inserted into the scapula and humerus of 12 asymptomatic and 10 symptomatic participants for direct bone-fixed tracking using electromagnetic sensors. Glenohumeral joint angular positions and linear translations were calculated during active shoulder flexion, abduction, and scapular plane abduction.

Results.—Differences between groups in angular positions were limited to glenohumeral elevation, coinciding with a reduction in scapulothoracic upward rotation. Symptomatic participants demonstrated 1.4 mm more anterior glenohumeral translation between 90° and 120° of shoulder flexion and an average of 1 mm more inferior glenohumeral translation throughout shoulder abduction.

Conclusion.—Differences in glenohumeral kinematics exist between symptomatic and asymptomatic individuals. The clinical implications of these differences are not yet understood, and more research is needed to understand the relationship between abnormal kinematics, shoulder pain, and pathoanatomy.

▶ This interesting report investigates the alterations in motion and kinematics in patients with shoulder pain over normal controls. Two cohorts of patients (those with asymptomatic shoulders and those with shoulder pain) underwent evaluation of glenohumeral and scapulothoracic motion using electromagnetic sensors. Statistically significant differences in the motion patterns were seen in patients with and without shoulder pain, which were related to differences in the scapulothoracic kinematics. This and the companion report suggest that the mechanics of the sternoclavicular, acromioclavicular, and scapulothoracic joints influence glenohumeral joint kinematics when positioning the hand in space. Moreover, there may be compensatory mechanisms in the setting of shoulder pain, in which shoulder pain results in or results from altered kinematics of the shoulder complex.

J. E. Adams, MD

Collateral Ligament Laxity of the Finger Metacarpophalangeal Joints: An *In Vivo* Study

Lutsky K, Matzon J, Walinchus L, et al (Rothman Inst, Philadelphia, PA)
J Hand Surg Am 39:1088-1093, 2014

Purpose.—To assess the normal degree of laxity of the collateral ligaments (CLs) of the finger metacarpophalangeal (MCP) joints and to compare side-to-side differences in CL laxity.

Methods.—One hundred subjects had measurements of the degree of laxity in the radial (RCL) and ulnar (UCL) collateral ligaments of the MCP joints of each digit on both hands with the joints at neutral and at 30° and 90° of flexion using a custom-made measuring device. Statistical analysis was performed to assess both the difference in laxity for each ligament at each position of flexion and between sides for analogous ligaments (eg, the right index RCL at neutral compared to the left index RCL at neutral).

Results.—There was a significant decrease in laxity for all ligaments between neutral (mean, 24° laxity) and 90° of flexion (mean, 15° laxity). There was a side-to-side difference between the RCL of all digits in extension (mean, 3°) and the index RCL in flexion (2°). These differences were statistically significant but clinically minimal. There were no side-to-side differences between any of the other ligaments at any position.

Conclusions.—Finger MCP joint CL stability increases with increasing flexion of the joint. There is little to no difference between analogous ligaments on either hand of the subject when tested in the same position of MCP joint flexion. Knowledge of the average degree of MCP joint CL laxity can be helpful in assessing a potentially injured joint. A patient's contralateral, uninjured side can be used to determine that individual's normal laxity and a substantial increase from this on an injured digit can indicate CL rupture.

Type of Study/Level of Evidence.—Diagnostic II.

▶ The present paper provides hand surgeons with data on the "normal" laxity of metacarpophalangeal (MCP) joints of fingers except the thumb. Even though data for thumb MCP joint angulation are available and widely used as a criterion for treatment decisions, knowledge of the normal range of MCP angulation of the other fingers in a healthy person has been sparse thus far. The authors also provide a recommendation for the investigation of an injured joint: examination in neutral position and in 90 degrees of flexion.

A possible weakness of this study, which is not discussed by the authors, is the selection of the study pool: The authors investigated patients who visited a hand surgery office. Even though they did their best to exclude patients whose MCP mobility might have been influenced by the underlying hand problem, it remains unclear if they really investigated only "normal hands."

Nevertheless, the data presented in this publication will serve as a useful reference for the diagnosis and treatment of collateral ligament injuries or diseases.

M. Choi, MD

Return to Football and Long-Term Clinical Outcomes After Thumb Ulnar Collateral Ligament Suture Anchor Repair in Collegiate Athletes

Werner BC, Hadeed MM, Lyons ML, et al (Univ of Virginia Health System, Charlottesville)

J Hand Surg Am 39:1992-1998, 2014

Purpose.—To evaluate return to play after complete thumb ulnar collateral ligament (UCL) injury treated with suture anchor repair for both skill position and non–skill position collegiate football athletes and report minimum 2-year clinical outcomes in this population.

Methods.—For this retrospective study, inclusion criteria were complete rupture of the thumb UCL and suture anchor repair in a collegiate football athlete performed by a single surgeon who used an identical technique for all patients. Data collection included chart review, determination of return to play, and Quick Disabilities of the Arm, Shoulder, and Hand (*Quick*-DASH) outcomes.

Results.—A total of 18 collegiate football athletes were identified, all of whom were evaluated for follow-up by telephone, e-mail, or regular mail at an average 6-year follow-up. Nine were skill position players; the remaining 9 played in nonskill positions. All players returned to at least the same level of play. The average *Quick*DASH score for the entire cohort was 1 out of 100; *Quick*DASH work score, 0 out of 100; and sport score, 1 out of 100. Average time to surgery for skill position players was 12 days compared with 43 for non–skill position players. Average return to play for skill position players was 7 weeks postoperatively compared with 4 weeks for non–skill position players. There was no difference in average *Quick*DASH overall scores or subgroup scores between cohorts.

Conclusions.—Collegiate football athletes treated for thumb UCL injuries with suture anchor repair had quick return to play, reliable return to the same level of activity, and excellent long-term clinical outcomes. Skill position players had surgery sooner after injury and returned to play later than non–skill position players, with no differences in final level of play or clinical outcomes. Management of thumb UCL injuries in collegiate football athletes can be safely and effectively tailored according to the demands of the player's football position.

Type of Study/Level of Evidence.—Therapeutic IV

▶ The authors present a retrospective series of collegiate football athletes that had repair of a thumb metacarpophalangeal joint ulnar collateral ligament using bone anchors. In their series, return to play was on average 7 weeks for skill players and 4 weeks for nonskill players. Unfortunately, no clinical assessment has been performed at long-term follow-up; however, excellent Quick Disabilities of the Arm, Shoulder, and Hand (*Quick*DASH) scores suggest that the athletes are functioning well. My personal experience in dealing with elite athletes using a bone anchor repair has also been similarly favorable. My rehabilitation differs in that early flexion and extension exercises within 10 days are encouraged and a protective low-profile splint is worn between exercises. The splint is worn to play and train for protection until the ligament has healed, usually somewhere between 8 and 10 weeks. We have noticed some of our athletes like the protective splint so much that they have had them custom-made prophylactically for the noninjured thumb.

M. Hayton, MD

Comparison of the Anatomical Dimensions and Mechanical Properties of the Dorsoradial and Anterior Oblique Ligaments of the Trapeziometacarpal Joint

D'Agostino P, Kerkhof FD, Shahabpour M, et al (KU Leuven, Kortrijk, Belgium; Louise Med Ctr, Kortrijk, Belgium; St-Elisabeth Clinic, Kortrijk, Belgium; et al)
J Hand Surg Am 39:1098-1107, 2014

Purpose.—The respective roles of the dorsoradial (DRL) and anterior oblique (AOL) ligaments in stability of the highly mobile trapeziometacarpal (TMC) joint remain disputed. Earlier publications have pointed to the

AOL as the key stabilizing structure; yet, more recent publications have challenged the stabilizing role of the AOL, favoring the DRL as the main TMC joint stabilizer. We executed an anatomical study of the ligaments, including detailed dissection to quantify the length, width, and thickness of the AOL and DRL and tested the material properties of these ligaments.

Methods.—Thirteen fresh frozen cadaveric thumbs from 9 specimens were used. Length, width, and thickness of the AOL and DRL were measured on magnetic resonance imaging and/or after dissection. Next, the first metacarpal and trapezium were isolated together with both ligaments, and both bones were cut sagittally to isolate a first metacarpal—AOL—trapezium and first metacarpal—DRL—trapezium complex from each thumb. These samples were subjected to cyclic loading in displacement-controlled tests. The obtained force-displacement curves were used to calculate stiffness and hysteresis of each sample.

Results.—Our results showed that the DRL is significantly shorter and thicker than the AOL, which is thin and ill-defined. Our results also indicate that the DRL has a higher stiffness than the AOL, making it a more likely candidate to provide joint stability.

Conclusions.—Although the AOL has been asserted to be the primary restraint to dorsoradial subluxation, this view has been challenged over the past 10 years by several studies. These studies have shown the AOL to be relatively weak and compliant compared with the intermetacarpal and dorsoradial ligaments and have demonstrated that the DRL is the strongest and stiffest ligament of the TMC joint. Our studies confirm these findings.

Clinical Relevance.—This study indicates that the DRL is relatively stiff and thick, suggesting it should be repaired or reconstructed when disrupted to restore stability of the TMC joint.

▶ The first carpometacarpal joint has a complex articular geometry and requires multiple ligamentous stabilizers to afford both mobility and stability.

Much work has been done to elucidate the various ligamentous structures that support and restrain this joint. This knowledge is important because the loss or injury to these structures has been associated with joint instability and joint degeneration.

As the authors point out, early work in this area has considered the anterior oblique ligament (AOL) to be the main restraint to dorsoradial subluxation.[1] However, some more recent work by Strauch,[2] Bettinger,[3] and others has not just refined previous work but also suggested that the AOL may not be the only key to the joint stability. The other candidate is the dorsoradial ligament (DRL).

In this study, 2 methods of measurements were used to assess the length and thickness of the ligaments. Both MRI and calipers were used. However, because of significant discrepancy between the 2 result sets, MRI was selected as the more accurate method and reported. Based on the physical characteristics and biomechanical properties of the AOL and DRL, the authors suggest that the DRL may be the primary restraint to dorsoradial subluxation.

There is consensus that the ligamentous structures afford the trapeziometacarpal joint much of its stability. Assessment of the relative contributions of various ligaments to joint stability have been done by assessing their physical dimensions, structural properties, tautness in various joint positions, and correlating the status of the ligaments in various stages of trapeziometacarpal joint arthritis.

The DRL is not affected in early-stage trapeziometacarpal osteoarthritis, and reconstruction of the AOL using the Eaton-Littler procedure has been clinically successful. Doyle and Botte[4] and others have pointed out that the Eaton procedure does to some extent reconstruct the dorsal ligamentous components.

Given the complexity of the joint, it is likely that both AOL and DRL, as well as other components of the ligamentous complex, contribute to the stability of the joint. Their relative contribution may differ, depending on the position of thumb and direction of force application. The verdict is still out as to which one is more important during common injury or use patterns.

A. Chong, MD

References

1. Pellegrini VD Jr. Pathomechanics of the thumb trapeziometacarpal joint. *Hand Clin.* 2001;17:175-184, vii-viii.
2. Strauch RJ, Behrman MJ, Rosenwasser MP. Acute dislocation of the carpometacarpal joint of the thumb: an anatomic and cadaver study. *J Hand Surg Am.* 1994;19:93-98.
3. Bettinger PC, Linscheid RL, Berger RA, Cooney WP 3rd, An K-N. An anatomic study of the stabilizing ligaments of the trapezium and trapeziometacarpal joint. *J Hand Surg Am.* 1999;24:786-798.
4. Doyle JR, Botte MJ. Hand. In: Doyle JR, Botte MJ, eds. *Surgical Anatomy of the Hand and Upper Extremity.* Philadelphia, PA: Lippincott Williams & Wilkins; 2003:204.

The Impact of Obesity on Complications of Elbow, Forearm, and Hand Surgeries

London DA, Stepan JG, Lalchandani GR, et al (Washington Univ in St. Louis School of Medicine; St. Louis Univ School of Medicine, MO; Case Western Reserve Univ, Cleveland, OH)

J Hand Surg Am 39:1578-1584, 2014

Purpose.—To compare the rates of postoperative complications in obese and nonobese patients following elbow, forearm, and hand surgeries.

Methods.—This case-control study examined 436 patients whose body mass index (BMI) was over 35 and who underwent hand, wrist, forearm, or elbow surgery between 2009 and 2013. Controls were patients (n = 433) with a BMI less than 30 who had similar surgeries over the same period, and who were frequency-matched by type of surgery (ie, bony, soft tissue, or nerve), age, and sex. Postoperative complications were defined as infection requiring antibiotic or reoperation, delayed incision healing, nerve dysfunction, wound dehiscence, hematoma, and other reoperation. Medical comorbidities (eg, hypertension, diabetes, stroke, vascular disease, kidney disease, and liver disease) were recorded. Chi-square analyses were performed to explore the association between obesity and postoperative complications. Similar analyses were performed stratified by surgery type and BMI classification. Logistic regression modeling was performed to identify predictors of postoperative complications accounting for surgery type, BMI, the presence of comorbidities, patient age, and patient sex. This same model was also run separately for case and control patients.

Results.—The overall complication rate was 8.7% with similar rates between obese and nonobese patients (8.5% vs 9.0%). Bony procedures resulted in the greatest risk of complication in both groups (15% each group). Multivariate analysis confirmed surgery type as the only significant predictor of complications for nonobese patients. However, among obese patients, both bony surgery and increasing BMI were associated with greater complication rates.

Conclusions.—Not all obese patients appear to be at any higher risk for complications after elbow, forearm, and hand surgery compared with nonobese patients. However, there appears to be a dose-dependent effect of BMI among obese patients such that increasing obesity heightens the risk of complications, especially for those with a BMI greater than 45.

Type of Study/Level of Evidence.—Prognostic II.

▶ This case-control study compared the rates of postoperative complications in an obese (body mass index [BMI] > 35, n = 346) vs nonobese (BMI < 30, n = 433) patient population that underwent hand, wrist, forearm, and elbow surgery at 1 institution between 2009 and 2013. Postoperative complications were defined as infection requiring antibiotic or reoperation, delayed incisional healing, nerve dysfunction, wound dehiscence, hematoma, and other reoperation. The complication rates were similar between the nonobese and the obese groups; however, bony surgery and increasing BMI (> 45) were associated with increased complication rates in the obese group. The authors discussed the potential reasons for the discrepancy between their upper extremity surgery data and the data presented in the lower extremity literature on complications associated with obesity.

The reasons for upper extremity preference may include shorter surgical duration, decreased thromboembolic risk, less subcutaneous fat, and more frequent use of regional anesthetics. In my practice, I will continue to counsel my patients about the general health risks associated with obesity and will continue to encourage weight loss. In the morbidly obese and super obese undergoing elective surgery, I will continue to delay elective surgery whenever possible.

J. Tueting, MD

Carpal Tunnel Syndrome: Assessment of Surgeon and Patient Preferences and Priorities for Decision-Making

Hageman MGJS, Science of Variation Group (Massachusetts General Hosp, Boston)

J Hand Surg Am 39:1799-1804.e1, 2014

Purpose.—This study tested the null hypothesis that there are no differences between the preferences of hand surgeons and those patients with carpal tunnel syndrome (CTS) facing decisions about management of CTS (ie, the preferred content of a decision aid).

Methods.—One hundred three hand surgeons of the Science of Variation Group and 79 patients with CTS completed a survey about their priorities and preferences in decision making regarding the management of CTS. The questionnaire was structured according the Ottawa Decision Support Framework for the development of a decision aid.

Results.—Important areas on which patient and hand surgeon interests differed included a preference for nonpainful, nonoperative treatment and confirmation of the diagnosis with electrodiagnostic testing. For patients, the main disadvantage of nonoperative treatment was that it was likely to be only palliative and temporary. Patients preferred, on average, to take the lead in decision making, whereas physicians preferred shared decision making. Patients and physicians agreed on the value of support from family and other physicians in the decision-making process.

Conclusions.—There were some differences between patient and surgeon priorities and preferences regarding decision making for CTS, particularly the risks and benefits of diagnostic and therapeutic procedures.

Clinical Relevance.—Information that helps inform patients of their options based on current best evidence might help patients understand their own preferences and values, reduce decisional conflict, limit surgeon-to-surgeon variations, and improve health.

▶ This project assessed patient and surgeon perspectives about carpal tunnel syndrome treatment. The goal is to identify areas of conflict and guide the development of decision aides. Not surprisingly, the authors found that patients and surgeons did differ, especially in areas such as the role of nerve diagnostics and the bother of orthoses. Interestingly, in regard to the disadvantages to surgery, patients were more concerned about painful scars than were the surgeons. Eighteen percent of the surgeons listed scar as the disadvantage of surgery, but what is it about the scar? If the surgeons are concerned about the pain in the scar, then the surgeons and patients are actually in more concordance than the percentages suggest. This lack of clarity highlights the challenges of these types of studies and the difficulty of face validity when working with 2 different populations. There is clearly a need to bridge the divide between the perspectives of surgeons and their patients, and studies exploring these issues are important first steps.

C. Curtin, MD

Evidence for safe tourniquet use in 500 consecutive upper extremity procedures

Drolet BC, Okhah Z, Phillips BZ, et al (Warren Alpert Med School of Brown Univ, Providence, RI; Washington Univ, St Louis, MO; et al)

Hand 9:494-498, 2014

Background.—Although pneumatic tourniquets are widely used in upper extremity surgery, further evidence is needed to support their safe use. Excessive pressure and prolonged ischemic time can cause soft-tissue injury. The purpose of this study was to determine the safety of tourniquet use in a yearlong, consecutive series of patients.

Methods.—A retrospective review of all patients who underwent upper extremity surgery by two board-certified hand surgeons over a 1-year period was performed. Demographic variables, comorbidities, and complications were noted along with tourniquet parameters, including application site, ischemic pressure, and time.

Results.—A total 505 patients were included in the study because a tourniquet was used during their operation. Patients ranged in age from 3 months to 90 years old (mean 40.1 years). More than half of the population was overweight (mean body mass index (BMI) 27.1), and 77.1% of adults had at least one cardiac risk factor. No immediate or delayed tourniquet-related injuries were identified. The average operative time was 35.9 min, with an average tourniquet time of 33.1 min. Tourniquet inflation pressure of 250 or 225 mm Hg was utilized in 78 and 21% of adult patients, respectively; no patients had a pressure setting exceeding 275 mm Hg.

Conclusion.—In this series of more than 500 operations, there were no immediate or delayed tourniquet-related events using parameters determined perioperatively by the attending surgeon. Tourniquet pressures of 250 mm Hg or less in adult patients with less than 2 h of ischemic time appear to be safe, even in the elderly and patients with multiple medical comorbidities.

▶ The use of tourniquets in hand surgery is pervasive. However, the evidence behind appropriate use is certainly lacking. The potential complications are worthy of a standardized approach to their use. This retrospective series is a valuable follow-up to the previous review done at the same institution in 2012.[1] Fittingly, the authors have departed from the basic science view to a clinical review. Their study has a reasonable number of patients with a wide range of ages, comorbidities, and other variables that are shown in the literature to be related to potential complications. Additionally, there is reassurance in the article's ability to substantiate the common parameters of tourniquet use accepted by most hand surgeons. Nevertheless, despite the sizable number of patients, the very short tourniquet times and lack of variation may not have been adequate to detect complications. Further, there were only 7 cases outside of the commonly accepted 120-minute window and 1 case exceeding 134 minutes. As the authors point out, the sample size would need to be increased and the variation in tourniquet time increased to detect complications in an area of already remarkably rare complications. This valuable article affirms my group's current practice, and we look forward to potential prospective reports.

J. C. Saillant, MD

Reference

1. Fitzgibbons PG, DiGiovanni C, Hares S, Akelman E. Safe tourniquet use: a review of the evidence. *J Am Acad Orthop Surg*. 2012;20:310-319.

Volar locking plate fixation of distal radius fractures: use of an intra-operative 'carpal shoot through' view to identify dorsal compartment and distal radioulnar joint screw penetration

Marsland D, Hobbs CM, Sauvé PS (Queen Alexandra Hosp, Portsmouth, UK)
Hand 9:516-521, 2014

Introduction.—We report our experience using a 'carpal shoot through' view of the distal radius to identify dorsal compartment screw penetration intra-operatively when performing volar plating of the distal radius.

Methods.—A prospective study of 42 patients (mean age 56 years) with acute distal radius fractures treated with open reduction internal fixation was undertaken. Surgical fixation was performed using a volar locking plate in all patients. After plate application, inclined posteroanterior and lateral radiographs were taken followed by the carpal shoot through view.

Results.—In six cases (14 %), the carpal shoot through view revealed dorsal screw protrusion, which was not detectable on standard PA and lateral views. In one case, a screw had penetrated the distal radioulnar joint (DRUJ), which was only apparent on the shoot through view. The overall screw exchange rate was 17 %.

Conclusions.—Using the hand and carpus to minimise the contrast in X-ray penetration, the dorsal cortex of the distal radius may be imaged intra-operatively and dorsal compartment screw penetration detected in cases with significant multifragmentation when screw measurement is difficult. This view potentially reduces the risk of post-operative pain and extensor tendon injury and also provides excellent visualisation of the DRUJ.

▶ To visualize the dorsal cortex to avoid dorsal compartment screw penetration when performing volar plating of the distal radius, the authors report their experience of what they describe as a "carpal shoot through view." In a prospective study of 42 patients with distal radius fractures all treated with open reduction and internal fixation using a volar locking plate, they performed an intraoperative radiologic examination. They state that conventional fluoroscopy (posteroanterior [PA] and lateral views) is unreliable because screw tips are often hidden by Lister's tubercle. Additional views, such as the dorsal skyline view, have been used; however, the authors describe difficulties with the latter view, as it requires palmar flexion of the wrist giving them unsatisfactory imaging caused by overexposure by the image intensifier. Thus, the authors describe the "carpal shoot view" in which the patient's forearm is supinated, the elbow flexed in approximately 70°, and the wrist dorsiflexed. The image intensifier beam is directed over the base of the thenar eminence, and by using this technique, views of the dorsal cortex and distal radial ulnar joint are obtained; the distal radius is visualized with the carpal bones overlying. Intraoperatively, the investigators checked the placement of the screws using PA and lateral fluoroscopy views; however, in 6 of 42 cases, these conventional views did not detect dorsal screw penetration visible using the above-described "carpal shoot through" view, and in one case penetration of distal radial ulnar joint was detected with this shoot through view.

Volar plating of distal radius fractures has gained popularity as more stable fixation of the bone is achieved and early mobilization is allowed. This treatment, however, may not properly address and avoid complications from the soft tissue. In volar plating, dorsal penetration of screws may lead to irritation, pain, tenosynovitis, and even tendon rupture. These complications may necessitate removal of hardware or tendon reconstruction. Although this usually has been true for the extensor tendons, reports indicate that volar plates may lead to rupture of flexor tendons (eg, the FPL), a complication that can be seen as late as 5 to 10 years after surgery. To avoid these complications, adequate placement of plate and screws is necessary, and this newly described technique may help surgeons. The authors claim that the learning curve to use the technique was short and that general orthopedic trauma surgeons and trainee specialist registrars easily obtained the shoot through view.

In my practice, I've used PA, lateral, and skyline views to check for dorsal penetration of screws. However, I will add this new shoot through view in the future. Good views intraoperatively depend on the fluoroscope as well as the experience of the surgeon, and I'm anxious to see if the learning curve is as short as the authors say. Measurement of the screw lengths is often difficult, and I always try to stay as short as possible. Unicortical fixation is also an option. I inform the patients of potential risks for tendon rupture and do not recommend hardware removal in all patients. However, for younger patients I do recommend removal of plate and screws.

J.-R. Haugstvedt, MD

Health-Related Quality of Life in Patients Undergoing Palmar Fasciectomy for Dupuytren's Disease

Thoma A, Kaur MN, Ignacy TA, et al (McMaster Univ, Hamilton, Ontario, Canada; Univ of Toronto, Ontario, Canada)
Plast Reconstr Surg 133:1411-1419, 2014

Background.—The present study was undertaken to assess the health-related quality of life in patients with Dupuytren's disease who undergo palmar fasciectomy.

Methods.—A prospective cohort of patients with Dupuytren's disease undergoing palmar and/or digital fasciectomy was recruited from the practice of three plastic surgeons in Hamilton, Ontario, Canada. After written informed consent was obtained, participants were asked to complete three health-related quality-of-life questionnaires (i.e., Short Form-36, Michigan Hand Outcomes Questionnaire, and Health Utility Index Mark 3) at five time points: at 1 week and 1 day preoperatively, and at 1, 3, 6, and 12 months postoperatively. Ranges of motion and grip strength measurement were also recorded.

Results.—For the 26 patients in the study, the multiattribute scores of the Health Utility Index Mark 3 improved from 0.80 before surgery to 0.83 at 12 months postoperatively ($p > 0.05$). There was no difference in the Short Form-36 scores, but the Michigan Hand Outcomes Questionnaire scores improved from 74 at 1 week preoperatively to 90 at the 12-month postoperative visit ($p < 0.001$).

Conclusions.—Patients who undergo palmar fasciectomy for Dupuytren's disease experience a substantial improvement in their health-related quality of life 12 months after surgery. In the authors' study population, a benefit of 0.85 quality-adjusted life-year within 12 months was observed. This can be translated as follows: the average patient who undergoes palmar fasciectomy gains the equivalent of approximately 14.4 days (0.48 months) in perfect health by undergoing palmar fasciectomy.

Clinical Question/Level of Evidence.—Therapeutic, IV.

▶ In this study, the investigators wanted to assess the health-related quality of life in patients with Dupuytren's disease who were treated with palmar or digital fasciectomy. From the practice of 3 plastic surgeons, the authors recruited patients who were asked to complete 3 health-related quality-of-life questionnaires (Short Form-36 [SF-36], Michigan Hand Outcomes Questionnaire [MHOQ], and Health Utility Index Mark 3 [HUIM 3]) at 5 time points: 8 days preoperatively and 1, 3, 6, and 12 months postoperatively. Twenty-six patients were enrolled in the study. The results showed no difference in the SF-36 scores at 12 months, but the MHOQ improved from one week preoperatively(74) to 12 months postoperatively (90) ($P < .001$). As for the HUIM 3, the score improved from 0.80 before surgery to 0.83 at 12 months postoperatively ($P > .05$).

The HUIM 3 provides, according to the authors, utilities that can be transformed to quality-adjusted life-years, "a health outcome measurement unit that integrates quality and quantity of life." They say furthermore, "quality-adjusted life-years form an important component of cost-utility analysis, a variant of cost-effectiveness analysis." Quality-adjusted life-years were calculated by multiplying the difference in quality of life from before and after surgery by the remaining years of life of the average patient. In this study, the authors found that the patients enrolled in the study gained a benefit of 0.85 quality-adjusted life-year within 12 months, or "translated as follows: the average patient who undergoes palmar fasciectomy gains the equivalent of approximately 14.4 days

(0.48 months) in perfect health by undergoing palmar fasciectomy." It could be added that the authors had calculated a sample size of 33 patients to have the power needed to show the change they hypothesized; however, 7 patients were lost to follow-up, which weakens the study.

Cost-benefit, or cost-effectiveness analysis, is becoming more popular and important to evaluate a treatment in question. For evaluation of the outcome after treatment of Dupuytren's disease, many evaluation forms have been used, some of which concentrate on hand function, whereas others include the function of the hand and arm or the patient's own perception of the total health status. Not all evaluation forms used are perfect for Dupuytren's disease. The evaluation form described in this report, HUIM 3, is a form that has been used for different conditions and is a form that might gain popularity in the future, especially when cost effectiveness is taken into consideration.

In my practice, I see lots of patients with Dupuytren's disease, and the treatment offered has varied from needle fasciotomy, fasciectomy with or without removal of the skin followed by open secondary healing or skin transplant, free vascular flaps to cover the defect, or treatment with collagenase *Clostridium histolyticum*. The patients come for treatment because they cannot put on a glove, they cannot wash their face without putting one finger in an eye, they cannot shake hands or clap their hands, or they cannot work because the "finger is in the way." I tell my patients that the recurrence rate varies depending on the joint involved and the time passed after surgery or that for collagenase, approximately 75% of the patients are satisfied 1 year after treatment. This does not reflect the position of the finger and the patient's own expectations and satisfaction. I have not yet told my patients that they can expect 14 days of perfect health after treatment.

J.-R. Haugstvedt, MD

The operative treatment of fractures of the distal radius is increasing: results from a nationwide Swedish study

Mellstrand-Navarro C, Pettersson HJ, Tornqvist H, et al (Karolinska Inst, Stockholm, Sweden)

Bone Joint J 96-B:963-969, 2014

The aim of this study was to investigate the epidemiology of fractures of the distal radius in the Swedish population and to review the methods used to treat them between 2005 and 2010.

The study population consisted of every patient in Sweden who was diagnosed with a fracture of the wrist between 1 January 2005 and 31 December 2010. There were 177 893 fractures of the distal radius. The incidence rate in the total population was 32 per 10 000 person-years. The mean age of the patients was 44 years (0 to 104). The proportion of fractures treated operatively increased from 16% in 2005 to 20% in 2010. The incidence rate for plate fixation in the adult population increased 3.61 fold. The incidence rate for external fixation decreased by 67%. The change was greatest in the 50 years to 74 years age group.

In Sweden, there is an increasing tendency to operate on fractures of the distal radius. The previously reported increase in the use of plating is confirmed: it has increased more than threefold over a five-year period.

▶ The authors present an epidemiologic study of fractures of the distal radius in the Swedish population. Every patient in Sweden who had a fracture of the wrist diagnosed between 2005 and 2010 was recorded in a nationwide registry to see the incidence of the injury and focus on the treatment methods for this kind of fracture. All age groups and all fractures treated operatively and nonoperatively were included.

The authors found that the incidence rate for fractures of the distal radius in the whole population (32 per 10 000 person-years) did not change during the study period, although there were minor changes within the different age groups. The proportion of patients treated operatively changed from 16% in 2005 to 20% in 2010, with the largest increase seen in the 50- to 74-years age group. The use of plate fixation increased more than 3-fold between 2005 and 2010. The mean number of in- and out-patient visits for a fracture of the distal radius was 2.25; for a fracture treated operatively the mean number of visits was 3.8, for nonoperative treatment it was 1.9.

Over the last few years, specially designed plates for fixation of fractures of the distal radius have been made and improved. In this study, specification of dorsal or volar plates has not been recorded; however, there are reasons to believe that volar plating is becoming the most popular and widely used method. Whether this is a change owing to better hardware and fracture fixation or to better outcomes of this form of fracture treatment is yet to be proven. To answer this question, a nationwide study in which the total population is included, like in this study, could be of great value. However, one would need to register other lesions such as soft tissue and ligament lesions (if an arthroscopy was performed to diagnose these lesions), whether the patient had postoperative casting, and if so for how long, and one would also need to register the number of follow-ups and complications such as tendon ruptures, surgery for carpal tunnel syndrome, and need for hardware removal. We know that more than 50% of patients with a fracture of the distal radius have concomitant soft tissue (ligament, triangular fibrocartilage complex) lesions. When the patients were treated using a cast, the soft tissue lesions were allowed to heal. When a fracture is fixed using a plate and screws to allow early mobilization, the soft tissue lesions may not be given time to heal. However, it is still unclear if this will influence the long-term results. The question remains: What will patients benefit from acute treatment of the concomitant soft tissue lesion? If more attention is paid to the different parameters recorded in such a nationwide register, we could probably gain lots of valuable information.

In our practice, we will look at the fracture type, the mechanism of injury, the age, and the demands of the patients to choose the best treatment. If surgery is found to be the treatment of choice, volar plating is preferred; however, dorsal plating or column-specific plates are also used. If possible, I prefer to perform arthroscopy to diagnose the soft tissue lesions and would, if found, treat them accordingly with k-wire stabilization (carpal instability) or sutures (triangular fibrocartilage complex lesions). If soft tissue lesions were found, I would immobilize the wrist in a cast.

J.-R. Haugstvedt, MD

An open-label comparison of local anesthesia with or without sedation for minor hand surgery

Rozanski M, Neuhaus V, Reddy R, et al (Massachusetts General Hosp, Boston)
Hand 9:399-405, 2014

Background.—The purpose of this study was to assess satisfaction and pain intensity in patients undergoing minor hand surgery under local anesthesia (LA) with or without sedation.

Methods.—Seventy-three adult patients presenting to two hand surgeons were enrolled in this prospective observational study in 2012. They completed questionnaires prior to surgery (current pain intensity, Patient Health Questionnaire-2 (PHQ-2) to measure symptoms of depression, Pain Self-Efficacy Questionnaire (PSEQ) to assess the effective coping strategy of pain self-efficacy) and within 48 h after surgery (satisfaction with surgery, satisfaction with anesthesia, pain during the injection, and pain during the procedure). Thirty-seven patients had carpal tunnel release (bilateral in 3), 22 had release of one or more trigger digits, and 12 had excision of a benign tumor, gouty tophus (1 patient), or foreign body (1 patient). Forty-six patients chose LA and 27 chose LA with sedation.

Results.—There was no difference in satisfaction with surgery or anesthesia by the type of anesthesia. Satisfaction with surgery was associated with older age alone. Satisfaction with anesthesia was associated with no prior surgery for the same condition. Pain during injection and during the procedure were significantly higher without sedation. Pain during injection was associated with younger age and LA. No factors were associated with pain during the procedure.

Conclusions.—Patients that had local anesthesia immediately prior to incision with tourniquet use during surgery had more pain during the procedure but were equally satisfied on average with surgery and with anesthesia compared to patients that had sedation.

▶ The authors present a study assessing satisfaction and pain intensity in patients undergoing minor hand surgery under local anesthesia (LA) with or without sedation. Seventy-three adult patients (operated on for *carpal tunnel syndrome*, trigger-finger, benign tumors, gouty tophus, or foreign body) were included in a prospective study in which the patients completed the Patient Health Questionnaire-2 to measure symptoms of depression and the Pain Self-Efficacy Questionnaire to assess the effective coping strategy of pain self-efficacy. The questionnaires were completed prior to surgery. Within 48 hours after surgery, the patients were contacted by phone to rate satisfaction with the treating surgeon, surgery, and anesthesia, and to rate the pain during injection of anesthesia and pain during the procedure. The authors conclude that patients having local anesthesia immediately prior to incision with tourniquet use during surgery had more pain during the procedure compared with patients that had sedation. The groups were equally satisfied on average with surgery and anesthesia.

The study design describes, "patients were allowed to choose between LA alone and LA with intravenous sedation." The investigators enrolled 101 consecutive patients; however, for different reasons the final cohort consisted of 73 patients. Forty-six patients chose LA alone and 27 LA with sedation. Statistical analysis was performed using different tests to compare the groups. After enrollment of 20 patients, a power analysis was performed to calculate the number needed for a given effect size. The results show that there was a significant positive correlation between satisfaction with surgery and satisfaction with anesthesia. Satisfaction with anesthesia was not related to choice of anesthesia but was associated with no prior surgery for the same condition. In this study, the procedures were short, less than 20 minutes, and the tourniquet time was less than 14 minutes for all patients. It should be noted that the decision for anesthesia "was meant to be the patients'"; however, there was a difference in the use of sedation, suggesting that the 2 surgeons presented the options differently.

Wide-awake surgery has gained popularity and is now widely used. Depending on the facilities and availability of the different resources, patients coming for minor surgery may have the surgery performed under LA or general anesthesia. I try to use the best for the patient, which I often think is "as simple as possible." For certain procedures, like tendon transfers, it is of great value that the patient can move the hand while surgery is being performed to check the result, thus, I want to use LA. However, I am aware that I, as in the referred article, am able to influence the choice of my patients. LA should be injected at least 30 minutes prior to surgery; the choice of anesthesia (with or without epinephrine, warm or cold), the size of the needle, and the technique of the injection are factors that all should be considered; however, they are not taken into account in this study.

J.-R. Haugstvedt, MD

Litigation relating to conditions affecting the shoulder and elbow: an analysis of claims against the National Health Service

Talbot CL, Ring J, Holt EM (Univ Hosp of South Manchester NHS Foundation Trust, Manchester, UK; Royal Blackburn Hospital, UK)

Bone Joint J 96-B:574-579, 2014

We present a review of claims made to the NHS Litigation Authority (NHSLA) by patients with conditions affecting the shoulder and elbow, and identify areas of dissatisfaction and potential improvement. Between 1995 and 2012, the NHSLA recorded 811 claims related to the shoulder and elbow, 581 of which were settled. This comprised 364 shoulder (64%), and 217 elbow (36%) claims. A total of £18.2 million was paid out in settled claims. Overall diagnosis, mismanagement and intra-operative nerve injury were the most common reasons for litigation. The highest cost paid out resulted from claims dealing with incorrect, missed or delayed diagnosis, with just under £6 million paid out overall. Fractures and dislocations around the shoulder and elbow were common injuries in this category. All 11 claims following wrong-site surgery that were settled led to successful payouts.

This study highlights the diagnoses and procedures that need to be treated with particular vigilance. Having an awareness of the areas that lead to litigation in shoulder and elbow surgery will help to reduce inadvertent risks to patients and prevent dissatisfaction and possible litigation.

▶ This report is an analysis/review of litigation related to conditions affecting the shoulder and elbow. The authors analyze all data related to claims made to the National Health Service Litigation Authority in the United Kingdom between 1995 and 2012. Over this timeframe, 811 claims were made, of which 581 were settled. A total of 18.2 million pounds (roughly $28 million US) were paid in settlement claims.

The study is useful in that the authors highlight the most common causes of litigation, which include errors in diagnoses (including delayed, missed, and incorrect diagnoses). Of the settled claims lost, 43% of the errors in diagnosis occurred in the emergency department, 31% in orthopedic outpatient clinics, and 26% in another clinical area. Failure to diagnose or late diagnoses of fractures and dislocations were the most common reasons for claims in the diagnosis group. The second most common reason for claims was alleged mismanagement, including delays to referrals to specialists, incorrect treatment choice, and postoperative complications. Neurologic defect was the third most common area for litigation in all claims. Wrong side surgery accounted for 1.9% of all total claims.

This study highlights the most common causes of litigation related to shoulder and elbow conditions in a developed society. Although the authors correctly point out there is no single way to reduce litigation associated with shoulder and elbow conditions, they provide health care providers valuable information regarding the most common reasons for litigation claims. Table 6 in the original article is particularly useful, as the authors offer strategies to avoid claims by patients presenting with conditions affecting the shoulder and elbow, which include (1) adequate radiographs, (2) senior review of radiographs, (3) discussion with relevant specialists, (4) appropriate use of further imaging, (5) clear patient counseling/consenting, and (6) clear preoperative marking.

S. M. Jacoby, MD

Upper Extremity Orthoses Use in Amyotrophic Lateral Sclerosis/Motor Neuron Disease: Three Case Reports

Ivy CC, Smith SM, Materi MM (Mayo Clinic in Arizona, Phoenix)
Hand 9:543-550, 2014

Background.—Central to the armamentarium of a hand therapist is evaluation for successful orthotic use. Orthoses can have a profound effect on quality of life in persons with amyotrophic lateral sclerosis (ALS)/ motor neuron disease (MND). The purposes of orthoses are to decrease the effects of muscle imbalance, provide assistance in performance of activities of daily living (ADLs), prevent joint contracture, and relieve pain. There are few published accounts on the usefulness of orthoses and ALS. The purpose of this paper is to expand the body of literature by describing three successful cases.

Methods.—Three cases illustrate effects on weakened proximal muscles, wrist extensors, thenar musculature, and intrinsic muscles. The primary outcome measure is patient report, but functional rating scales, goniometry, quality of life scores, and pinch strength when obtainable are described.

Results.—Due to the progressive nature of the disease, outcome measures can be inconclusive. Patient report of increased life satisfaction and ability to participate in daily life is the critical outcome in these case examples. In all cases, satisfaction increased. Some of the stated changes include the following: ability to manipulate objects, grip, eat, wipe face, hold phone, use iPad®, and adjust hat.

Conclusions.—Upper extremity orthotic use can be a beneficial adjunct contributing to the quality of life for individuals with ALS/MND. We have observed positive responses in pain control, contracture management, functional positioning, and increased independence with the use of orthoses. Designing appropriate means of studying effects of orthosis intervention is deficient in the current scientific literature.

▶ This article not only reports on a comprehensive literature review for the process of decision making in orthotic use with persons who have amyotrophic lateral sclerosis (ALS) and other motor neuron diseases (MND), but also provides 3 case reports of functional orthoses for 3 persons with ALS/MND, and also contributes to and expands the literature for the effective use of orthoses to improve function and quality of life.

This population, because of incidence and nonconformity of expression of the disease, most likely would not warrant a randomized approach in the study of the best clinical orthotic. The literature found in their comprehensive search ranged from expert opinion to case reports, all lower levels of evidence. Therefore, focusing on the decision-making process of orthotic intervention was appropriate. The clinical reasoning presented in this article in the customized orthotic intervention was based on various physical symptoms of each person: pain, weakness, joint contracture intervention and prevention, muscle spasticity, nerve compression, and joint instability. The article also reports on the importance of keeping sensibility for the occupational task as a part of the decision-making process in the orthotic intervention. Of the literature reviewed and case reports presented by the authors, the theme of the process of orthotic intervention was based on each person's needs, which were important to their occupations of life and the enhancement and maintenance of their quality of life as well as the biomechanical knowledge of functional hand positioning. This article notes well that each person's needs must be analyzed with regard to their individual occupational functional importance, which is the science of occupational therapy and hand therapy, so well delineated in this article.

Another notable theme of this article is outcome tools. None of the studies reviewed reported use of an outcome tool. Although the diagnosis-specific ALS Functional Rating Scale[1] is specific to show changes in the disease, it is not sensitive enough to detect change in quality of life as a result of important orthotic intervention. The Canadian Occupational Performance Measure[2] and the McGill quality of life questionnaire[3] are discussed with the potentials for use in this population and for this intervention.

The authors present good visuals of the orthotic interventions and adaptive techniques used in the case reports, which will be informative to guide the physician and hand therapist to stir the creative juices for interventions to improve the quality of life for other persons with this and other progressive diseases. As well, we are stirred to complete further research of the importance of the process of orthotic intervention and to measure its outcome.

V. H. O'Brien, OTD, OTR/L, CHT

References

1. Maier A, Holm T, Wicks P, et al. Online assessment of ALS functional rating scale compares well to in-clinic evaluation: a prospective trial. *Amyotroph Lateral Scler.* 2012;13:210-216.
2. Carswell A, McColl MA, Baptiste S, Law M, Polatajko H, Pollock N. The Canadian occupational performance measure: a research and clinical literature review. *Can J Occup Ther.* 2004;71:210-222.
3. Cohen SR, Mount BM, Strobel MG, Bui F. The McGill quality of life questionnaire: a measure of quality of life appropriate for people with advanced disease. A preliminary study of validity and acceptability. *Palliat Med.* 1995;9:207-219.

Factors Used by Program Directors to Select Hand Surgery Fellows

Nies MS, Bollinger AJ, Cassidy C, et al (Michigan State Univ, Grand Rapids; Grand Rapids Med Education Partners, MI; Tufts-New England Med Ctr, Boston, MA)

J Hand Surg Am 39:2285-2288, 2014

Purpose.—To identify factors and attributes hand surgery fellowship program directors consider important in selecting applicants for interview and ranking.

Methods.—A web-based questionnaire was sent to all hand fellowship program directors in the United States. The questionnaire was designed to identify the most important criteria in granting an interview, sources of letters of recommendation, the interview process, and factors used to rank a candidate. Each criterion was ranked in importance on a 1 to 5 Likert scale, with 1 being not important and 5 being critical. All responses were anonymous. The most important criterion for each section of the survey was determined by comparing the average Likert scores.

Results.—Fifty-two of 76 program directors responded (68%). The criteria with the highest mean Likert scores for offering an applicant an interview were, in order, quality letters of recommendation from hand surgeons, completion of an orthopedic surgery residency, comments regarding the applicant's technical competence, applicant having an MD degree (as opposed to a DO degree), and residency program reputation. The letters of recommendation with the highest value were from the division chief of hand surgery and another hand surgeon in the division/department. The most important features of the interview were maturity of applicant, ability of applicant to articulate thoughts, ability to listen well, self-confidence, and relevant questions asked. The most important factors in ranking a candidate were applicant integrity, commitment to hard work, quality of letters of recommendation, quality of the interview, and ability to work well with other members of the hand surgery team.

Conclusions.—There are identifiable factors considered important by hand surgery fellowship directors when selecting and ranking an applicant. This information may be valuable to medical students and residents contemplating careers in hand surgery.

▶ Nies et al's article explores an interesting topic: what factors do hand surgery program directors consider important in an application. Using a web-based questionnaire and a 1 to 5 Likert scale, more than two-thirds of hand fellowship directors responded. The highest average scores were seen for highly supportive recommendation letters from hand surgery faculty, orthopedic surgery residency training, comments regarding technical competence, Doctor of Medicine degree (vs Doctor of Osteopathy), and residency program reputation. The least important factors were applicant sex, ethnicity, geographical location, and microsurgical experience. The article also addresses which factors program directors felt were important in an interview and which faculty members' recommendation letters were most influential. The major strength of this study was (for a web-based survey) the high rate of response. There was moderate disagreement (standard deviation >1)[1] among a number of factors that were in the most and least influential categories. The other major issue is that the answers are the program directors self-reported sense of what factors are important or unimportant; there is no check that program directors' actual behaviors follow these suggestions.

This study is of value to potential applicants in understanding the process from the perspective of a program director. It is also of value as a baseline, which should be repeated in the future as the process of fellowship matching evolves. As programs and surgical education incorporate more simulated learning and interview tactics such as structured interviews, it will be interesting to see if the important factors in granting interviews shift over time.

P. Blazar, MD

Reference

1. Sclove SL. Notes on Likert Scales. University of Illinois at Chicago. Available at: https://www.uic.edu/classes/idsc/ids270sls/likert. Accessed 2/1/15.

Patient-centered care and distal radius fracture outcomes: A prospective cohort study analysis

Constand MK, MacDermid JC, Law M, et al (McMaster Univ, Hamilton, ON)

J Hand Ther 27:177-184, 2014

Study design.—Prospective cohort.

Introduction.—Effects of patient-centered care on distal radius fracture recovery lacks evidence.

Purpose of the Study.—To understand from the perspective of a patient with a distal radius fracture: if the Patient Perception of Patient-Centeredness Questionnaire (PPPC) subscales apply to distal radius fracture populations; the strongest and weakest areas of patient-centered care; changes in patient perceptions of patient-centeredness during recovery; and, correlations between aspects of patient-centered care and patient reported pain and disability.

Methods.—Patients with distal radius fractures ($n = 129$; mean age = 54.03, SD = 14.63) completed the Patient Rated Wrist Evaluation (PRWE) and PPPC, at baseline (less than 10 days post-fracture) and at three months post-injury. Outcome measure responses were factor analyzed and tested for correlations.

Results.—Factors identified were titled Clinician-Patient Dialogue, representing communication components of patient-centered care, and Clinician-Patient Alliance, representing partnership components of patient-centered care. Small significant correlations ($r = 0.22$) between PRWE and PPPC responses were observed with Clinician-Patient Alliance more correlated at baseline and Clinician-Patient Dialogue at follow-up.

Discussion.—Important aspects of the patient-clinician dynamic were identified.

Conclusions.—Communication between clinician and patient was perceived most favorably at baseline; and partnership improved by three months.

Level of Evidence.—1b.

▶ Patient-centered care is an important aspect of health care that has been getting increased attention with advocacy to develop care plans that include patient input. Using the Patient Perception of Patient-Centeredness Questionnaire that was developed for family practice, the authors examined how this might relate to the acute orthopedic population by developing a prospective cohort study with a patient population comprising those with acute distal radius fractures. This was a well-designed study with 129 patients identified and analyzed less than 10 days after fracture and 3 months after injury. The authors found small significant correlations between the patients' perceptions of patient-centered care and pain reduction and functional recovery.

It is well stated in the discussion that clinicians should focus on developing good communication and relationships with their patients from the beginning so that patients understand they will have an active part in determining their care. Since the authors' findings indicate that patient-centered care does have an impact on improving patient outcomes after distal radius fracture, this study supports the need for surgeons and therapists to include components of patient-centered care in their practice. Enhancing the patient experience and providing the best outcomes possible after fracture is our goal as clinicians. We now have evidence that supports having our patients play an active role in their care.

S. J. Clark, OTR/L, CHT

Discrepancies Between Meeting Abstracts and Subsequent Full Text Publications in Hand Surgery

Theman TA, Labow BI, Taghinia A (Boston Children's Hosp and Harvard Med School, MA)

J Hand Surg Am 39:1585-1590.e3, 2014

Purpose.—Research abstracts presented during the proceedings of an annual meeting are often cited and can influence clinical practice. Prior studies show that roughly 50% of abstracts at American Society for Surgery of the Hand meetings are eventually published. Yet, it is unknown how often the results or conclusions of published studies differ from the podium presentation. The objective of this study was to quantify the differences between abstracts presented during the annual meeting of the American Society for Surgery of the Hand and the resulting manuscripts.

Methods.—We retrospectively reviewed every abstract delivered as a podium presentation at the American Society for Surgery of the Hand annual meeting from 2000 to 2010. We searched the PubMed database for matching publications and compared authorship, country of origin, hypothesis, study design and methodology, changes in study groups or populations, results, and conclusions.

Results.—Of 798 total abstracts, we analyzed 719 involving the hand, wrist, and brachial plexus. Fifty-six different journals published 393 of the abstracts, for a 49% publication rate. Mean time to publication was 18 months with a median of 14 and maximum of 122 months. There were inconsistencies between the results and/or conclusions in 14% of full-length articles compared with the abstract presented at the meeting. A total of 9% of articles were published with fewer subjects. Authorships changes were noted in 54% of publications.

Conclusions.—Abstracts represent preliminary investigations and major and minor changes occur before subsequent publication. Caution should be exercised in referencing abstracts or altering clinical practice based on their content.

Type of Study/Level of Evidence.—Economic/decision analysis IV.

▶ This article brings to light several issues that should be considered after hearing a podium presentation. It should be remembered that podium presentations are only preliminary data and that a limited peer-review process occurs, if at all, for a presentation. Frequently, when abstracts are submitted, the full data from the study are not yet available, being made ready only in time for the meeting itself. Therefore, incorrect calculations and conclusions can be identified when more closely examined.

The finding that 14% of final papers had substantial changes in their conclusions points to the importance of understanding the limits of presentations. Changes in clinical practice should be made slowly and are better made in response to peer-reviewed papers in high-quality journals. If clinical information obtained from a podium presentation is to shape clinical practice, frequent review of personal outcomes and review of the literature for additional support for that change should be made routinely.

The study also showed that more abstracts have been published over the past decade and that they have been in a greater number of journals. The American Society for Surgery of the Hand meeting is a high-quality meeting, at which high-quality studies are likely to be presented. If the studies are rejected by the *Journal of Bone and Joint Surgery* or *Journal of Hand Surgery*, there is a greater chance of publication in the next tier of journals. Additionally, there are more journals available in which to publish.

We are all likely guilty of adapting a new technology based on early data (ie, volar plating of distal radius fractures). A year ago, I changed my practice on the timing of manipulation of Dupytren's contracture after collagenase injection based on a podium presentation. Fortunately, this has been borne out in the published literature, but I probably should have waited for those publications before making a change.

T. Hughes, MD

Ethical and Educational Considerations in Coding Hand Surgeries

Lifchez SD, Leinberry CF, Rivlin M, et al (Thomas Jefferson Univ, Philadelphia, PA; Johns Hopkins/Univ of Maryland, Baltimore; Harvard Univ, Boston, MA; et al)

J Hand Surg Am 39:1370-1377, 2014

Purpose.—To assess treatment coding knowledge and practices among residents, fellows, and attending hand surgeons.

Methods.—Through the use of 6 hypothetical cases, we developed a coding survey to assess coding knowledge and practices. We e-mailed this survey to residents, fellows, and attending hand surgeons. In additionally, we asked 2 professional coders to code these cases.

Results.—A total of 71 participants completed the survey out of 134 people to whom the survey was sent (response rate = 53%). We observed marked disparity in codes chosen among surgeons and among professional coders.

Conclusions.—Results of this study indicate that coding knowledge, not just its ethical application, had a major role in coding procedures accurately. Surgical coding is an essential part of a hand surgeon's practice and is not well learned during residency or fellowship. Whereas ethical issues such as deliberate unbundling and upcoding may have a role in inaccurate coding, lack of knowledge among surgeons and coders has a major role as well.

Clinical Relevance.—Coding has a critical role in every hand surgery practice. Inconstancies among those polled in this study reveal that an increase in education on coding during training and improvement in the clarity and consistency of the Current Procedural Terminology coding rules themselves are needed.

▶ The authors report the results of a survey completed by a total of 71 participants of 134 who were contacted and asked to participate. The respondents included 44 residents ranging from PGY-2 to PGY-6, 5 fellows, 22 attendings, and 2 professional coders. There were 64 orthopedic surgeons, 6 plastic surgeons, and 1 general surgeon. They proposed 6 common case scenarios and charged each individual with providing common procedural terminology codes for each case. Not surprisingly, there was great variability from individual to individual, including the professional coders. The authors appropriately point out that residency and fellowship education spends little to no time on the topic of coding.

This study is both interesting and not surprising. Coding is an art rather than a science, although some guidelines are clearly available and I do recommend the American Society for Surgery of the Hand "coding corner" as a resource. From my own experience, and after having coded all of my own cases for more than 20 years, I can say that coding is both personal and controversial at times. What some may consider "unbundling" is perceived as proper billing by others. Everyone has a different comfort level when it comes to billing behavior, and I advise our fellows to follow both published guidelines and their conscience. I do agree that there should be more education on a resident/fellow level for this critical topic, and we do dedicate time to this topic during our fellowship training.

D. Zelouf, MD

Second Toe Metatarsophalangeal Joint Transfer for Sternoclavicular Joint Reconstruction

Bendon CL, Giele HP (Oxford Univ Hosps NHS Trust, UK; Univ of Oxford, UK)
J Hand Surg Am 39:1327-1332, 2014

Purpose.—We describe the anatomical basis for microsurgical reconstruction of the sternoclavicular joint using a vascularized, innervated second metatarsophalangeal joint, the surgical technique, and outcomes in 2 patients.

Methods.—We harvested the second metatarsophalangeal joint along with the joint capsule, portions of the metatarsal and phalanx, the flexor sheath and flexor tendon, the extensor sheath and tendon, the first metatarsal artery, and the deep peroneal nerve. This composite tissue was used for reconstruction of an excised sternoclavicular joint following infection or chondrosarcoma. The proximal phalanx was dowel-jointed into the manubrium and fixed with 1 or 2 screws; the metatarsal was plated to the remaining clavicle. The joint was oriented to allow maximal elevation and restricted depression, and the normal mediolateral laxity allowed anterior and posterior movement. Vascular anastomoses were performed to branches of the thoracoacromial axis vessels, and digital nerves were connected to a supraclavicular nerve.

Results.—Two patients had their excised sternoclavicular joints reconstructed using this technique. Both achieved union at the clavicular and sternal junctions. Both obtained restoration of movement of the sternoclavicular joint and upper limb. One patient developed joint subluxation and pain requiring tendon graft reconstruction of the costoclavicular ligament.

Conclusions.—In these 2 cases, the vascularized second toe metatarsophalangeal joint satisfactorily reconstructed the widely excised sternoclavicular joint and costoclavicular ligament and restored function.

Type of Study/Level of Evidence.—Therapeutic IV.

▶ Bendon and Giele describe a technique for reconstruction of the sternoclavicular joint using a vascularized innervated free second metatarsophalangeal joint transfer. Their technique provides a simple but elegant solution for treatment of sternoclavicular joint defects. The majority of hand surgeons will never encounter this problem, and the surgical technique is technically complex. Hence, the utility of this article is limited, but it provides a valuable guide to a useful technique for reconstruction of this difficult problem.

H. Chim, MD

Forearm Bier Block: A New Regional Anesthetic Technique for Upper Extremity Surgery

Arslanian B, Mehrzad R, Kramer T, et al (Beth Israel Deaconess Med Ctr, Boston, MA; Univ of Gothenburg, Sweden; Univ of Massachusetts Med School, Worcester; et al)

Ann Plast Surg 73:156-157, 2014

Purpose.—This study aimed to introduce the technique and results of a forearm Bier block for upper extremity surgery.

Introduction.—Various techniques of anesthesia are used for hand surgery. Intravenous regional anesthesia, the Bier block, is an effective anesthetic technique. However, there exist several disadvantages and potential complications. We present our technique and results using the forearm Bier block.

Materials and Method.—A retrospective review was performed studying our experience using forearm Bier block from May to December of 2010. The technique involves exsanguination of the forearm and inflation of a pneumatic tourniquet placed distal to the elbow joint. Twenty-five milliliter of 0.5% lidocaine is injected intravenously. One hundred five patients underwent hand surgery using this technique. There were 53 females and 52 males with a median age of 56 years. In total, 121 procedures were performed. Patients were interviewed by telephone 24 hours postoperatively.

Results.—All patients received adequate anesthesia from the block. There were no intraoperative and no postoperative complications. There were no mechanical or tourniquet problems. Average tourniquet time was 10.1 minutes. Total operating time was less than 30 minutes.

Discussion.—Forearm Bier block presents several advantages over standard upper arm technique. Conventional Bier block involves a double tourniquet and a significant amount of lidocaine, which has potential cardiac and neurologic toxicity. Consequently, minimum tourniquet inflation time is 30 minutes. The dosage of lidocaine needed to provide analgesia using the forearm Bier block is significantly reduced, thereby minimizing the potential for these complications. This lower dose allows for shorter tourniquet time rather than the standard 30 minutes. This shorter tourniquet time in itself presents several advantages. Tourniquet pain and risk of ischemic problems are minimized, and efficiency is increased. This efficiency has practical and financial implications such as decreased total operating and recovery room times, decreased cost of medicines, and decreased operating time for the surgeon. Lastly, this technique might also be used for lower extremity surgeries.

Conclusions.—Forearm Bier block is a safe and efficient method for upper extremity surgery. It significantly reduces the risk of complications and increases the efficiency of the surgeon and surgery facility.

▶ The use of Bier block for anesthesia in hand surgery has fallen out of favor secondary to concerns of potential systemic effects of the anesthetic agent as well as technical concerns such as the need to wait 30 minutes before tourniquet deflation in cases that often take much less time to complete. Nonetheless, there are also numerous advantages. The authors of this study report on use of a forearm Bier block protocol, and endorse the potential advantages of decreased pain associated with a forearm tourniquet and the ability to use lower doses of anesthesia, thus allowing deflation of the tourniquet sooner than upper arm tourniquet Bier blocks.

This article is one of the few to report on forearm tourniquet safety. The authors have standardized their protocol and notably had an average tourniquet time of 10.1 minutes. They also had adequate follow-up because any complications would be realized by the time of a first postoperative visit. Although they have the largest series of patients in the current literature, their numbers are lacking to detect the rare complications associated with the use of a Bier block. Furthermore, the use of less lidocaine (25 mL) in their protocol would make these rare complications less likely. The concept of a Bier block providing a wide anesthetic field and maintaining the surgical planes that are often disrupted with subcutaneous injections is attractive. These benefits, while allowing early release of the tourniquet, make this technique appealing. Nevertheless, knowledge regarding the amount of anesthetic seen systemically with an earlier tourniquet release is critical to the assessment of this technique modification. Forearm Bier block and early tourniquet release is potentially a valuable tool, and I suspect further evidence regarding its safety would change some surgeons' practice.

J. C. Saillant, MD

Cytotoxic Effects of Ropivacaine, Bupivacaine, and Lidocaine on Rotator Cuff Tenofibroblasts

Sung C-M, Hah Y-S, Kim J-S, et al (Gyeongsang Natl Univ, Jinju, Korea; Eulji Univ, Seoul, Korea; et al)

Am J Sports Med 42:2888-2896, 2014

Background.—Concern has recently arisen over the safety of local anesthetics used on human tissues.

Hypothesis.—Aminoamide local anesthetics have cytotoxic effects on human rotator cuff tenofibroblasts.

Study Design.—Controlled laboratory study.

Methods.—Cultured human rotator cuff tenofibroblasts were divided into control, phosphate buffered saline (PBS), and local anesthetic study groups; the PBS study group was further subdivided by pH level (pH 7.4, 6.0, and 4.4). The 6 local anesthetic subgroups (0.2% and 0.75% ropivacaine, 0.25% and 0.5% bupivacaine, and 1% and 2% lidocaine) were also studied at 10% dilutions of their original concentrations. Exposure times were 5, 10, 20, 40, or 60 minutes for the higher concentrations and 2, 6, 12, 24, 48, or 72 hours for the lower concentrations. Cell viability was evaluated through live, apoptotic, and necrotic cell rates using the annexin V—propidium iodide double-staining method. Intracellular reactive oxygen species (ROS) and the activity of mitogen-activated protein kinases (MAPKs) and caspase-3/7 were investigated.

Results.—The control and PBS groups showed no significant differences in cell viability ($P > .999$). In the local anesthetic study groups, cell viability decreased significantly with increases in anesthetic concentrations ($P < .001$) and exposure times ($P < .001$), with the exception of the lidocaine subgroups, where this effect was masked by the very high cytotoxicity of even low concentrations. Among the studied local anesthetic subgroups, 0.2% ropivacaine was the least toxic. The levels of intracellular ROS of each local anesthetic subgroup also increased significantly ($P < .05$). The studied local anesthetics showed increases in the phosphorylation of extracellular signal—regulated kinase 1/2 (ERK1/2), c-Jun N-terminal kinase (JNK), and p38 as well as in levels of caspase-3/7 activity ($P < .001$).

Conclusion.—The cytotoxicity of the anesthetics studied to tenofibroblasts is dependent on exposure time and concentration. Of the evaluated anesthetics, ropivacaine is the least toxic in the clinically used concentration. The studied anesthetics induce tenofibroblast cell death, mediated by the increased production of ROS, by the increased activation of ERK1/2, JNK, and p38 and by the activation of caspase-3/7.

Clinical Relevance.—This study identified the cytotoxic mechanisms of aminoamide local anesthetics acting on rotator cuff tenofibroblasts. The greatest margin of safety was found in lower anesthetic concentrations in general and more specifically in the use of ropivacaine.

▶ Aminoamide local anesthetics (eg, lidocaine, bupivacaine, and ropivacaine) are commonly used in many physicians' practices to help administer analgesia to injection sites and perioperative surgical sites, as well as in combination with steroid solutions for the treatment of inflammation in and around joints. This article, in conjunction with other recently reported studies, brings several safety concerns to the forefront of these routinely used drugs. Although the article is lengthy and complex in nature, it is a must read for physicians. Strengths of the study include the in vitro basic science design, blinded data collection, sound methods with good experimental and control groups, and clinically relevant drug dosages. Some of the weaknesses include the complex technical terminology used, as well as the question of potential clinical applicability.

The article demonstrates that in this in vitro model, the cytotoxic effects of the studied aminoamide local anesthetics on tenofibroblasts are dependent on exposure time and concentration. Of the evaluated anesthetics, ropivacaine is the least toxic in the clinically used concentration.

For the reviewer, there are several questions that should be asked. First, do these drugs behave in vivo as they do in vitro? Second, how long do these drugs remain active in vivo? The article tests several time points of exposure from 2 hours to 72 hours. This may not be clinically relevant given that the half-lives of these medications in vivo are 1.5 hours for lidocaine, 2.7 hours for bupivacaine, and 5 to 7 hours for ropivacaine, which are substantially shorter than the length of exposure times noted in the article. As the authors mentioned, these drugs were once used for intraarticular pain pumps after arthroscopy, but this practice has since been discontinued. It is likely that more studies will surface looking at the safety and efficacy of recently released anesthetics such as liposomal bupivacaine. This article, in conjunction with other recently published articles noting the cytotoxicity of these drugs on chondrocytes, has made the medical community more judicious in the use of these drugs in clinical practice.

M. B. Gottschalk, MD
J. T. Capo, MD

Thrombin and Topical Local Anesthetic for Postoperative Pain Management

Haddock NT, Weinstein AL, Sinno S, et al (New York Univ)
Ann Plast Surg 73:30-32, 2014

Purpose.—Local anesthetic is often used for perioperative pain control. Thrombin serves as a carrying medium for sustained release of antibiotics, chemotherapy, and growth factors. We tested the hypothesis that local anesthetic pain relief can be prolonged with the adjunct use of thrombin.

Methods.—A prospective single-blinded clinical study was performed. Patients undergoing elective hand surgery inclusive of carpal tunnel release, excision of ganglion cyst, trigger finger release, and excision of mucous cyst under local block were enlisted. Before closure, patients received 1 of the following combinations: (1) control with oral analgesics, (2) 5 mL of 2% xylocaine, (3) 5 mL of 0.5% bupivacaine, (4) 2.5 mL of 2% xylocaine with 2.5 mL of 0.5% bupivacaine (XB), (5) thrombin with 5 mL of 2% xylocaine (XT), (6) thrombin with 5 mL of 0.5% bupivacaine (BT), and (7) thrombin with 2.5 mL of 2% xylocaine and 2.5 mL of 0.5% bupivacaine (XBT). There were 7 patients in each group, and patient demographics were similar between groups. Outcome measures included postanesthesia care unit (PACU) time, pain level, and number of pain pills required.

Results.—Compared with oral analgesics alone, mean (SD) postoperative pain levels were reduced by 33.3% (8.9%) by xylocaine, 69.1% (8.7%) by bupivacaine, and 45.7% (9.4%) by XB. When thrombin was added, pain levels were further reduced by 69.9% by XT ($P < 0.001$), 23.1% by BT ($P = 0.071$), and 50.5% by XBT ($P < 0.001$) compared with their nonthrombin counterparts. In addition, PACU time was decreased by 34.8% by XT ($P = 0.003$) and 19.7% by XBT ($P = 0.013$) compared with xylocaine and XB, respectively. However, there was no difference in total pain pills needed between xylocaine, bupivacaine, and XB when administered with and without thrombin.

Conclusions.—The addition of topical thrombin to local anesthetic at the end of elective hand surgery provides for sustained postoperative pain control. Patients in this study who received thrombin and local anesthetic before wound closure had lower pain levels and were discharged from the PACU sooner than those who received local anesthetic alone.

Level of Evidence.—Therapeutic level 2.

► This is single-blinded prospective study on thrombin as an agent prolonging the anesthetic effect of locally used xylocaine or bupivacaine. The authors divided patients undergoing minor hand surgery procedures into 7 groups, each having a different combination of anesthetics. Although it gives a clear comparison and answers regarding postanesthesia care unit (PACU) time, number of oral narcotics used, and pain levels in several postoperative periods, it is still unclear how long the anesthesia is effective in the investigated groups. For sure, looking at all the results provided, it seems that thrombin makes local anesthesia more effective. A weakness of this study is the number of patients enrolled in each group (n = 7), which makes statistical analysis less trustful. I also doubt that PACU time is a good measure of local anesthetic effectiveness. The authors also do not give information on adverse reactions to the drugs administered, taking into account that thrombin can be an allergen because of its bovine origin.

Still, this study proves that thrombin should be considered as an additional and beneficial factor when using local anesthesia. I have no personal experience with use of thrombin, but after reading this research I am more convinced to give it a try in everyday practice.

P. Czarnecki, MD, PhD

Effect of Anxiety and Catastrophic Pain Ideation on Early Recovery After Surgery for Distal Radius Fractures

Roh YH, Lee BK, Noh JH, et al (Gachon Univ School of Medicine, Incheon, South Korea; Kangwon Natl Univ Hosp, Gangwon-do, South Korea; Seoul Natl Univ College of Medicine, South Korea)

J Hand Surg Am 39:2258-2264, 2014

Purpose.—To evaluate the effects of preoperative anxiety and catastrophic pain ideation on perceived disability and objective measures after distal radius fracture surgery.

Methods.—A total of 121 patients with distal radius fractures treated with volar plate fixation were enrolled. The wrist range of motion (ROM), grip strength, and perceived disability as measured by the Michigan Hand Questionnaire (MHQ) score were assessed 4, 12, and 24 weeks after surgery. To evaluate psychological factors related to pain, catastrophic pain ideation was measured using the Pain Catastrophizing Scale (PCS) and pain anxiety was measured using the Pain Anxiety Symptom Scale (PASS). Then relative contributions of pain anxiety and catastrophic pain ideation and other clinical parameters to functional recovery in terms of grip strength, ROM, and MHQ score were assessed.

Results.—An increase in the PCS score was associated with the wrist ROM and grip strength only at week 4, whereas an increase in the PASS score was associated with the wrist ROM at week 4 and grip strength at weeks 4 and 12. According to a multivariate regression analysis, an increase in the PCS score was associated with a decrease in grip strength, ROM, and MHQ score at week 4; and an increase in the PASS score was associated with a decrease in grip strength, ROM, and MHQ score at week 4 and grip strength and MHQ score at week 12. At week 24, only age and fracture severity were associated with the MHQ score. In addition, age was associated with grip strength and fracture type was associated with ROM.

Conclusions.—Preoperative PCS and PASS were significantly associated with delayed recovery as evidenced by scores on both objective and subjective measures of function. Given these relationships, it becomes important to assess preoperative PCS and PASS and address issues for patients at risk with brief psychosocial intervention early in the recovery process.

Type of Study/Level of Evidence.—Prognostic II.

▶ The authors have conducted a well-designed study to look at the effects of pain and anxiety on recovery after surgical treatment of distal radius fractures. It is appropriately powered, and they used both subjective and objective outcomes measures. As our understanding of the effects of psychological factors and their effect on recovery after injury or surgery increases, it becomes clear that these conditions are an important but often underappreciated part of recovery and likely are responsible for some of the variation in outcomes. Fortunately, these factors become less important as time from injury increases and by 6 months appear to have minimal effect.

The initial evaluation is after the injury and before surgery, so it is difficult to determine the baseline levels of pain catastrophizing and anxiety. Further research to determine a minimum score that will negatively affect outcomes will be helpful and, perhaps, most importantly, aid in determining an algorithm or method to address the pain and anxiety when identified to improve the short-term outcomes.

Many practitioners do not have access to behavioral psychologists and other practitioners who are more experienced than hand surgeons in treating these conditions. My current approach is merely to spend extra time with these patients, reassuring them that what they are experiencing is normal after an injury while being empathetic and reassuring them that their condition will improve. We set short-term goals for subjective and objective function and work together to meet our long-term goals.

W. C. Hammert, MD

Article Index

Chapter 1: Hand and Wrist Arthritis

Chapter 2: Dupuytren's Contracture

Chapter 3: Tendon

Chapter 4: Wrist Arthroscopy

Chapter 5: Carpus

Chapter 6: Distal Radius Fractures

Chapter 7: Elbow: Trauma

Chapter 8: Elbow: Miscellaneous

Chapter 9: Brachial Plexus

Chapter 10: Shoulder: Rotator Cuff

Chapter 11: Shoulder: Miscellaneous

Chapter 12: Diagnostic Imaging

Chapter 13: Compressive Neuropathies

Chapter 14: Nerve

Chapter 15: Microsurgery

Chapter 16: Trauma

Chapter 17: Pediatric/Congenital

Chapter 18: Rehabilitation

Chapter 19: Miscellaneous

Author Index

M

N

O

P

X

Y

Z

FSC
www.fsc.org
MIX
Papier | Fördert
gute Waldnutzung
FSC® C083411

Kolibri 360 GmbH
Ferdinand-Jühlke-Straße 7
99095 Erfurt, Deutschland
produktsicherheit@kolibri360.de